New Aspects in Thyroid Diseases

New Aspects in Thyroid Diseases

Medullary Thyroid Carcinoma, Thyroiditis, Peripheral Thyroid Hormone Metabolism

IV. Multilateral Symposium on Thyroid
Reinhardsbrunn — Thuringia 1991

Edited by
H. F. Deckart · E. Strehlau

Walter de Gruyter
Berlin · New York 1992

Editors
Prof. Dr. H. F. Deckart
Dr. E. Strehlau
Nuklearmedizinische Klinik
Städtisches Klinikum Berlin-Buch
Wiltbergstraße 50
O-1115 Berlin-Buch

This publication has been made possible by the kind support of
E. Merck, Darmstadt.

The project has also benefited from the support of
Isocommerz, Leipzig

Die Deutsche Bibliothek — Cataloging-in-Publication Data

New aspects in thyroid diseases: medullary thyroid carcinoma, thyroiditis, peripheral thyroid hormone metabolism / 4. Multilateral Symposium on Thyroid, Reinhardsbrunn — Thuringia, 1991. Ed. by H. F. Deckart ; E. Strehlau. — Berlin ; New York : de Gruyter, 1992
ISBN 3-11-013731-3
NE: Deckart, Harald [Hrsg.]; Multilateral Symposium on Thyroid <04, 1991, Reinhardsbrunn>

Medical science is constantly developing. Research and clinical experience expand our knowledge, especially with regard to treatment and medication. For dosages and applications mentioned in this work, the reader may rely on the authors, editors and publisher having taken great pains to ensure that these indications reflect the standard of knowledge at the time this work was completed.
Nevertheless, all users are requested to check the package leaflet of the medication, in order to determine for themselves whether the recommentations given for the dosages or the likely contraindications differ from those given in this book. This is especially true for medication which is seldom used or has recently been put on the market and for medication whose application has been restricted by the German Ministry of Health.
The quotation of registered names, trade names, trade marks, etc. in this copy does not imply, even in the absence of a specific statement that such names are exempt from laws and regulations protecting trade marks, etc. and therefore free for general use.
Printing: Gerike GmbH, Berlin. — Binding: Dieter Mikolai, Berlin. — Cover design: R. Hübler. — Printed in Germany.

PREFACE

Since 1981, every third year, thyroidologists have met together with specialists in Nuclear Medicine, Radiology, Surgery, Pathology, Ophthalmology and Laboratory Medicine in Reinhardsbrunn. Experienced teams from Austria, Czechoslovakia, Poland, Yugoslavia and East-Germany discussed variant topics of diagnostic strategies and treatment procedures in functional thyroid disorders, thyroiditis, thyroid cancer and immunogenic endocrine orbitopathy.
The special atmosphere in the old hunting palace of the Dukes of Saxony Coburg-Gotha with remnants of Benedict monastery of the medivian ages with its lovely surroundings of the Thuringian forest were stimulating the scientific output.
The proceedings of the first three symposia were published in the Isocommerz-Series (ISSN 0233-1268 and -0466).
The Symposium was planned to be held in 1990. However because of the Basedow-Symposium in Halle-Merseburg, marking the 150th anniversary of the description of Basedow's disease, the Fourth Symposium on Thyroid was postponed to May 1991.
This volume includes papers and discussions presented in this Meeting held for the first time in unified Germany in Reinhardsbrunn. Topics were: Medullary Cancer, Parathyroid, Thyroiditis, Immunology and Peripheral Thyroid Metabolism.
The editors wish to express their sincere thanks to MERCK company and Isocommerz for their generous support. They also thank Dr. Radtke from Walter de Gruyter Publishers for promoting the editing of these Proceedings.

Berlin, January 1992

Harald F. Deckart
Ernst Strehlau

Contents

IMMUNOLOGY

Polyendocrine autoimmunity in thyroid disease (a preliminary report)
M. Gryczyńska, A. Baumann-Antczak, J. Kosowicz 1

The effect of anti-microsomal antibodies on thyroid peroxidase activity
E. Mezösi, S. Szücs, S. Sárközi, E. Fórizs, J. Szabó 8

Antithyroid antibodies in the synovial fluid in thyroiditis
K. Łacka, M. Gembicki 18

Immunological and genetical aspects in T_3-predominant Graves' disease
Sabine Gerlach, H.F. Deckart, Eva Deckart, Annemarie Blottner 23

Unexpected course in immunological pattern in Graves' Basedow's disease - Marine-Lenhart Syndrome?
H.F. Deckart, Eva Deckart, Annemarie Blottner, E. Strehlau, G. Mühr 32

Comparative investigations of sonography and TRAK - follow up of Graves' disease
Angelika Wünsche, Dietlind Sorger, G. Neumann, Susanne Schenk, L. Otto, G. Schneider 38

Guanyl nucleotide regulatory proteins and GTPase activity in normal and hyperthyroid human thyroid tissue and human polymorphonuclear granulocytes
E. Fórizs, A. Panyige, Zs. Jenei, T. Fülöp Jr., J. Szabó, E. Mezösi, I. Seres, A. Leövey 46

PERIPHERAL THYROID HORMONE METABOLISM

Peripheral thyroid hormone metabolism
H. Meinhold 54

Value of the estimation of peripheral serum T_3 and rT_3 for prognosis assessment in patients with liver cirrhosis - a prospective study

Chr. Rink, U. Siersleben, J. Haerting, T. Mende, R. Nilius 73

Thyroid hormones and TSH in acute myocardial infarction

J. Pechán, I. Vereš, J. Murín 83

Deiodination of thyroxine and reverse triiodothyronine in cells of human adipose tissue

Ch.-F. Wolf, J. Wieberneit, L. Duntas, F.S. Keck 89

Comparison of natural killer activity with thyroid function in Graves' disease

A. Sztankay, Gy. Bakó, E. Fórizs, E. Mezösi, A. Leövey 96

The influence of the calcium antagonist nitrendipine on thyroid hormone status in the baboon

J. Wieberneit, F.S. Keck, U. Loos, Ch.-F. Wolf 101

Effect of thyroid hormones on lipoprotein (a) level in hypothyroidism

S. Oravec 111

THYROIDITIS

Thyrotoxicosis due to thyroiditis

A. Leövey 118

Thyroiditis - a histopathological review

H.G. Peschel 127

Clinical and cytological classification of lymphocytic thyroiditis

Z. Limanová 134

The role of ultrasound investigation in the diagnosis and treatment of thyroiditis

Z. Novák, V. Zamrazil, J. Němec, P. Vlček 142

Subacute thyroiditis de Quervain in male subjects

P. Hnilica, J. Podoba, V. Štrbák, S. Nyulassy 145

Thyroid function in postpartum thyroiditis and its follow up
Nina Simova 152

Riedel's thyroiditis - positive therapeutic response to glucocorticoids
M. Ventz, G. Knappe, D. Ziegelitz 161

Management of chronic lymphocytic thyroiditis in children and adolescents
I. Hniková, J. Zikmund, M. Finková 165

Thyroiditis and thyroid hyperfunction
V. Zamrazil, J. Němec 172

Clinical and laboratory evaluations of patients with different types of thyroiditis
I. Sztojka, Zs. Karányi, A. Leövey 177

Hashimoto-thyroiditis with long-term negative auto-antibody determination: a case report
Marie-Luise Weiss, A. Blottner, H.F. Deckart 184

Combination of Hashimoto- and de Quervain thyroiditis
K.P. Schmidt, Eva Deckart, R. Pilz, E. Strehlau 193

Occurrence of goitre and diffuse lymphoid thyroiditis (DLT) in secondary school adolescents in Bratislava
J. Podoba, P. Hnilica, M. Srbecký 205

Spontaneous course of Graves' Basedow's disease into hypothyroidism (case report)
Eva Deckart 210

MEDULLARY CANCER

Epidemiology, clinical syndrome, follow up, and prognostic factors in medullary carcinoma
F. Raue 216

Neue Entwicklungen in der chirurgischen Therapie des Sipple-Syndroms: die Kompartment-orientierte systematische Mikrodissektion der Lymphknoten beim medullären Schilddrüsenkarzinom
H. Dralle, I. Damm, G.F.W. Scheumann 228

Medullary cancer in histopathological view
H.G. Peschel, T. Decker 241

Cytological view of medullary cancer
Marie-Luise Weiss 246

Imaging techniques in detection and follow up of MTC
H.F. Deckart, Katharina Djakowa, H. Marciniak, E. Strehlau, Marie-Luise Weiss 253

Positive scintigraphy in medullary thyroid cancer
V. Holub, M. Neradilová, J. Němec, M. Benová, T. Blažek, P. Vlček 265

I-131-uptake in medullary thyroid carcinoma
G. Riccabona, A. Stöger, D. Ladurner, K. Schmid 272

Our experiences with medullary carcinoma and MEN-syndrome
H.F. Deckart, S. Birke, E. Deckart, Ch. Koloc, W. Lobers, R. Pilz, E. Strehlau, C. Wardius, M.L. Weiss 280

Possibilities and limitations of tumor-scintigraphy for follow up of medullary thyroid cancer
Chr. Reiners 291

Thyroid cancer - differentiated and medullary: the aftercare system
J. Němec, M. Neradilová, V. Zamrazil 302

Medullary carcinoma of the thyroid - own experience
M. Neradilová, J. Němec, P. Vlček, V. Holub, J. Bednář, M. Soutorová 309

Prevalence of medullary thyroid cancer in the endemic goiter area
Z. Szybiński, E. Mazurek 316

Family screening in medullary thyroid carcinoma (MTC)
P. Groth, Ursula Zarmstorf, Irmtraud Stoll, R. Reincke 324

Results of therapy in patients with medullary carcinoma of thyroid gland
(Poster)
D. Gottschild, Gabriele Zinner, Carmen Luck, N.M. Granzow 330

The place of ultrasonography in the evaluation of medullary thyroid cancer
P. Vlček, M. Neradilová, J. Němec, J. Bednář, Z. Novák 333

Medullary thyroid carcinoma - results of some diagnostic procedures used at our institute
D. Bergant, M. Auersperg, M. Us-Krasovec, F. Pompe, J. Petric, T. Movrin, Z. Zemva, N. Bešič 337

FREE PAPERS

Tumor markers in thyroid disease
J. Bednář, J. Němec, M. Neradilová, M. Soutorová 345

Effects of Propranolol enantiomers in hyperthyroidism (Poster)
B. Obermayer-Pietsch, C. Stiegler, H. Warnkroß, G. Obermayer, S. Sager, W. Lindner, G. Leb 354

Thyroglobulin pattern in hyperthyroidism factitia (Case report)
Eva Deckart 355

Parameters of bone-metabolism in patients with hyperthyrosis (Poster)
P. Dietel, H.J. Heberling, D. Lohmann 360

PARATHYROID

Clinical experience in parathyroid carcinoma
G. Knappe, Helga Gerl, M. Ventz 362

Unusual course of primary hyperparathyroidism
R. Hehrmann 370

Long-term results operated hyperparathyroidism
U. Krause, Ch. Jeziorowski, Th. Olbricht 373

Diagnostik problems of primary hyperparathyroidism (pHPT) - own experiences
H.J. Heberling, B. Bierwolf, P. Dietel,
E. Kuhlmann, D. Lohmann 380

X-ray-morphologic and radiomorphometric results in patients with primary hyperparathyroidism
(Poster)
K.P. Schröder, P. Dietel, H.J. Heberling,
D. Lohmann 389

Authors' Index 391

Index 395

IMMUNOLOGY

Polyendocrine autoimmunity in thyroid disease

(a preliminary report)

M. Gryczyńska, A. Baumann-Antczak, J. Kosowicz
Department of Endocrinology, University School of Medicine, Poznań, Poland

Autoimmunity plays an essential role in the pathogenesis of a number of thyroid diseases such as Graves' disease, Hashimoto's thyroiditis and primary myxoedema. In autoimmune thyroid diseases various autoantibodies were detected anti-thyroglobulin, anti-thyroid peroxidase, anti-TSH receptor stimulating and blocking antibodies, anti-tubulin antibodies and:antibodies reacting with orbital muscles and connective tissues.

In other autoimmune diseases such as diabetes type I, Addison's disease, pernicious anaemia, and rheumatic disease the presence of thyroid antibodies was of much higher incidence than in control subjects /1,2/. In our study /3/ we found anti-thyroglobulin antibodies in 23 %, and anti-thyroid microsomal antibodies in 57 % of patients with Addison's disease.

In recent years we introduced a sensitive and simple radioimmunoassay for the detection of antiadrenal antibodies by solid phase technique in tubes coated with solubilised microsomal fraction of adrenal cortex /3/.

The aim of the study was to examine the occurence of adrenal and pituitary antibodies in blood sera of patients with autoimmune thyroid disease.

Material and methods

Blood samples were taken in 45 patients with autoimmune thyroid diseases: 25 (20 females, 5 males) with autoimmune hyperthyroidism, and 20 patients (18 females, 2 males) with autoimmune hypothyroidism. The diagnosis was based on typical clinical manifestations supported by hormones concentration and on the presence of anti-thyroid antibodies. The patients had no evident clinical symptoms and signs of adrenal or pituitary dysfunction. Serum blood samples of 30 healthy young volunteers served as a control group.

Blood samples were collected after overnight fast at 8 a.m., and serum samples were frozen at -20 °C until the assay.

The adrenal and pituitary antibodies were determined by solid phase radioimmunoassay as previously described /3/. For preliminary screening serum samples were diluted 1:600. The binding of I-125-Protein A exceeding two standard deviations (SD) obtained for control samples were considered as weakly positive (+), those exceeding 3 SD - as positive (++) and those exceeding 4 SD as strongly positive (+++). The positive sera were subsequently examined at the dilutions 1:1200, 1:4800, 1:19200, 1:76800, 1:307200 and compared with control sera at the same dilution.

Results

Solid phase RIA for adrenal and pituitary antibodies were performed in 25 cases with autoimmune hyperthyroidism and 20 cases with autoimmune hypothyroidism.

In the group with autoimmune hyperthyroidism in 19 cases (76 %) the results were positive for adrenal antibodies. Eight patients had very high titer adrenal antibodies (1:307200), in five patients the titer was 1:76800, in the other four was 1:19200, one patient had the antibodies titer 1:4800 and another one 1:1200.

The pituitary antibodies were found in 19 (76 %) hyperthyroid patients. The titer of the antibodies was 1:307200 in twelve cases, in four cases it was 1:76800; two patients had the titer 1:19200 and one had 1:1200. The presence of adrenal antibodies without pituitary antibodies was found in two patients only. In other two cases we detected pituitary antibodies in the absence of adrenal antibodies. Only four patients (16 %) had neither pituitary nor adrenal antibodies.

Among patients with autoimmune hypothyroidism 13 (65 %) had adrenal antibodies. The titre of the antibodies was 1:307200 in four cases, 1:76800 in other four, in another four was 1:19200 and 1:4800 in one case. Pituitary antibodies were found in 12 (60%) patients. Seven of these patients had wery high antibodies titre 1:307200, in three cases the titre was 1:76800 and in two cases 1:4800. Two patients had adrenal antibodies in the absence of pituitary antibodies and one patient had pituitary but no adrenal antibodies. In six cases (30 %) neither adrenal nor pituitary antibodies were found.

Detailed results of adrenal and pituitary antibodies solid phase RIA in both groups of patients with autoimmune thyroid diseases are listed in Table 1 and 2. In the control group no adrenal antibodies were detected and only in one case the pituitary antibodies at 1:600 serum dilution was found.

Conclusions

1. In majority of patients with autoimmune thyroid diseases we detected by solid phase radioimmunoassay adrenal and pituitary antibodies.
2. In autoimmune hypothyroidism among 20 patients 13 (65 %) had adrenal antibodies and 12 (60 %) had pituitary antibodies. In 6 patients (30 %) adrenal and pituitary antibodies were not detected.
3. In 25 patients with autoimmune thyrotoxicosis we found the presence of adrenal antibodies in 19 (76 %) patients, and of pituitary antibodies in 19 (76 %) patients. Only in 4 (16 %) patients neither adrenal nor pituitary antibodies were detected.
4. In the majority of autoimmune thyroid diseases the titres of anti-adrenal and anti-pituitary antibodies were high although the patients did not present clinical manifestations of adrenal or pituitary dysfunction.
5. Results of our study indicate that autoimmune thyroid diseases constitute a part of a more generalized autoimmune process.

References

1. Scherbaum, W.A.: Acta Endocrinol. (Kbh), Suppl. **281** (1987), 325. - 2. Batterle, C., G. Callegari, F. Presotto, F. Zanette, B. Pedini, T. Rampazzo, R.S. Slack, M.E. Girelli, B. Busnardo: Acta Endocrinol. (Kbh), **114** (1987), 321. - 3. Kosowicz, J., M. Gryczyńska, G.F. Bottazzo: Clin. Exp. Immunol. **63** (1986), 671.

Table 1
Autoimmune Hyperthyroidism

No.	Patient	Sex F/M	Autoantibodies adrenal		pituitary	
1.	H.M.	F	+	1: 19200	++	1: 76800
2.	K.M.	F	+	1:307200	++	1:307200
3.	K.E.	F	-		-	
4.	R.B.	F	+++	1: 19200	++	1:307200
5.	S.M.	F	+++	1:307200	+++	1:307200
6.	P.E.	F	+++	1: 19200	+++	1: 76800
7.	Z.K.	F	+++	1: 4800	+++	1: 76800
8.	K.I.	F	+	1: 19200	++	1:307200
9.	S.K.	F	+++	1: 76800	+	1: 19200
10.	S.E.	F	-		-	
11.	O.M.	F	+++	1:307200	+++	1:307200
12.	B.M.	F	+	1: 76800	-	
13.	K.S.	F	+++	1:307200	+++	1:307200
14.	T.S.	F	+++	1:307200	+++	1:307200
15.	L.D.	F	-		-	
16.	S.D.	F	+	1: 1200	+	1: 76800
17.	S.M.	F	-		-	
18.	M.B.	F	+++	1: 76800	++	1: 19200
19.	R.W.	F	-		+	1:307200
20.	N.B.	M	+++	1:307200	+	1: 1200
21.	R.F.	M	+++	1:307200	+++	1:307200
22.	K.F.	M	++	1.: 76800	++	1:307200
23.	A.K.	M	+++	1:307200	+++	1:307200
24.	L.W.	M	-		+++	1:307200
25.	S.H.	M	+++	1: 76800	-	

Table 2

Autoimmune Hypothyroidism

No.	Patient	Sex F/M	Autoantibodies adrenal		pituitary	
1.	P.R.	F	+	1: 19200	+	1:307200
2.	G.E.	F	-		-	
3.	M.M.	F	++	1: 19200	+	1: 4800
4.	M.I.	F	+++	1:307200	-	
5.	M.M.	F	+	1: 76800	+	1: 4800
6.	M.U.	F	-		-	
7.	W.M.	F	+++	1:307200	+++	1:307200
8.	P.J.	F	-		-	
9.	G.A.	F	+++	1: 76800	-	
10.	P.M.	F	-		-	
11.	K.C.	F	++	1:307200	++	1: 76800
12.	T.A.	F	+++	1: 19200	+++	1:307200
13.	K.L.	F	-		-	
14.	B.B.	F	-		+	1:307200
15.	G.D.	F	+	1: 76200	+++	1:307200
16.	K.E.	F	+	1: 76800	+++	1:307200
17.	D.M.	F	+++	1:307200	+++	1:307200
18.	N.J.	F	++	1: 19200	+	1: 76800
19.	T.M.	M	+	1: 4800	++	1: 76800
20.	S.M.	M	-		-	

Discussion

Benker: 1. What is the prevalence of adrenal autoantibodies in Addison's disease, using your assay system? 2. Can you comment as to the nature of the microsomal antigen which is recognized by your assay?

Remark: We have once studied adrenal autoantibodies in autoimmune Addison's disease using immunofluorescence where the prevalence was only 50 %.

Lacka: The prevalence in autoimmune Addison's disease is about

85 % using our assay system, solid phase immunoassay. And for the pituitary antibodies only immunofluorescence technique was used up to now. Radioimmunoassay is more sensitive than immunofluorescence. And of course it depends on the purification of the antigens and we used very pure microsomes. And to the second question: I think there is no information about the characterisation.

Limanova: We highly appreciate your paper, it will be used in the diagnosis of endocrinopathies in future.

One question. As far as the adrenal glands are infiltrated by lymphocytes in a large amount of autopsies, are there any correlations between the histological findings of adrenal from autopsie or from surgery you used for antibody method and the results you found in your studies? - I.E. don't you think that the adrenal material can influence the antibodies you got from patients?

Lacka: The adrenals are from patients with Cushing syndrome.

Gembicki: Material is taken from these cases, not from the autopsies. It is taken from patients treated by surgery.

Simova: 1. Is there a difference in the titre of antiadrenal antibodies in autoimmune thyroiditis and in Addison's disease? 2. Whether all functional tests for adrenal and pituitary functions have been applied to exclude a dysfunction of these glands?

Gembicki: The answer for the second question is: yes, all of them were controlled according to the functional status of adrenals and pituitary.

Lacka: This method is developed at our department and they have got the antigens, it means microsomes. They obtain microsomes for human pituitary gland and adrenal pituitary gland obtained from operated patients. Everything was prepared by the laboratory of our department. Only protein which can bind F_C-fragment of immunoglobuline, IGG is commercial.

Gembicki: I just would like to make a short comment: Since many years our department is working on different determination of different antibodies to different organs. And this is some kind of conclusion that with the progress of the methods whith possibility of the determination of different antibodies against pituitary, against thyroid, suprarenal gland and so on, we come to the conclusion that probably most of the endocrinopathies have multiimmune process as the basis for pathological changes. Of course some of the directions, some of ways are connected more or less with one organ, but usually we have several autoantibodies to several organs detected if we have autoimmunity process in some endocrine cases.

The effect of anti-microsomal antibodies on thyroid peroxidase activity

E. Mezösi, S. Szücs, S. Sárközi, E. Fórizs, J. Szabó and A. Leövey
University Medical School, I. Department of Medicine, Debrecen, Hungary

Thyroid microsomal antibodies (MAbs) are detectable in the serum of most patients with autoimmune thyroid disease (AITD). The nature of microsomal antigen (M-ag) remained unknown for more than twenty years after its discovery. Recently, it has become evident that the M-ag is very closely related to, if not identical with thyroid peroxidase (TPO) /2,4,5,11,12/. The TPO is a glycosilated hemoprotein bound to membranes with a mol. wt. of about 100-110 kD /2,5/. It is involved in two major steps of thyroid hormone biosynthesis: iodination of tyrosine residues on thyroglobulin and coupling of iodotyrosines into T_4 and T_3. The M-ag/TPO is expressed on the apical surface of thyroid cells /1/. The expression of M-ag is TSH dependent both on the surface and in the cytoplasm of the cells. By this time the complete cDNA and protein sequence of both human and porcine TPO has been revealed and a homology of 72 % was found /7/.

The presence of circulating anti-TPO antibodies in patients with AITD was independently identified by many investigators using different techniques /3,7,9,10,11/. It is well known since 1986 from Kohno's experiments that MAbs can inhibit TPO activity /8/.

The aim of our study was to investigate the effect of a relative large series of sera and IgG fractions from patients with AITD on TPO acticity.

Materials and Methods

82 untreated patients with Graves-Basedow disease (aged 16-64 yr, mean 39 yr, 69 women and 13 men) and 23 normal subjects (aged 20-72 yr, mean 43,4 yr, 16 women and 7 men) were included in the study.

The globulin fraction of sera was isolated by precipitation with ammonium-sulphate. In the first part of our work we prepared IgG fractions from 25 patients and 6 controls using ion exchange chromatography on DEAE-Sephacel column.

Microsomal antibodies were assayed with Boyden's passive haemagglutination.

Porcine TPO was prepared and purified according to A. Taurog et al. /15/. Briefly after homogenization the material was solubilised by sodium-cholate (1 % final concentration), precipitated by acetone and ammonium-sulphate and then we used ion exchange DEAE-cellulose column chromatography and gel filtration (Sephadex G-75) for purification of the enzyme. The specific activity was 14.1 GU/mg protein, the ratio A_{413}/A_{280} was 0.11.

The catalytic activity was measured by guaiacol and iodide assay according to Hosoya et al. /6/. The guaiacol assay was followed by the change in absorbance at 470 nm, the iodide substrate was measured at 350 nm. One unit was defined as the amount of enzyme required to produce an optical density change of 1.0/min. 20 μl of TPO was incubated with different amount of sera or IgG fractions (20-80 μl) at room temperature for one hour. The percent inhibition of TPO activity was calculated as follows:

$$\% \text{ inhibition} = 1 - \frac{A_{1\ min} \text{ with TPO + serum}}{A_{1\ min} \text{ with TPO alone}} \times 100$$

Results

In the first part of our work we compared the effect of globulin fractions and purified IgG fractions from 25 G-B patients and 6 controls using guaiacol and iodide substrates. The inhibitory effect was dose-dependent in every cases. In the iodine assays both the patients' and controls' sera inhibited the activity of TPO, we didn't find any difference between the two groups. Fig. 1 shows the effect of graded amount (20-80μl) of IgG fractions. There is a significant difference between the mean values. The normal IgG didn't decrease TPO activity, IgG fractions from 13 out of 25 patients (52 %) showed inhibitory effect in varying degree (10-52%, mean 14.9±16.6 %). Sera from all the 25 patients inhibited the peroxidation of guaiacol. Using 80 µl sera the inhibition ranged from 30-100 % (Mean 53±18 %) control sera caused a moderate decrease of encymatic activity (less than 20 %), which seems to be a nonspecific effect (Fig. 2). Using IgG fractions in the guaiacol assay, IgG from 22 out of 25 patients (88 %) inhibited TPO activity. The inhibition was less than in the case of sera, ranged from 15 to 45 %, mean 34±14 %. No inhibitory effect of control IgG was detected (less than 5 %) (Fig. 3).

In the second part of our work we examined sera from 82 patients suffered from G-B disease and 23 normal subjects using guaiacol assay. Fig. 4 demonstrates our results. The majority of patients' sera inhibited TPO activity. The mean of patient group was 49.5 %, ranged from -15 to 100 %. The value of control group was 18.3±15.3 %. 85 % of patients showed significant inhibition when we defined the positive value as more than the mean + SD of control group.

Finally, we investigated the relationship between the inhibitory effect of sera and microsomal antibodies measured by passive haemagglutination (Fig. 5). We found a correlation characterized by the following parameters: $r = 0.359$, $p = 0.0008$, $y = 4.1*\log_2 X + 18.87$. This provided further evidence of the relationship between the M-ag and TPO.

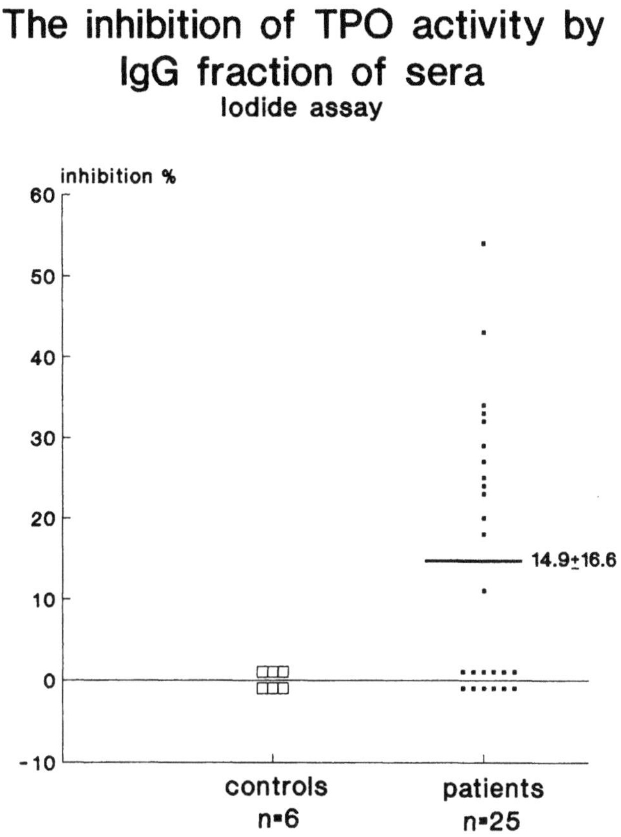

Figure 1
The IgG fraction from 13 out of 25 G-B patients (52 %) showed inhibitory effect on TPO activity using iodide assay. The inhibition ranged from 10 to 52 %, mean 14.9±16.6 %. The IgG fractions from other patients and controls didn't inhibit the TPO activity. Each pint is the mean of triplicate assays.

The inhibition of TPO activity by sera from patients and controls
Guaiacol assay

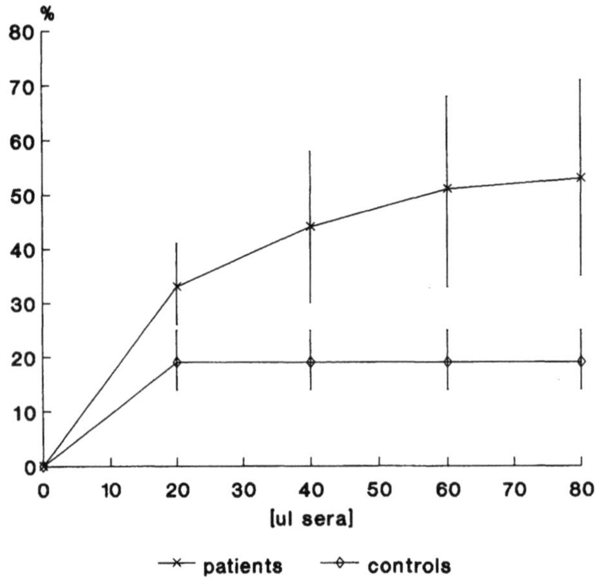

Mean (+SD) of 25 patients
Mean (+SD) of 6 controlls
p‹0,05

Figure 2
In the guaiacol assay all the 25 patients' sera caused inhibition of TPO. Using 80 /ul serum, the inhibitory effect ranged from 30 to 100 %, the mean ± S.D. was 53±18 %. All the sera from controls showed a nonspecific inhibition less than 20 %.

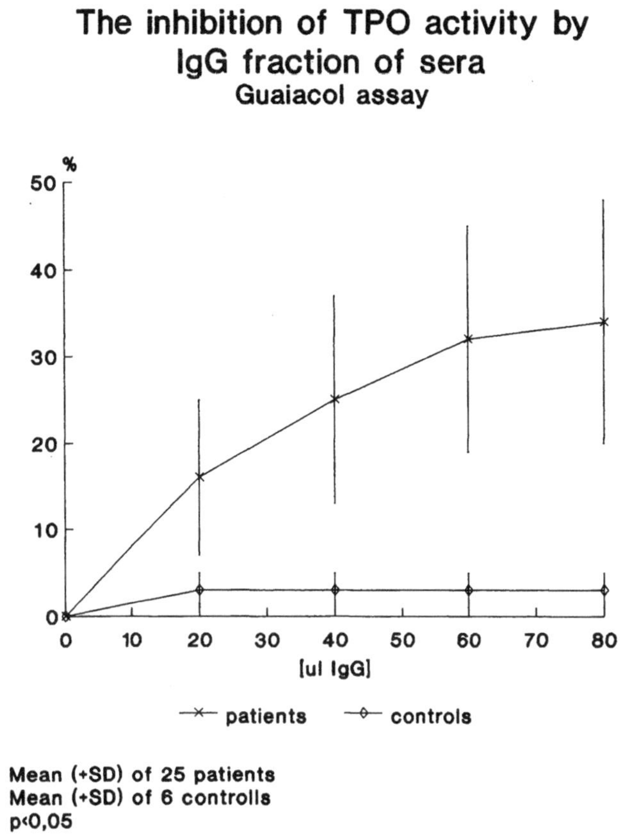

Figure 3
The IgG fraction from 22 out of 25 G-B patients (88 %) inhibited the TPO activity using guaiacol assay. Mean 34±14 %, ranged from 15 to 45 %. No inhibitory effect of controls' IgG was detected (less than 5 %).

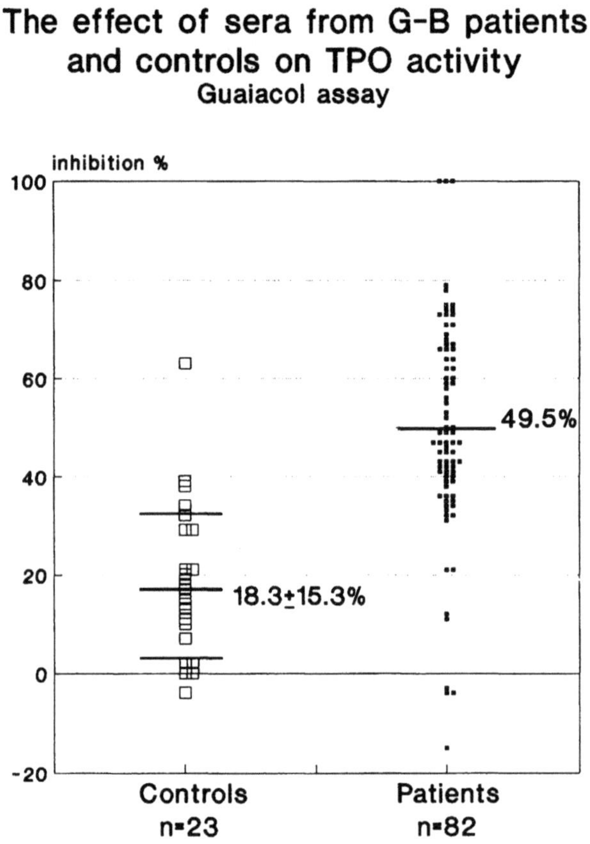

Figure 4
The majority of patients' sera inhibited TPO activity. The mean of patient group was 49.5 %, ranged from -15 to 100 %. The value of control group was 18.3±15.3 %. Defining the positive value as more than the mean + S.D. of control group, 85 % of patients showed significant inhibition. Each point is the mean of triplicate assays.

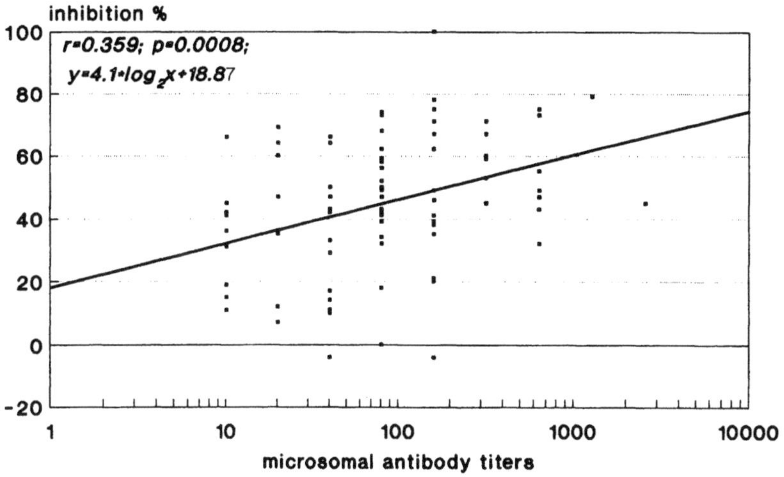

Figure 5
The inhibition of TPO activity by sera from patients and controls correlate with the microsomal antibody titers measured by Boyden' passive haemagglutination.

Discussion

In this study we investigated the effect of MAbs from patients with AITD on porcine TPO activity. Reports from several laboratories have established that TPO is very closely related to M-ag /3-11/. We used partially purified porcine TPO as antigen, which is accepted in the literature. The catalytic activity was measured by two substrates: iodide and guaiacol. According to recently published studies /3,16,17/ we observed that the majority of Basedow patients' sera decreased the peroxidation of guaiacol (85 %), but only 52 % of patients show inhibitory effect in the iodide assay. Data from immunoblot experiments /3-5,14/ support that the catalytic site dealing with peroxidation of guaiacol is the most potent autoantigenic epitope of TOP. There is not consensus according to the numbers of epitopes of TPO, some authors found 6, others 7 epitopes which can provoke immune reactivity /3,14/. This results in a large heterogenity of anti-TPO antibodies, which can explain the variability of inhibitory capacity. Our findings confirm this theory. An alternative explanation for antibody interference with TPO enzymatic activity would be a change in the conformation of TPO, which would lead to masking or exposure of catalytic sites and results in decreased or increased activity.

Comparing the effect of serum and IgG fractions on TPO we found that the serum had a nonspecific, which caused about 20 % inhibition in the guaiacol assay and disturbed the evaluation of iodide assay. We didn't observed this phenomenon using IgG fractions. Experiments with IgG provide more accurate results, but routinely the serum is suitable for the guaiacol assay,

We found a correlation between the inhibition of TPO activity and MAbs titres. We join the observations of Yokoyama and Okamoto, who reported similar results /13,16,17/. Using more sensitive methods for detecting MAbs the correlation might become closer.

So far many details about TPO has been revealed, but in vivo importance of enzyme inhibition remained unclear and further investigations are required.

References

1. Chiovato, L., P. Vitti et al.: Clin. Exp. Immunol. **76** (1989), 47. - 2. Czarnocka, B., J. Ruf et al.: FEBS Letts **190** (1985), 147. - 3. Doble, N.D., J.P. Banga et al.: Immunology **64** (1988), 23. - 4. Hamada, N., N. Jaeduck et al.: J. Clin. Endocrinol. Metab. **64** (1987), 230. - 5. Hamada, N., L. Portman et al.: J. Clin. Invest. **79** (1987), 8/9. - 6. Hosoya, T., I. Sato et al.: J. Biochem. **98** (1985), 637. - 7. Kimura, S., T. Kotani et al.: Proc. Natl. Acad. Sci. USA **84** (1987), 5555. - 8. Kohno, Y., Y. Hiyama et al.: Clin. Exp. Immunol. **65** (1986), 534. - 9. Kotani, T., K. Umeki et al.: J. Clin. Endocrinol. Metab. **62** (1986),928. - 10. Mariotti, S. et al.: J. Clin. Endocrinol. Metab. **65** (1987), 987. - 11. Portman, L., N. Hamada et al.: J. Clin. Endocrinol. Metab. **61** (1985), 1001. - 12. Portman, L., F. Fitch et al.: J. Clin. Invest. **81** (1988), 1217. - 13. Okamoto, Y.,N. Hamada et al.: J. Clin. Endocrinol. Metab. **68** (1989), 730. - 14. Ruf, J., N. Toubert et al.: Endocrinology **125** (1989), 1211. - 15. Taurog, A. et al.: Arch. Biochemist. Biophysic. **139** (1970), 221. - 16. Yokoyama, N., A. Taurog et al.: J. Clin. Endocrinol. Metab. **68** (1989), 766. - 17. Yokoyama, N., A. Taurog et al.: Clin. Endocrinol. Metab. **70** (1990), 758.

Discussion

Benker: I wonder if antibody has ever shown that the requirement for antithyroid drugs is lower in patients with a high titer of anti-TPO antibodies - due to a kind of self - inhibition of thyroid function in these patients; provided, of course, that these antibodies can, somehow, reach the enzyme within the thyrocytes.

Mezösi: I think it is the most important question about the enzyme inhibition at the recent level of our knowledge, that in the group of patients suffered from AITD with high titer of anti-TPO-antibodies would be expected more severe hypothyroidism. It was reported in the literature, but only one article delt with this problem so far as I know. So further follow-up studies are required in this area.

Antithyroid antibodies in the synovial fluid in thyroiditis

K. Łacka, M. Gembicki
University School of Medicine, Department of Endocrinology, Poznań, Poland

Hashimoto's thyroiditis, the most common clinical type of thyroiditis is characterized by the presence of specific antithyroid antibodies in patients serum as well as the infiltration of the thyroid gland by lymphocytes or plasma cells. Antithyroglobulin and antimicrosomal antibodies are detectable in the serum of nearly all these patients, often with very high titer /4/.

In this paper there are described two unrelated patients with Hashimoto's thyroiditis and elevated antithyroid antibodies in the synovial fluid aspirated from the elbow cyst.

Material and methods

Case report

The first patient, H.S., is a 47-yr old man with Hashimoto's disease. His thyroid was enlarged /III° according to WHO classification/ and diffuse with the presence of a pyramidal lobe. Goiter developed during the last 3 years. Thyroid radioisotope scan showed an uneven distribution of isotope. Thyroid radioactive iodine uptake was 28 % at 24 h. Serum TSH was 6.5 μU/ml (normal range: 0.35-5.0 μU/ml), serum total thyroxine: 5.5 μg/dl (normal range: 4-12 μg/dl), serum total triiodothyronine: 122 ng/dl (normal range: 80-200 ng/dl). Histological examination of the thyroid needle biopsy specimen revealed an infiltration of the gland with plasma cells and lymphocytes and follicular destruction. A. cyst located in the elbow area, painfree and without motor limitation was observed. There is no records of rheumatoid disease of this patient.

Second patient, A.C., 52-yr old woman was admitted to the Department of Endocrinology with a large /III° according to WHO classification/, painfull thyroid and the presence of the elbow cyst also painfree and without motor limitation. Enlargement of the thyroid was noted for six last months, the elbow cyst for 3 last days. As in the first case no records of rheumatoid disease was present. She appeared euthyroid: serum total thyroxine was 4.2 /ug/dl, serum total triiodothyronine: 92 ng/dl and serum TSH was 2.5 /uU/ml, radioactive iodine uptake by the thyroid was 35 % at 24 h. The scan showed the asymetric thyroid gland and in biopsy material the infiltration with lymphocytes and plasma cells in focal areas was described.

Methods

Blood samples and synovial fluid were taken for determination of antithyroid antibodies and specific antibodies against various structures. Synovial fluid was aspirated from the elbow cyst. Samples were mixed with EDTA for white cells contents and were centrifuged at 1500 x g for 10 min. The supernatant was stored at -40 °C.

Antithyroglobulin and antimicrosomal antibodies in serum and synovial fluid were measured by solid-phase radioimmuniassay, immunofluorescence and tanned red cell haemagglutination test /1,3,5,6,7/. Antibodies to antinuclear factor, mitochondria, smooth muscle, gastric parietal cells, biliaris ductuli were determined with an immunifluorescence technique /5/. Rheumatoid factor was detected by haemagglutination test /5/.

Results

Table 1 show the results of the various antibodies detected in serum and synovial fluid. In both serum and synovial fluid antibodies to antinuclear factor, gastric parietal cells,mitochondria, smooth muscle and biliaris ductuli as well as rheumatoid factor were not found.

The occurence of antithyroglobulin and antimicrosomal antibodies determined by solid-phase radioimmunoassay as well as haemagglutination and immunofluorescence test in serum of investigated patients have not been detected.
However these antibodies were present in synovial fluid in both cases using all three methods (table 1 and 2).

Table 1: Results of haemagglutination and immunofluorescence tests for various antibodies in serum and synovial fluid of two patients with Hashimoto's disease

antibody	serum n = 2	synovial fluid n = 2
rheumatoid factor > 1:32	negative	negative
antinuclear factor > 1:20	"	"
gastric parietal cells	"	"
mitochondrial	"	"
smooth-muscle	"	"
biliaris ductuli	"	"

Table 2: Occurence of antithyroglobulin / anti-Tg / and antimicrosomal / anti-Mo / antibodies in serum and synovial fluid of two patients with Hashimoto's thyroiditis / detected by solid-phase RIA, haemagglutination / Hg / and immunofluorescence / IF / test

		Anti-Mc			Anti-Tg		
		RIA	Hg	IF	RIA	Hg	IF
case 1	serum	neg	neg	neg	neg	neg	neg
	synovial fluid	60 %	1:25600	+	55 %	1:25600	+
case 2	serum	neg	neg	neg	neg	neg	neg
	synovial fluid	36 %	1:640	+	20 %	1:640	4

Discussion

The diagnosis of Hashimoto's thyroiditis can be confirmed by biochemical test showing euthyroidism or mild hypothyroidism, by estimation of the thyroid antibodies in serum and by thyroid gland biopsy examination. According to our knowledge there are no patients described with Hashimoto's disease with elevated antithyroid antibodies in their synovial·fluid. Blake and al. showed the presence of thyroid antibodies in the synovial fluid aspirated from the knees in patients with various rheumatoid diseases /2/.

The presence of antithyroid antibodies detected in the synovial fluid without elevated antithyroglobulin and antimicrosomal antibodies in serum in two patients described in this paper seems to be the result of local production of antithyroid antibodies by synovial leucocytes /2,4/.

Conclusion

Antithyroglobulin and antimicrosomal antibodies in synovial fluid aspirated from the elbow cyst in patients with Hashimoto's disease were found.

References

1. Amino, N. et al. Clin. Endocrinol. **5** (1976), 115. - 2. Blake, D.R. et al. Lancet **II** (1979), 224. - 3. Cayzer, I. et al. J. Clin. Pathol. **31** (1978), 1147. - 4. De Groot, L.J. et al. Endocrine Reviews **10** (1989), 537. - 5. Johnson, J.D. et al. Hand book of experimental immunology. Immunochemistry. Oxford: Blackwell 1/1973, chap. 18. - 6. Kosowicz, J. et al. Pol. Arch. Med. Wewn. **67** (1982), 225. - 7. Lacka, K. et al. Radiob. Radioth. **25** (1984), 729.

Discussion

Benker: Did your patients have other clinical signs of rheumatic diseases?

Lacka: No, they have no signs, only we have observed the elbow-cyst without motor-limitation, without pain. And they have no recourse of rheunatoid disease. And we have aspirated the synovial fluid and have given to this patients steroids, 100 mg

of hydrocortison and afterwards till for weeks we have no observed cysts.
Benker: Did you have the chance to study aspirates of synovial fluid from patients with rheumatoid arthritis?
Lacka; According our knowledge we have no patients with thyroiditis disease and elevated antithyroglobuline and antimicrosomal antibodies in synovial fluid. But there is one paper about the occurrence of antithyroglobuline and antimicrosomal antibodies in synovial fluid aspirated from the nees in patients with rheumatoid diseases, not with thyroid diseases. And there are no problems to detect antithyroid antibodies in synovial fluid. It is the same method.
Gembicki: We did not investigate that rheumatoid cases, we know only the information from the literature that some cases were investigated. But we could not find any information about the thyroiditis and any kind of cyst investigated for this antibodies.
Lacka: We have measured the cytosis comparence in the synovial fluid, aspirated from this patient and in first case there were about 4500 cells per one milliliter. And in the second patient there were 5200 cells per ml. It means that it was inflammatory fluid. But we have not measured viscosis.
Leövey: Did you check the lymphocytes in synovial fluids?
Lacka: We have measured only the cells in the synovial fluid, we have not measured population of lymphocytes. But I think it should be the result of the production of subpopulation there in the synovial fluid.
Leövey: May be, that these locally produced antibodies play an important role in the cell-mediated cytotoxic immunity?

Immunological and genetical aspects in T_3-predominant Graves' disease

Sabine Gerlach, H.F. Deckart, Eva Deckart and Annemarie Blottner
Klinik für Innere Medizin Universität Leipzig, Klinik für Nuklearmedizin und Endokrinologie im Klinikum Berlin-Buch, Germany

Nowadays it is undisputed that the special entity or biochemical feature termed T_3-predominant hyperthyroidism may appear in association with toxic multinodular goiter, toxic adenoma, but also Graves' disease /1/. T_3-predominant hyperthyroidism may be a short-time state in the course of a thyrotoxicosis or in some cases the forerunner of the usual form of thyrotoxicosis in which both T_3 and T_4 production are increased, whereas in other patients it may persist as such /2,3/. The aim of our study was to find out, if there is any special immunologic or genetic background in patients with T_3-predominant Graves' disease.

Patients and methods

We investigated 106 patients with Graves' disease (11 males, 95 females, mean age 46 years) in the first onset or in relapse of the disease - minimum three months and maximum one year after cessation of drug treatment. They were compared with a control group (n = 40, 22 males, 18 females, mean age 40 years).
The differentiation between immunogenic and non immunogenic hyperthyroidism was carried out in the usual clinical way and by determination of thyroid antibodies /4/ and ultrasound investigation. We used a RIA for the determination of TAb, the passive haemagglutination method for determination of MAb (Wellcome) and a radioligand receptor assay (Henning) for TRAb measurement. HLA antigens were estimated by a microlymphocyte-toxicity-test.

Results

22.6 % of our patients were suffering from a T_3-predominant disease (table 1). The real and exact prevalence of T_3-toxicosis found by the most other authors is uncertain, but may be as high as 10 percents or even a little higher in areas of iodine deficiency without selection of autoimmune disease /1/.

It was very surprising for us, that 71.1 % of our patients with T_3-predominant Graves' disease showed relapses, whereas this portion was only 29.2 % in patients with combined T_3/T_4-hyperthyroidism (table 1).

Table 1: T_3-predominant and T_3/T_4-combined hyperthyroidism and relapses

patients	T_3-predominant G.d.	combined T_3/T_4 G.d.
n	24	82
%	22.6	77.4
relapses %	71.1	29.2

We observed the following interesting results in the distribution of TAb and MAb in T_3-predominant and combined T_3/T_4-Graves' disease (table 2): The patients with selective T_3-hyperthyroidism showed positive TAb in nearly 50 % and positive MAb in 100 % contrary to positive TAb in 17 % and positive MAb in 83 % of our patients with combined T_3/T_4-hyperthyroidism. Nearly 50 % of the patients with T_3-predominant hyperthyroidism showed both TAb and MAb, whereas this antibody pattern was found only in 16 % of the patients with combined T_3/T_4-hyperthyroidism (table 2).

Table 3 demonstrates a comparison of higher and lower antibody levels, a method used by many other authors, too. We summarized three titer or concentration steps into one group at least because of possible differences in the antibody secretion rate of the thyroid. Patients with T_3-hyperthyroidism were found to have significant higher levels of MAb in 75 % in contrast to 37 % of the patients with T_3/T_4-hyperthyroidism (table 3).

The patients with Graves' disease (total group) showed a significantly higher distribution of HLAB8 (31 %) in comparison with the control group (table 4).

Table 2: Distribution of autoantibodies
Graves' disease (n = 106)

antibodies TAb, MAb, TRAb	T_3-hyperthyroidism n	%	T_3/T_4-hyperthyroidism n	%	significance p <
TAb positive MAb pos. and negative	11	46	14	17	0.01
MAb positive TAb pos. and negative	24	100	68	83	0.05
TAb positive MAb positive	11	46	13	16	0.01
at least 1 antibody pos. MAb or TAb	24	100	69	84	0.05
TAb negative MAb negative	0	0	13	16	0.05
TAb positive MAb negative	0	0	1	1	n.s.
TRAb positive	22	92	72	88	n.s.

Table 3: Comparison of antibody titers and concentrations (Graves' disease, n = 106)

antibodies	levels or titer steps	T_3-hyperthyroidism positive n	%	significance p <	T_3/T_4-hyperthyroidism positive n	%	significance p <	significance between both groups p <
TAb (mg/l)	positive	11	100		14	100		
	> 0.1-25 > 25 - > 40	9 2	82 18	0.01	8 6	57 43	n.s.	n.s.
MAb (titer steps)	positive	24	100		68	100		
	1:400-1:25600 1:102400-1:6.5 Mio	6	25	0.01	43	63	0.01	0.01
TRAb (U/l)	positive	22	100		72	100		
	10-180 >180->405	16 6	71 29	0.01	50 22	70 30	0.01	n.s.

Table 4: HLA-B8 in Graves' disease and control group

patients	n	HLA-B8 n	HLA-B8 %	significance p <
control group*	3000	540	18	0.01
Graves' disease	61	19	31	

*Schleusener 1984

The most HLAB8 positive patients (47 %) were found in the group with T_3-hyperthyroidism (table 5),

Table 5: HLA-B8 and comparison of patients with T_3-predominant and T_3/T_4-combined Graves' disease

patients	n	HLA-B8 n	HLA-B8 %	significance p <	
control group*	3000	540	18	0.01	
T_3-hyper-thyroidism	15	7	47		n.s.
T_3/T_4-hyper-thyroidism	46	13	28	n.s.	

*Schleusener 1984

Discussion

The relatively high prevalence of T_3-predominant Graves' disease in our patients (22.6 %) may be due to a special situation in iodine supply in the area of the former GDR in 1987, when the study was performed /5,6/. The iodine salt prophylaxis showed its top effects just in this time /7/ and also in immunogenic hyperthyroidism /5,8/.
The results of high prevalence of relapses in our patients with T_3-predominant Graves' disease are compatible with those of Takamatsu in 1986 /9/. One could conclude, that remissions possibly not really occured in our patients if taking account of the short time after cessation of antithyroid drug treatment in some patients, the special situation of iodine supply in that time and the finding of autonomously functioning areas also in Graves' goiters recently reported /10-12/.

To explain the high prevalence of TAb and MAb and the higher MAb titers of our patients with T_3-predominant Graves' disease we considered the following hypotheses: 1. special immunological activity, special affinity or specifity of the antibodies; 2. higher "overflow" of the antibodies; 3. altered and enhanced iodine metabolism via TPO in iodine deficient Graves' goiter.
We prefer the last hypothesis regarding the results reported by Takamatsu in 1988 /13/, who observed a lower iodine content in the thyroglobulin, increased titers of microsomal antibodies with positive correlation with higher antibody levels against TPO and a higher activity of TPO in patients with T_3-predominant Graves' disease. It has to be discussed if there exists an altered and enhanced iodine metabolism via TPO in iodine deficient Graves' goiters.
A high prevalence of relapses in HLAB8 positive patients with Graves' disease (without differentiation into T_3- and T_3/T_4-hyperthyroidism) has been discussed /14,15/. It's a new finding by us that HLAB8-positivity is mostly found in patients with T_3-predominant hyperthyroidism and in patients showing relapses. Thus T_3-hyperthyroidism may possibly be a predictor of relapses in HLAB8 positive patients with Graves' disease.

Further investigations will be required to define the structure of microsomal antibodies and antigen-that means of the TPO and its different epitopes /18/ under the special circumstances of T_3-hyperthyroidism. And it remains to be clarified the question, if there exist autonomously functioning areas in Graves' goiters tending to T_3-predominant hyperthyroidism in iodine deficiency areas.

Conclusions

The high prevalence of T_3-predominant Graves' disease in our patients may be the result of iodine prophylaxis in 1987. The high prevalence of TAb and MAb and higher MAb titers in T_3-predominant patients with Graves' disease can only be explained by hypotheses. May be these findings are expression of an altered iodine metabolism via TPO in iodine deficient Graves' goiters. We observed T_3-hyperthyroidism preferentially in HLAB8 positive patients and in patients with relapses. Thus T_3-hyperthyroidism may possibly be a predictor of relapses, above all in HLAB8 positive patients with Graves' disease.

References

1. Ingbar, S.H. in: Williams: Textbook of Endocrinology, 7. Aufl., Saunders Co. 1985, S. 719. - 2. Oberdisse, K., E. Klein and D. Reinwein: Die Krankheiten der Schilddrüse, 2. Aufl., Thieme Stuttgart 1980, S. 311. - 3. Loos, U., F. Konrad and E.F. Pfeiffer: Klin. Wochenschr. (1981), 495. - 4. Schumm-Draeger, H.J., C. Wenisch: Akt. Endokr. Stoff. **10** (1989), 90. - 5. Deckart, H., E. Deckart and F. Behringer: Acta Med. Austriaca, 39. - 6. Spaulding, S.W. and H. Lippes: Med. Clinics of North Amer. **69** (1985), 937. - 7. Bauch, K., W. Seitz, S. Förster and U. Keil: Z. gesamte inn. Med. **45** (1990), 8. - 8. Schicha, R. and D. Emrich: Dt. med. Wochenschr. **108** (1983), 6. - 9. Takamatsu, J., K. Kuma and T. Mozai: J. Clin. Endocrinol. Metab. **62** (1986), 980. - 10. Studer, H., H.J. Peter and H. Gerber: Clin. Endocrinol. Metab. **14** (1985), 351. - 11. Schleusener, H., H. Schwander, C. Fischer et al.: Acta Endocrinol. **120** (1989), 689. - 12. Kraiem, Z., B. Glaser, M. Yigla et al.: J. Clin. Endocrinol. Metab. **65** (1987), 659. -13. Takamatsu, J., T. Hosoya, N. Naito

et al.: J. Clin. Endocrinol. Metab. **66** (1988), 147. - 14. Jahnke, K.A., M. Kinner and D. Reinwein:Münchener med. Wochenschr. **125** (1983), 385. - 15. Preus, M., M.F. Frecker, V. Stensky et al.: Clin. Endocrinol. **23** (1985), 653. - 16. Furmaniak, J. and B. Rees Smith: Autoimmunity **7** (1990), 63.

Discussion

Gembicki: May I ask you kindly for explanation, what do you mean speaking on "T_3-predominant Graves' disease", is that situation when only T_3 is elevated and T_4 normal?

Gerlach: That's right, I think it is only a laboratory status, a biochemical finding and not a special disease.

Gembicki: We know that T_3 in significant number of thyroid diseases is first higher and than after some time T_4 rise is observed. This is the normal course of the development. How it was in your predominant T_3 cases, are they all in the time T_3 predominant or later on they had T_3 and T_4 elevated?

Gerlach: I have to say that these results were found accidently. We performed another study and this was only retrospective study, we have not performed a follow-up study of these patients. That's why I can't answer if this patients any time changed into the normal course of Graves' disease.

Gembicki: My last question concerns your information that this T_3-predomination may be connected with more intensive iodine prophylaxis you had in 1987. Why the year 1987 was so special and influencing the course of the disease in your country?

Gerlach: We had a special situation in the former GDR, we performed a special iodine prophylaxis. This prophylaxis started in 1983. At first it was performed in human beings and since 1985 we started with animal feeding. Animals were feeded with iodine and the first positive result in iodine excretion of patients was found in March 1986. In 1987 we had the top-effect of this prophylaxis and accidently we performed the study in this time in 1987. The influence of iodine excess was very great in that time.

Gembicki: If you mentioned that you got the first positive results in iodine prophylaxis in March 1986, you are very lucky because it was just before the Tschernobyl catastrophe and it means that your population was relatively well secured.

Simova: Did you find any disorders in TSAb?

Gerlach: No, there were not significant differences in comparison of TSAb between patients with T_3- and T_4-hyperthyroidism.

Leövey: Did you find an increased radioiodine uptake in your patients with T_3-hyperthyroidism?

Deckart: We have not the iodine uptake curve but we performed the trapping.

Benker: To avoid confusion, there is not a definition of T_3-predominance in hyperthyroidism and it is related to a subgroup of patients who are usually young and have large goiters and usually endocrinologically activ. When they are treated with antithyroid drugs they tend to go down with the T_4 and stay way up with the T_3. So they have hyperthyroid T_4 values and thyrotoxic T_3 values. Thats another definition of T_3-predominance and they have a very poor prognosis when they are treated with drugs. But that is not what you mean, you mean hyperthyroidism presenting only with a raced T_3, a normal T_3?

Gerlach: Thats right, in literature are very different definitions of this T_3-hyperthyroidism. Some say selective T_3-hyperthyroidism other say predominant T_3-hyperthyroidism.

Hnikova: How was the TSH-TRH test in the so called predominant T_3-hyperthyroidism?

Gerlach: It has no significance.

Leb: As you suggest the effect of iodine prophylaxis as one of the causes of the high incidence of T_3-hyperthyroidism, did you perform iodine excretion measurements in this patients?

Gerlach: No, we didn't, because it was not the aim of the study we performed in 1987 and these results were found later.

Unexpected course in immunological pattern in Graves' Basedow's disease - Marine-Lenhart Syndrome?

H.F. Deckart, Eva Deckart, Annemarie Blottner, E. Strehlau, G. Mühr
Klinikum Berlin-Buch, Clinic for Nuclear Medicine and Endocrinology

The immunogenic hyperthyroidism, Graves'-Basedow's disease, is characterized by typical diagnostic criteria: increased iodine clearance of the thyroid represented by high pertechnetate trapping (as clearance equivalent), diffuse echopoor pattern in ultrasound as result of microfollicular tissue structure and lymphocytic infiltration, increase of thyroid extension in the depth, detectability of thyrotropin binding inhibiting antibodies (TBIAb) and increase antimicrosomal antibodies (MsAb), to a lower extent antithyroglobulin antibodies (TgAb).

Within our series of 579 patients with Graves'-Basedow's disease we observed 84 cases (14.5 %) with lack of serum-positive immunological parameter at onset of the disease or at time of first investigation or with discrepancies in the follow up.
These results are reported here in addition to our first notice in 1987 /1/.

Methods

Determination of antimicrosomal antibodies (MgAb) by hemagglutination test, of antithyroglobulin antibodies (TgAb) by radioligand assay, of TSH-binding inhibiting antibodies (TIAb) by TRAK^{R}-assay (Henning). Evaluation of clinical criteria together with hormone concentration measurements of TT_4, TT_3 and TSH and scintigraphy with pertechnetate Tc-99m, calculation of pertechnetate uptake or trapping in the thyroid, high resolution real time ultrasonography.

Patients

84 patients, 77 females, 11 males, male:female ratio 1:7, aged between 16 and 80 years. Mean 44.4 years of age: 4 patients were less than 20 years, 10 out of the third decade of life, 19 of fourth, 35 of fifth, 10 of sixth and 6 of the seventh decade.

52 out of 84 patients had an immunogenic-endocrine orbitopathy (61.9 %). Patients were treated with methimazole over a period of 2.6 years in mean, some up to 7 years. In 16 patients (19 %) recurrence after successful treatment and euthyroid state more than one year let to new thyrostatic drug therapy followed by definitive treatment with I-131 therapy in 11 patients, and surgery in 6, combination of both in 1 case.

Follow up investigation

At onset of the disease 83 out of 84 patients had the typical diffuse echopoor ultrasonographic pattern of the thyroid gland.

During treatment 56 % of patients changed to echonormal pattern, but 44 % persisted echopoor even in an euthyroid metabolic state.

Immune parameter at onset hyperthyroidism were:

TRAK positive, MsAb/TgAb negative in 58 patients
TRAK negative, MsAb/TgAb positive in 23 patients
TRAK negative, MsAb/TgAb negative in 3 patients

The behaviour of immune parameter was changing during treatment in the following manner, categorized into five groups (e.O. = patients with endocrine orbitopathy):

	before	during	after treatment
Group I			
N 38 (22 e.O.)			
TRAK	38 positive	38 decrease	26 pos./12 neg.
MsAB/TgAb	38 negative		38 neg.

	before	during	after treatment
Group II			
N 21 (14 e.O.)			
TRAK	21 positive	21 decrease	6 pos./15 neg.
MsAb	21 negative	21 positive	20 pos./ 1 neg.
TgAb	21 negative	6 positive	6 pos./16 neg.
Group IV			
N 3 (2 e.O.)			
TRAK	3 negative	3 positive	3 positive
MsAb	3 negative	3 positive	3 positive
TgAb	3 negative	3 positive	3 positive
Group III			
N 9 (5 e.O.)			
TRAK	9 negative	9 negative	9 negative
MsAb	9 positive	9 positive	9 positive
TgAb	1 positive		1 positive
	8 negative		8 negative
Group V			
N 14 (7 e.O.)			
TRAK	14 negative		14 positive
MsAb	14 positive	positive increased	14 positive increased titer
TgAb	6 negative		6 negative
	8 positive		8 positive

In comparison to the course of ultrasound pattern and immune reaction we may give the results of another series of 172 patients with immunogenic hyperthyroidism diagnosed and treated in our clinic in table 1.

Table 1: Course of ultrasound pattern and immune serum parameter in 172 patients with Graves'-Basedow's disease at onset and follow up under treatment with methimazole

Ultrasound pattern:			
at onset before treatment	diffuse echopoor	171	99.42 %
	echonormal	1	
18 months after treatment	diffuse echopoor	46	67.9 %
	less echopoor	68	
	echonormal	57	33.1 %
Immune parameter:			
before treatment		%	
TRAK ≥ 10 U/L	166	(96.5)	
MsAb ≥ 1:400	130	(75.6)	
TgAb ≥ 200 IE/L	46	(26.7)	
after treatment:			
TRAK ≥ 10 U/L	47	(36.6)	
MsAb ≥ 1:400	109	(63.4)	
TgAb ≥ 200 IE/L	39	(22.7)	

Results and discussion

The titer of serum antibody level may depend from the thyroid tissue volume - but we have observed no correlation between ultrasonographically determined thyroid volume and the course or activity of immune parameter.
The discrepancy of immune parameter course was found in 84 out of 579 cases of immune hyperthyroidism beeing detected and treated in our clinic - this are 14.5 %.
In 19 out of 84 patients micronodules were seen ultrasonographically within the diffuse echopoor pattern of thyroid -

these are 22.6 % of all: Studer et al. /2/ have observed the development of multiple hyperplasia and even macroscopic nodules with autonomous function growing even after the decrease of immunostimulation, resulting from longtime immunogenic stimulation of the gland. Marine and Lenhart described this observation in patients with Basedow's disease pathological-anatomically first in 1911 /3/. In one fourth of our patients the discrepancy of immune parameter behaviour can be declared in this way.

The negative results of TRAK-assay in an active immunogenic hyperthyroidism may by caused on the other hand from the so called "overflow phenomenon": since Kendall-Taylor described the production of TBIAb by B-lymphocytes within the thyroid gland in 1984 /4/ the concentration may be sometimes not high enough to be measured in the peripheral blood /5/, despite in overflow-situation. Thirdly one may see the discrepancy in detectable TBIAb and undetectable MsAb/TgAb-titer in serum by a prefered follicle cell stimulation without cell destruction (group I and II). Finally, the negative TBIAb serum level is discussed to be caused by antiidiotypic antibodies /6/, which we didn't investigate or by different stimulation respectively binding-inhibiting activity of TBIAb, which cannot be analyzed with the used radioligand assay.
One should take into account that the immunological process in Graves'-Basedow's disease is a dynamic process, in which one might bot find positive serum criteria at any time: within the course phases of activity with maximum stimulation and cell destruction change with those of decreased activity, as we know even from clinical symptomatology in this self-perpetuing process (group I, II, IV, V). This one should consider in regarding the immune parameter as in first diagnosis at onset as in the follow up of the disease.

Conclusion

1. Ultrasound diffuse echopoor pattern has been the most sensitive diagnostic parameter in the differentiation of immunogenic hyperthyroidism.
2. The absence or low titer of immune parameter (TBIAb, MsAb, TgAb) don't exclude an active immunogenic process in Graves'-Basedow's disease.
3. Only the complexity of clinical, morphological, functional criteria can lead to clear final diagnosis.
4. The discrepancy of behaviour of immune parameter may have several causes, which are discussed in the paper.

References

1. Deckart, E., A. Blottner, H. Deckart, W. Lobers, R. Pilz: Radiobiol. Radiother. **28** (1987), 607. - 2. Studer, H., G. Huber, M. Derwall: Akt. Endokr. Stoffw. **10** (1989), 110 (Sonderheft): P. Frey, Schweiz. Med. Wochenschr. **119** (1989), 203. - 3. Marine, D., C.H. Lenhart: Arch. Int. Med. **3** (1911), 265. - 4. Kendall, Taylor, P., A.J. Knox, N.R.Steel, S. Atkinson: Lancet I (1984), 654. - 5. Schatz, H., I. Ludwig, F. Wiss, P.E. Goretzki: Acta Endocrinol. Suppl. **281** (1987), 334. - 6. Hensen, J., P. Kotulla, R. Finke et al.: J. Endocrinol. Invest. **7** (1984), 215.

Comparative investigations of sonography and TRAK - follow-up of Graves' disease

Angelika Wünsche, Dietlind Sorger, G. Neumann, Susanne Schenk, L. Otto, G. Schneider
Department of Nuclear Medicine, Clinic of Radiology, University Leipzig, Germany

The aim of our comparative study is the test of suitability of typical echopoor pattern in sonography and TSH-receptor-antibody (TRAK) levels in diagnosis and follow-up of Graves' disease in addition to the hormone levels before and during a thiamazole-therapy /1/ and before and after Radioiodine.

Material and methods

Before any therapy we investigated 135 patients, 70 suspected Graves' disease and 65 suspected thyroidal autonomies. Follow-up studies of thiamazole treatment before, 3, 6, 12, 18 and 24 months after begin of therapy we performed in 57 patients. Preconditions of these patients' selection were clinical symptoms of Graves' disease, increased hormone levels and also a homogeneous activity enrichment in scintigraphy.
41 patients we checked before, 3 and 9 months after a single-I-131-therapy. We selected the intervals after the end of reaction time of Radioiodine and a half year later. Preconditions for these patient selection were unsuccessful thiamazole treatment of recidivation of Graves' disease and a homogeneous activity enrichment in scintigraphy.
As a long time follow-up we checked also 100 patients from 1-15 years after Radioiodine-therapy. For representative results we divided patients in five-year-interval-groups. Real-time sonography was performed by a Toshiba-Sonolayer C SAC 12 A with a "3 M"-precursor, scintigraphy as usually by Tc-99m only before therapy.
For the in vitro-diagnostic we took commercial kits, for hormone levels radioimmunoassay of the Academy of Sciences in Berlin (T_3-RIA, T_4-RIA, TSH-RIA) and for TRAK-values the TRAK-ASSAY of Henning - Berlin.

Results

Diagnosis of Graves' disease:

Before any treatment of Graves' disease, sonography and TRAK-values are good parameters to distinguish between immunogenic and non immunogenic hyperthyroidism. 86 % of patients suspected Graves' disease showed the typical echopoor thyroid pattern in sonography and 91 % increased TRAK-values. . TRAK-values were a bit more exactly than sonography (figure 1).

From 65 patients with thyroid nodules suspected thyroidal autonomy 6 showed an echopoor pattern in sonography, 4 in connection with an autonomous adenoma. All of these four patients had increased TRAK-values. The other 61 patients were TRAK-negative and 59 were echonormal. From 135 hyperthyroid patients we could not classify sonographically 16 (12 %) and with TRAK-Assay 10 (7 %).

Before iodine-therapy sonographical thyroid patterns are better for diagnosis of immunogenic hyperthyroidism. 88 % of patients showed the typical echopoor pattern. Only 68 % of TRAK levels were increased (figure 2). We think it is caused by immunosuppressive effect of thiamazole.

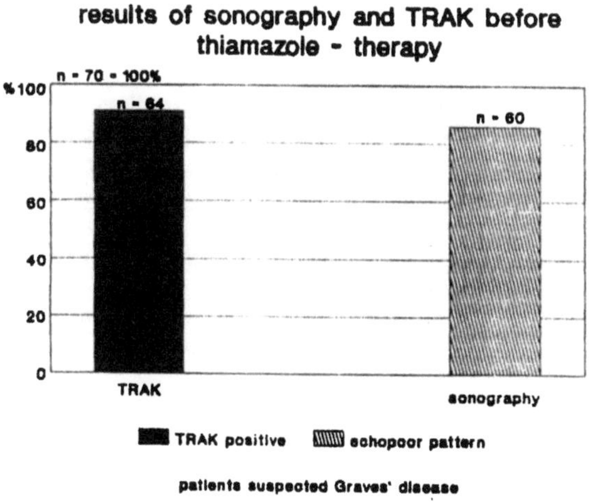

Figure 1

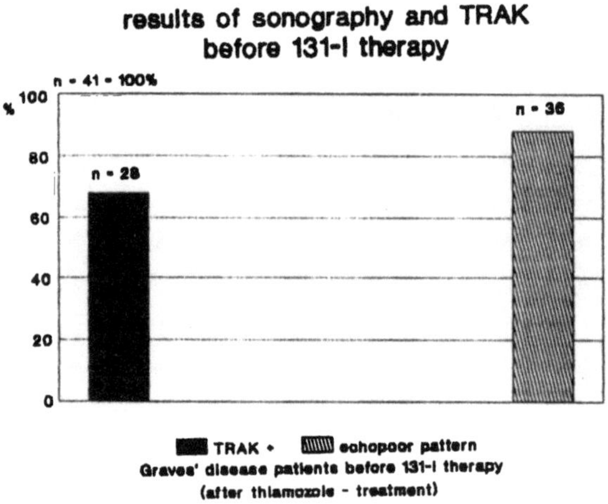

Figure 2

Follow-up:

Thiamazole-treatment:

During thiamazole treatment we found a good correlation between normalization of sonographical thyroid pattern, TRAK values and hormone levels after 12 months. In the therapy follow-up sonography and thyroid function showed a little better correlation, than function and TRAK-values (figure 3 and 4).

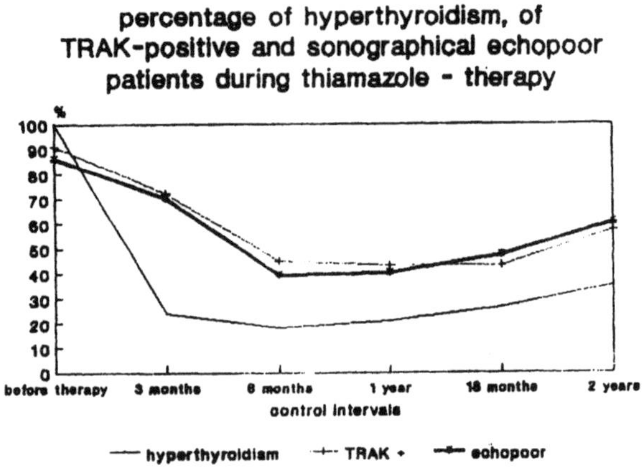

Figure 3

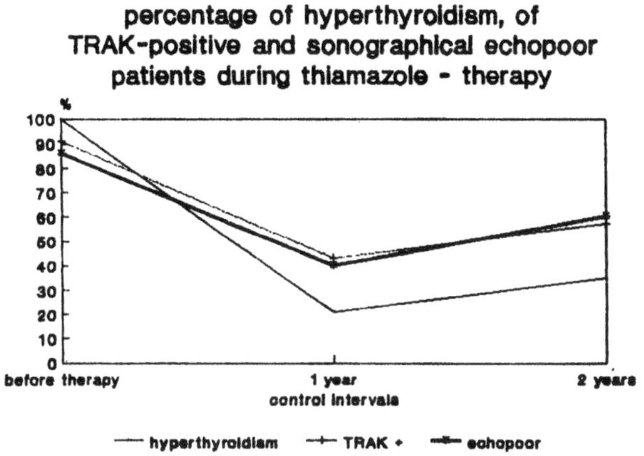

Figure 4

Only in very successful therapy sonographical structure normalizes a bit later than TRAK-values after returning of normal hormone levels (figure 5).

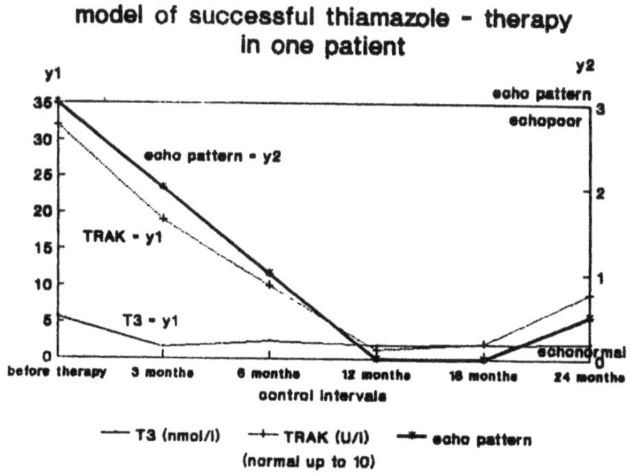

Figure 5

These ideal follow-up we saw seldom.
After one year we stopped therapy in patients with a normal thyroid function. Increasing of hyperthyroidism, echopoor

I-131-therapy:

After Iodine-therapy both methods sonography and TRAK evaluations were unfavourable for the follow-up. They did not correlate with thyroid functions. TRAK values were in 33 % higher than before therapy. May be it is caused by a higher release of antibodies in annihilation of thyroid tissue. Diminished but not normal TRAK values we only see in 7 % after 3 months and in 29 % after 6 months. Sonographical echopoor pattern of thyroids were nearly constant (figure 6).

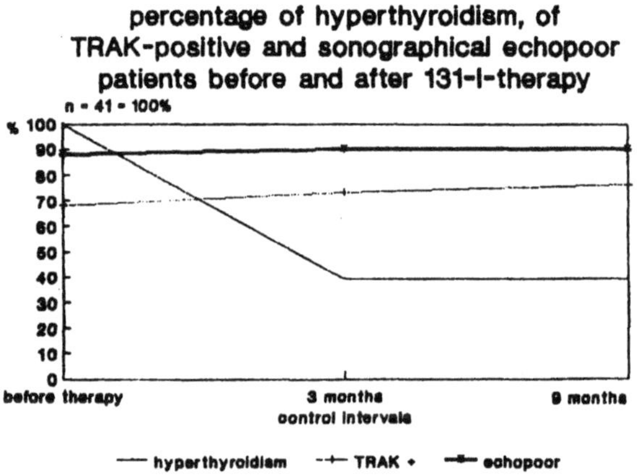

Figure 6

Most of our patients showed an individual diminuation of thyroid volume. Here we can not see a correlation with thyroid functions. Overlay of volume differences (volume before therapy - volume after therapy) do not allow a differentiation between thyroid functions (figure 7).

Also in long time follow-up we did not found a correlation between thyroid function, sonographical pattern and TRAK-values.

10 years after Radioiodine therapy TRAK-positive patients were decreasing and there with activity of autoimmunity. Sonographical structure and thyroid morphology are nearly constant (figure 8).

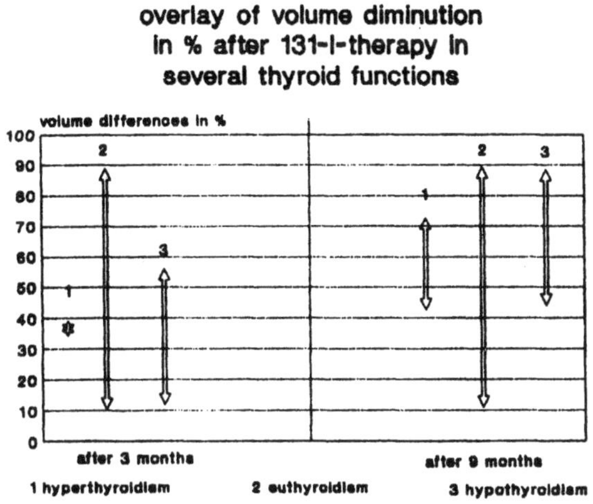

Figure 7

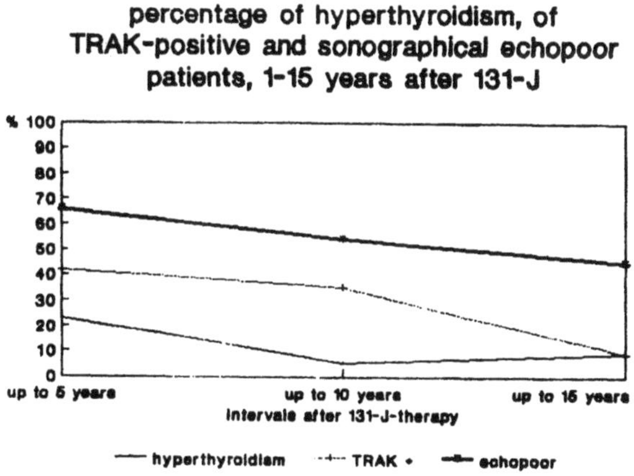

Figure 8

Conclusions

Diagnosis:

- Sonography and TRAK-values are suitable to differentiate between Graves' disease and thyroidal autonomy before any therapy. Sonography as a simple method should be the first step of investigations. The more expensive TRAK-evaluations should be especially for problem patients.

- Before radioiodine in complicated hyperthyroidism sonography is the better method to differentiate between Graves' disease and autonomy, may be because of the immunsuppression of thiamazole.

Follow-up:

thiamazole therapy:

Typical echopoor thyroid pattern and TRAK-values are normalizing during a successful therapy. Thiamazole influences autoimmune process. Antibodies decrease during therapy. In successful treatment also follicle size normalizes and therewith sonographical structure. The best results we got with both methods after 1 year of therapy. Sonography shows better results than TRAK-values in addition to hormone levels. We can recognize recidivations. But both methods are unsuitable for long time statements about further development of illness.

I-131-therapy:

After I-131-therapy sonography and TRAK evaluation can not give us additional informations about our patients. Most of thyroids show a volume diminution independent of the function. Only clinical symptoms and hormone levels should decide further therapy. Clinical feeling is important here not high techniques.
With I-131-iodine we do not influence the autoimmune process, only thyroid size. Because of the constant echopoor pattern we think that follicles remain small.

References

1. Wünsche, A., H.-J. Heberling, K. Hartung et al.: Radiol. diagn. **28** (1987), 832.

Discussion

Leövey: Among the patients who were treated with I-131 after 15 years you found TRAK positivity in relatively high percentage. How it is possible, what is your opinion about this problem?
Wünsche: The receptor assay was very often positiv. All patients had a normal function, but not all had this without treatment with drugs. A lot of patients got L-Thyroxin or Thyreotom. I think that autoimmunity of this patients is relatively constant and we can't influence this and we can only influence the size of thyroid.

Deckart: This presentation seems to me a little bit mechanistically theory to refuse the size only by iodine treatment; with iodine you even influence the immunopathy. You stop the target and the activation of immunogenic process. Of course you decrease the size but you stop the function too.
Nemec: According to our knowledge the behavior of TRAK-assay following iodine treatment is unpredictable. We have seen in some of our patients with endocrine orbitopathy where we use sometimes total thyroid destruction that in majority of patients the TRAK-levels decrease in the course of one or two years. But we have patients who are hypothyroid with no remainders of thyroid that could be detected by radioiodine. They are hypothyroid and they have still very high TRAK-levels. In the evaluation of the effect of iodine the TRAK plays not an important role.
Deckart: But it depends on the dose you get in the organ. If you give a high dose of radioiodine, 100 Gray or 150 Gray to 200 Gray you will stop the immunogenic process.
Novak: What frequency of ultrasound did you use and what type of transducer?
Wünsche: 5 MHz and now 7.5 MHz transducer in the last year.
Novak: Did you see any differences?
Wünsche: Also with 3.5 MHz transducer we got excellent pictures, and with the new transducers too, included the 7.5 MHz transducer.

Guanyl nucleotide regulatory proteins and GTPase activity in normal and hyperthyroid human thyroid tissue and human polymorphonuclear granulocytes

E. Fórizs, A. Panyige, Zs. Jenei, T. Fülöp Jr., J. Szabó, E. Mezösi, I. Seres, A. Leövey
First Department of Medicine, Institut of Biology, University Medical School of Debrecen, Debrecen, Hungary

The G proteins are a family of heterotrimeric guanine nucleotide-binding membrane proteins that are involved in transmembrane signaling /1/. Information from hormone receptors that stimulate adenylate cyclase is mediated by G_s, whereas negative impulses are transduced by G_i protein /2/. Activation occures when GDP bound to the alpha-subunit of the heterotrimer is exchanged for GTP. On binding of GTP, the alpha-subunit (G_a-GTP dissociates from the beta and gamma chains and directly modifies the activity of the target effector, e.g. adenylate cyclase. Activation is terminated by the conversion of GTP to GDP by the endogeneous GTPase activity of the alpha subunit /2/.

Several methods are used in G-proteins identification:
1. Bacterial toxins (Pertussis toxin (PT) and Cholera toxin (CT)). The alpha subunit of G_s can be ADP ribosylated by CT, similar ADP-ribosylation of the G_i alpha subunit is catalyzed by PT.
2. Radiolabelled nonhydrolyzable analogues of GTP;
3. Antibodies raised against native G proteins individual subunits and
4. cDNA probes /3/.

The aim of our present study was to investigate the patterns of G proteins in normal and hyperfunctional human thyroid tissues. We also measured the GTPase activity in resting conditions and under stimulation in human thyroid tissue and human polymophonuclear granulocytes (PMNLs).

Materials and methods

Thyroid tissue was obtained from 8 patients suffering from Graves'-Basedow disease undergoing thyroid surgery. As control normal thyroid tissue was used from 4 patients having surgery for thyroid cysts.

PMNLs were obtained from 12 untreated female Graves'-Basedow patients. As controls, 6 healthy volunteers were used. In the case of 7 patients (< 35 years) the disease lasted for less than 3 months, while in case of 5 patients (> 59 years) the disease was in a relapsed phase. The PMNLs were separated as it was described earlier /4/.

GTPase activity was measured by (gamma-P-32) GTP according to the method of Kikuchi et al. /5/. In brief: the thyroid was cut into slices and homogenized, then pottered. The samples were centrifuged at 4000 g for 10' at 4 ^{o}C. The protein content of the supernatant was determined by the method of Lowry et al. /6/. The separated PMNLs were centrifuged at 10000 g for 5' and the pellets were ultrasonificated in 0.5 ml PBS, than the suspensions were centrifuged again for separating the nucleus from the membrane fractions, which were used for GTPase activity determinations.

CT and PT catalyzed G proteins ADP ribosylation: Cholera and pertussis toxins were activated in 5 mM dithiotreitol. Crude extracts of thyreocytes were than labelled in the presence of the activated toxin and (P-32)NAD as described by Gill et al. /7/. After toxin labelling, the membrane proteins were subjected to SDS polyacrylamid gel electrophoresis as described by Laemmli /8/ and than proteins were electroblotted to nitrocellulose paper, and the pattern of ADP-ribosylated proteins were analyzed by autoradiography.

Results

We first determined the GTPase activity of normal and hyperfunctional (Graves'-Basedow disease) thyroid tissues in basic condition and also after TSH stimulation (table 1). We found that the TSH was able to stimulate the GTPase activity of normal human thyroid tissue. In contrast the TSH was not able to stimulate the GTPase activity in hyperfunctional thyroid tissue. It is interesting to note that the basic activity of hyperfunctional thyroid tissue is markedly lower than that of normal tissue.

Table 1: Effects of TSH stimulation on GTPase activity of normal and hyperfunctional (Graves'-Basedow disease) thyroid tissue

Sample	Basic activity	TSH (5 mU/ml) stimulation
	pM hydrolysed GTP/min/mg protein	
Graves'-Basedow	1.43 ± 0.19	1.38 ± 0.21
Control tissue	2.48 ± 0.19	3.00 ± 0.20

Each value represents the mean of at least 5 determinations ± S.D.

When we stimulated the PMNLs by TSH an increase in GTPase activity was found in case of PMNLs originating from healthy individuals, while in the case of PMNLs, obtained from young patients suffering from Graves'-Basedow disease, the GTPase activity could be only slightly stimulated (table 2). The GTPase activity could not be activated by TSH in case of PMNLs obtained from elderly persons suffering from Graves'-Basedow disease.

Table 2: Effects of TSH (5 mU/ml) stimulation on GTPase activity of polymorphonuclear granulocytes (PMNLs) obtained from healthy subjects and patients suffering of Graves'-Basedow disease

Sample	Age years	Basic activity	TSH (5 mU/ml) stimulation
		pM hydrolysed GTP/min/mg	
Graves'-Basedow	< 35	76.52 ± 4.80	86.20 ± 7.80
	> 59	86.72 ± 2.32	53.28 ± 4.24
Control	< 35	40.40 ± 3.60	74.24 ± 7.20

Each value represents the mean of at least 5 determinations ± S.D.

We were also interested how the GTPase activity is changing in thyroid disease by using an other stimulus than TSH e.g. FMLP. FMLP stimulated the GTPase acticity in PMNLs /4/ and in our experiments we could confirm this effect (table 3). In case of PMNLs of hyperthyroid patients the same phenomenon was found under FMLP stimulation than under TSH stimulation.

Table 3: Effects of FMLP (10^{-8}) stimulation on GTPase activity of polymorphonuclear granulocytes (PMNLs) obtained from healthy subjects and patients suffering of Graves'-Basedow disease

Sample	Age years	Basic activity	FMLP (10^{-8}) stimulation
		pM hydrolysed GTP/min/mg protein	
Graves'-Basedow	< 35	17.70 ± 1.08	21.56 ± 0.86
	> 59	29.12 ± 2.96	21.12 ± 3.36
Control	< 35	31.68 ± 4.40	43.36 ± 5.44

Each value represents the mean of at least 5 determinations ± S.D.

The spontaneous GTPase activity of PMNLs from healthy and hyperthyroid persons was rather different (figure 1). The GTPase activity of hyperthyroid patients' PMNLs is less than that of normal PMNLs.

During CT catalyzed ADP ribosylation of membrane proteins of normal and hyperfunctional thyroid tissue, we found in normal tissue a 45 kDa protein, while in hyperthyroid tissue a 45, a 52 and a low molecular weight protein (figure 2). When using PT catalyzed ADP ribosylation a 40 kDa protein could be demonstrated in normal and hyperthyroid tissue (figure 3).

Time course of GTPase activity of crude extracts of granulocytes of healthy and Graves'-Basedow patients

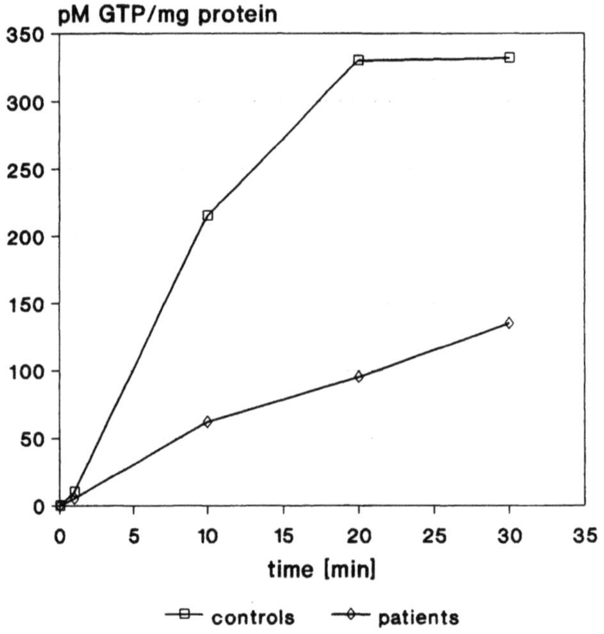

Figure 1

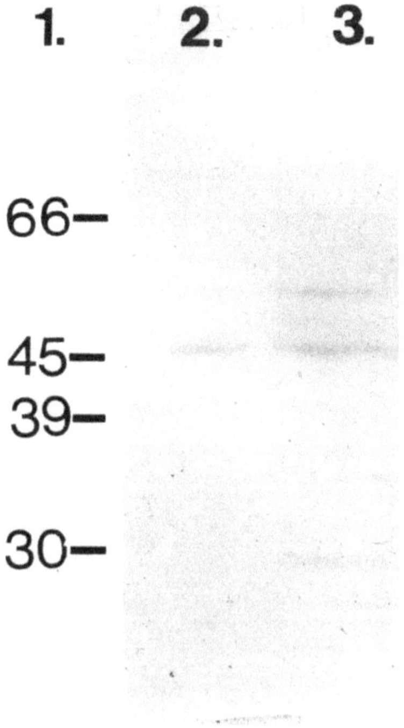

Figure 2

Cholera toxin catalyzed ADP-ribosylation of G_{Sa} in thyroid tissue
Lane 1.: Molecular weight standards
Lane 2.: Control
Lane 3.: Graves'-Basedow patient

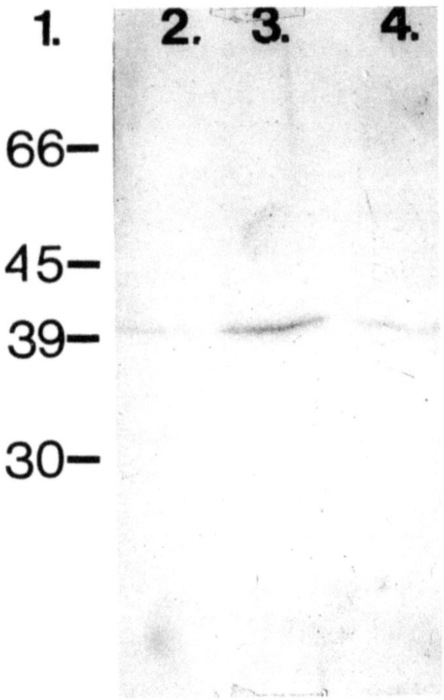

Figure 3

Pertussis toxin catalyzed ADP-ribosylation of G_{ia} in thyroid tissue
Lane 1.: Molecular weight standards
Lane 2.: Control
Lane 3.: Graves'-Basedow patient
Lane 4.: Graves'-Basedow patient

Discussion

The G proteins and the GTPase are playing a fundamental role in the cellular signal transduction. This was the reason why we were interested to determine the G proteins' pattern and the GTPase activity in thyroid tissue. The GTPase activity was not only determined in thyroid tissue, but also in PMNLs.

The G proteins' pattern seems not to change when ADP is ribosylated by PT. The G proteins' pattern seems to change under CT catalyzed ADP ribosylation. In the case of hyperfunctional thyroid tissue more CT labelled proteins could be demonstrated. We do not have the exact quantities of Gs proteins, but it seems that they are increased in hyperthyroidism. This seems to correlate with the findings that in hypothyroidism the Gi proteins tend to increase in quantity /9/. This finding is in accordance with the fact that c AMP increase is necessary for thyroid hormone secretion.

The GTPase activity determination is very important to analyse the regulation of signal transmission by G proteins /10/. The GTPase activity is an intrinsic characteristic of each G protein. We found that no stimuli was able to stimulate the GTPase activity of cells of hyperthyroid patients. This might signify that these cells are under a continuous stimulation which can not be further stimulated or that these cells ensure by this decreased stimulation a continuous activated state for hormone production.

The changes in Gs proteins and the dysregulation of GTPase activity might to some extent explain the hyperfunctional state of thyroid tissue and could provide some new way to try to modulate this hyperactivity.

References

1. Freissmuth, M.: FASEB J.: **3** (1982), 2125. - 2. Gilman, A.G.: Ann. Rev. Biochem. **56** (1987), 615. - 3. Harnett, N.M.: Immunology Today **9** (1988), 315. - 4. Fulop, T. Jr.: Klin. Exp. Immunol. **61** (1985), 425. - 5. Kikuchi, A.: J. Biol. Chem. **263**(1988), 2897. - 6. Lowry, O.H.: J. Biol. Chem. **193** (1951), 265. - 7. Gill, D.M.: Methods of Enzymol. **165**(1988), 235. - 8. Laemmli , U.K.: Nature **227** (1970), 680. - 9. Milligan, G.: Biochem. J. **247** (1987), 223. - 10. Landis, A.: Nature **340** (1989), 692.

PERIPHERAL THYROID HORMONE METABOLISM

Peripheral thyroid hormone metabolism

H. Meinhold
Department of Nuclear Medicine, Klinikum Steglitz,
Free University Berlin, Germany

The main secretory product of the thyroid gland, thyroxine (T_4), is metabolized extrathyroidally via the four well-known pathways: monodeiodination to 3,5,3'-triiodothyronine (T_3) and other thyronines iodinated to a lower degree, conjugation of the phenolic hydroxyl group to form glucuronides and sulfates, oxidative degradation of the alanine side-chain to yield tetrac and triac, the acetic-acid derivatives of T_4 and T_3, and, last but not least, cleavage of the T_4 molecule at its diphenyl ether bridge to form diiodothyrosine (DIT) and iodide (figure 1). These pathways are of different importance for providing the body with sufficient hormonal activity or for eliminating hormone excess in special situations.
The following survey will focus on the two pathways which ultimately lead to the formation of iodide: the hormone-activating process of sequential monodeiodination and the degradation of T_4 by ether link cleavage, a pathway which was not very attractive to researchers in the past.

A survey of studies dealing with thyroxine deiodination (table 1) clearly illustrates that a period of almost 20 years is spanned from the discovery of T_3 as a normal constituent of human plasma by Gross & Pitt-Rivers in 1952 to the demonstration of Braverman et al. (1970) that T_4 is peripherally converted to T_3 in athyreotic human subjects under T_4 substitution therapy. The development of radioimmunoassay for T_3 and reverse T_3 ushered in a 15 year-era of intensified studies on iodothyronine monodeiodination: its enzymatic nature was shown, and the clinical consequences of pathophysiologically altered T_4 deiodination were demonstrated for various nonthyroidal diseases referred to later as the low-T_4 syndrome. It is now only some months ago that type I of the three deiodinating isoenzymes was identified as a protein which contains the trace element selenium as an integral molecular component.

Table 1: Important steps in the research of metabolic thyroid hormone deiodination

1952	Gross & Pitt-Rivers Identification of T_3 in human plasma.
1970	Braverman, Ingbar & Sterling T_4 conversion to T_3 in athyreotic human subjects.
1970	Brown et al., Gharib et al. Radioimmunoassay of T_3.
1974	Chopra Radioimmunoassay of reverse T_3.
1975	Hesch et al., Visser et al. T_4 monodeiodination to T_3 in liver homogenates.
1975	Chopra et al., Vagenakis et al., Wenzel & Meinhold Reciprocal changes of T_3 and rT_3, Low-T_3 syndrom.
1978	Silva & Larsen Quantitation of intrapituitary T_4 conversion to T_3. T_4 is a prohormon.
1983	Visser, Mol & Otten Sulfation facilitates hepatic T_3 deiodination.
1987	Beckett, Arthur et al. Selenium deficiency inhibits hepatic T_4 deiodination.
1990	Köhrle et al. Affinity labelling of type I 5'-deiodinase.
1990	Behne, Kyriakopoulos, Meinhold & Köhrle Type I 5'-deiodinase is a selenoenzyme.
1991	Berry, Banu & Larsen Type I deiodinase contains selenocystenine.

The first step and key reaction of the sequential deiodination cascade is the conversion of T_4 to thyromimetically active T_3 by outer-ring and to hormonally inactive reverse T_3 by inner-ring deiodination (figure 2). The experimental investigations on the biochemical properties and behaviour of the enzyme system responsible for T_4 monodeiodination were accompanied and sometimes preceeded by clinical studies on alterations of

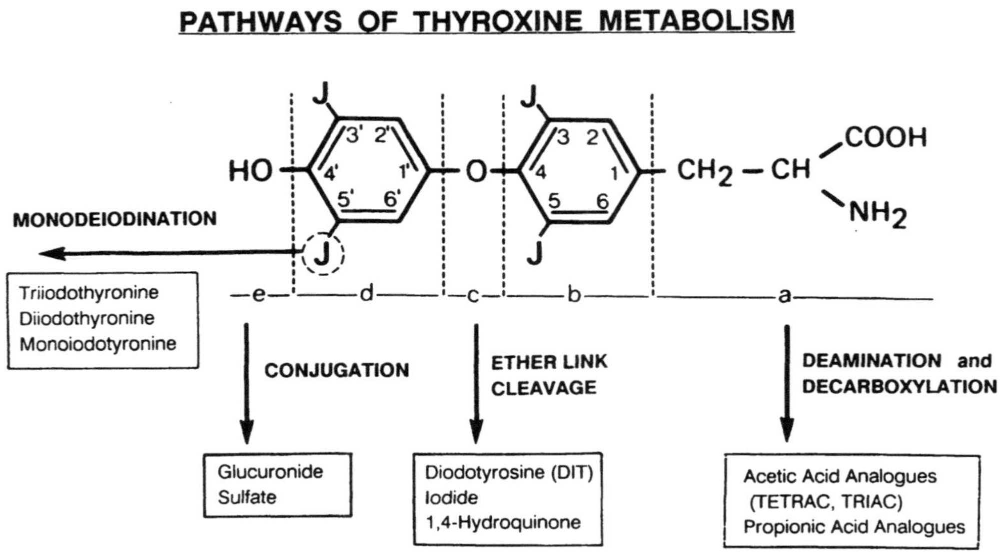

Figure 1
Pathways of thyroxine metabolism

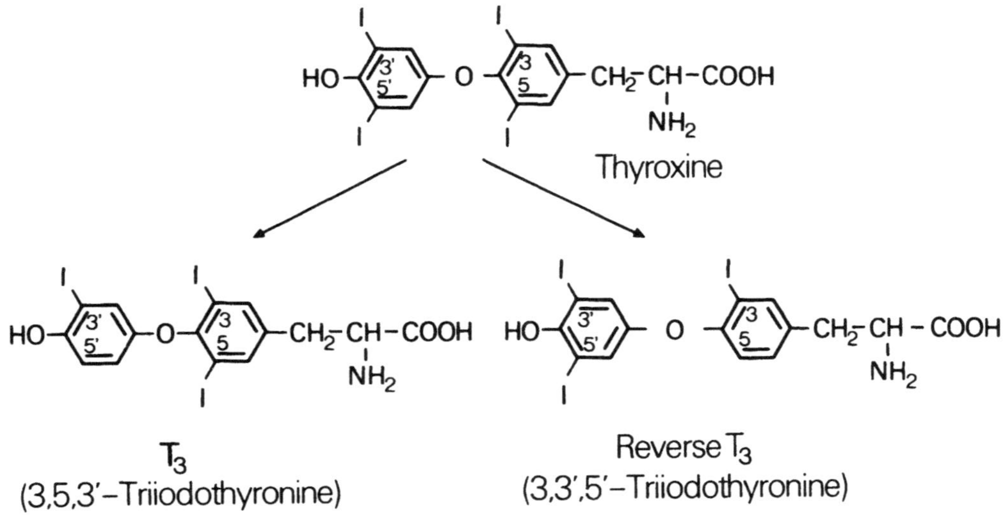

Figure 2

Monodeiodination of T_4 to T_3 and rT_3

circulating hormone levels under specific physiological conditions and in patients with various diseases. Table 2 shows one example of such phenomenological findings observed in newborn infants many years ago in our own laboratory.

Table 2: Serum concentrations of rT_3, 3,3'-T_2, T_3 and T_4 in normal adults, pregnant women and newborn infants (Data from Meinhold et al., 1979)

	Mean serum concentration (nmol/l)			
	rT_3	3,3'-T_2	T_3	T_4
normal subjects	0.36	< 0.018	2.21	115
pregnant women (24-40 weeks)	0.33	0.049	3.16	167
newborn infants	3.13	0.211	0.55	181

Comparison of rT_3 and T_3 serum levels in normal subjects and newborns shows a strong reduction of T_3 but an approximately tenfold increase of rT_3 and 3,3'-T_2 in newborn cordserum. A very similar pattern is found in amniotic fluid of pregnant women and, as will be discussed in the following three papers, in the serum of patients with severe nonthyroidal illnesses (NTI). Table 3 summarizes conditions involving such reciprocal changes of serum T_3 and rT_3 levels. Caloric deprivation by fasting was the first of these conditions for which increased serum rT_3 levels were reported in the literature. Besides various severe diseases, treatment with drugs like dexamethasone or application of radiographic contrast agents also produced this phenomenon. It was suggested that the observed serum T_3 and rT_3 alterations might be explained by an inhibition of enzymatic 5'-deiodination of T_4 and a metabolic switch to increased inner-ring deiodination yielding a higher rT_3 production. It now seems to be clear that the T_4-to-T_3-converting 5'-deiodinase is indeed suppressed, but the rT_3 production rate is unchanged, and several additional factors may help to determine the pattern of circulating iodothyronines in NTI patients.

Table 3: Reciprocal changes of T_3 and rT_3 serum levels (clinical observations)

T_3 ↓	rT_3 ↑
Fasting	
Surgical operation	
Myocardial infarction	
Liver cirrhosis	
severe infections	
Medications	
Dexamethasone	
Propranolol	
Radiographic contrast agents	

A complexity similar to that seen for hormone status, metabolism and regulation in critical illness is also found for the deiodinating enzyme system itself. Three types of membrane-bound iodothyronine deiodinases with different properties and tissue sites have so far been identified (table 4), type I beeing hitherto the best characterized isoenzyme. It catalyzes both 5'- and 5-deiodination of T_4 and rT_3, with highest substrate binding affinity for rT_3. Type I predominantly present in the liver and kidney. Its activity is decreased in hypothyroidism and in patients with the low-T_3 syndrome and is increased in hyperthyroidism. The properties of the type II deiodinase are quite different from those of the type I enzyme. Type II, which is predominantly located in the central nervous system, anterior pituitary, brown adipose tissue, and

Table 4: Characteristics of iodothyronine 5'- and 5-deiodinase isoenzymes (according to Köhrle and Hesch, 1989)

Type I	5'- and 5-deiodination (outer and inner ring) $rT_3 \rightarrow 3.3'-T_2$; $T_4 \rightarrow T_3$; $T_4 \rightarrow rT_3$ Substrate preference $rT_3 > T_4 > T_3$ Tissue: Liver, kidney, thyroid, pituitary,CNS Inhibitors: PTU, ipanoic acid Decreased: Hypothyroidism, low-T_3 syndrome Increased: Hyperthyroidism Biological function: rT_3 elimination. T_3 production for export
Type II	Only 5'-deiodination (outer ring) $T_4 \rightarrow T_3$, $rT_3 \rightarrow 3.3'-T_2$ Substrate preference: $T_4 > rT_3$ Tissue: CNS, pituitary, BAT, placenta Inhibitors: Ipanoic acid (not PTU); Decreased: Hyperthyroidism Increased: Hypothyroidism, low T_3 syndrome Biological function: Local T_3 neogenesis (auto supply in brain, cold adaptation)
Type III	Only 5-deiodination (inner ring) $T_3 \rightarrow 3.3'-T_2$, $T_4 \rightarrow rT_3$ (and sulfates) Substrate preference: $T_3 > T_4$ Tissue: Fetal membranes, various other tissues Biological function: T_3 prevention and degradation

placenta, deiodinates exclusively the 5'-iodine position and is therefore primarily responsible for the conversion of T_4 to T_3 in tissues with central functions. In contrast to type I, it is inhibited by PTU, decreased in hyperthyroidism and increased in hypothyroidism. - The type III isoenzyme deiodinates the inner ring only and catalyzes the bio-inactivating pathway of T_3 and T_4 degradation to their inactive metabolites 3.3'-T_3 and rT_3 which is of special importance in fetal tissues.

The hitherto recogniced physiological functions of the isoenzymes may be summarized as follows: Type I deiodinase is responsible for the systemic T_3 supply and, by T_4 conversion, produces approximately 70 % of the T_3 found in the circulation. Thus, type I supports the thyroid gland in providing sufficient hormonally active T_3 for its diverse actions in the body. - Produced from circulating T_4 type II is a local source of T_3 for organs requiring their own supply to maintain essential physiological functions like the pituitary and brain; for example, it is needed to maintain a euthyroid intracellular brain status in patients with incipient hypothyroidism or the low-T_3 syndrome. In brown adipose tissue, type II serves as a local source for thermogenic T_3 to protect against cold-included hypothermia. - Type III, finally, may prevent the inappropriate accumulation of energy-providing T_3 by its rapid 5-deiodination to 3.3'-T_2 during fetal development and maturation.

From the results of various turnover studies on the metabolic fate of T_4 in the whole body, it can be estimated that, in euthyroid subjects, roughly 75 % of the T_4 secreted by the thyroid gland is metabolized to T_3 and rT_3 by monodeiodination is the predominant pathway of T_4 disposal, but 25 % of the T_4 secreted is metabolized by other routes. This percentage of nondeiodinating T_4 disposal may be increased in pathophysiological situations and, as emphasized by Chopra et al. (1983), "we are left with the conclusion that routes of T_4 metabolism, other than through T_3 and rT_3, constitute a major pathway of T_4 disposal in nonthyroidal illness".

With this quotation let us proceed from monodeiodination to ether-link cleavage, a T_4-degrading pathway which seems to be

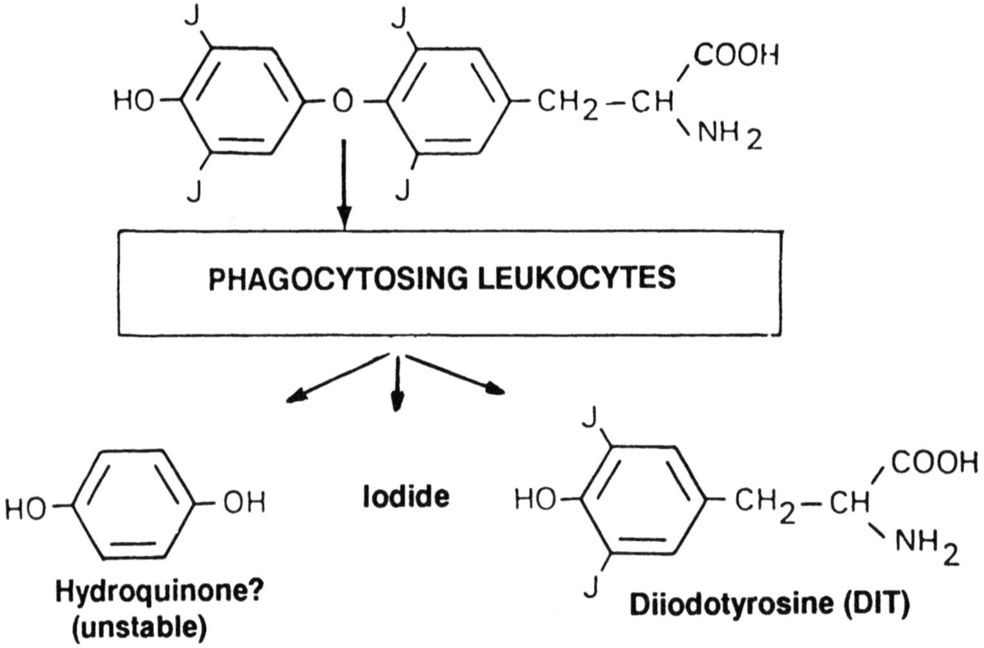

Figure 3

Ether link cleavage of T_4

of some importance in severe infections and sepsis. In vitro investigations by Burger et al. (1983) and by ourselfes (Schwander & Meinhold 1987) had shown that phagocytosing human leukocytes rapidly degrade T_4 by cleavage of its ether bridge between the two aromatic rings. This pathway, which plays a minor role under physiological conditions in vivo, leads to the formation of diiodothyrosine, iodide and an unstable hydroquinone compound (figure 3). The T_4 breakdown to DIT requires phagocytosis for T_4 uptake into the granulocyte and is catalyzed by peroxidases during the metabolic burst reaction of the cell.

A previously developed radioimmunoassay for measurement of DIT in human serum (Meinhold et al. 1981) provided us with an analytical tool for testing the following hypothesis: If ether link cleavage of T_4 by phagocytosing leukocytes occurs in vivo with characteristics similar to those observed in vitro, then sepsis and other infections associated with increased phagocytosis of white blood cells should enhance the metabolic production of DIT from T_4. This enhancement of cellular DIT production may be manifested as a measurable increase in the concentration of circulating DIT. Serial studies were performed to examine serum DIT and other thyroid parameters in critically ill patients with sepsis and other diseases who were treated at our Operative Intensive Care Unit. Some results of these studies, which have recently been published in detail (Meinhold et al. 1991a), are presented in figure 4 and 5 and in table 5.

The time course of DIT and iodothyronine serum levels in a patient who developed sepsis 7.5 days after severe head injury is shown in figure 4. The onset of septic shock was accompanied by a DIT and rT_3 increase which rapidly reached maximun levels some hours before the patient died, while T_4 and T_3 fell below the normal range. Figure 5 summarizes the results of DIT measurements in the four patient groups stu-

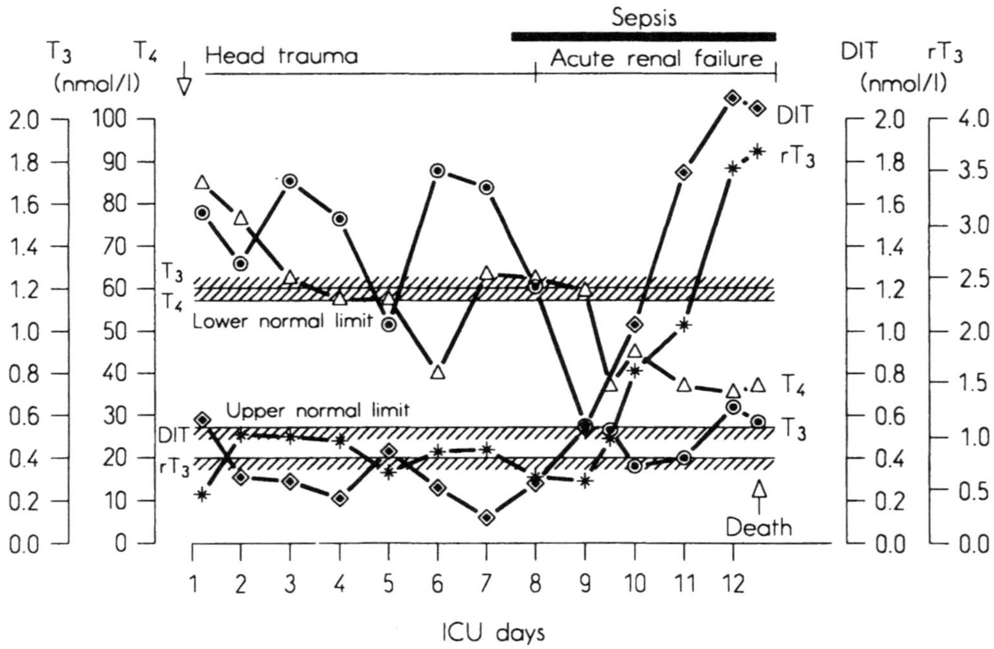

Figure 4

Serum levels of DIT, T_4, T_3 and rT_3 in a patient who developed sepsis after head trauma. The hatched lines indicate the lower normal limit of T_4 and T_3 and the upper normal limits of DIT and rT_3, respectively (Meinhold et al. (1991a)

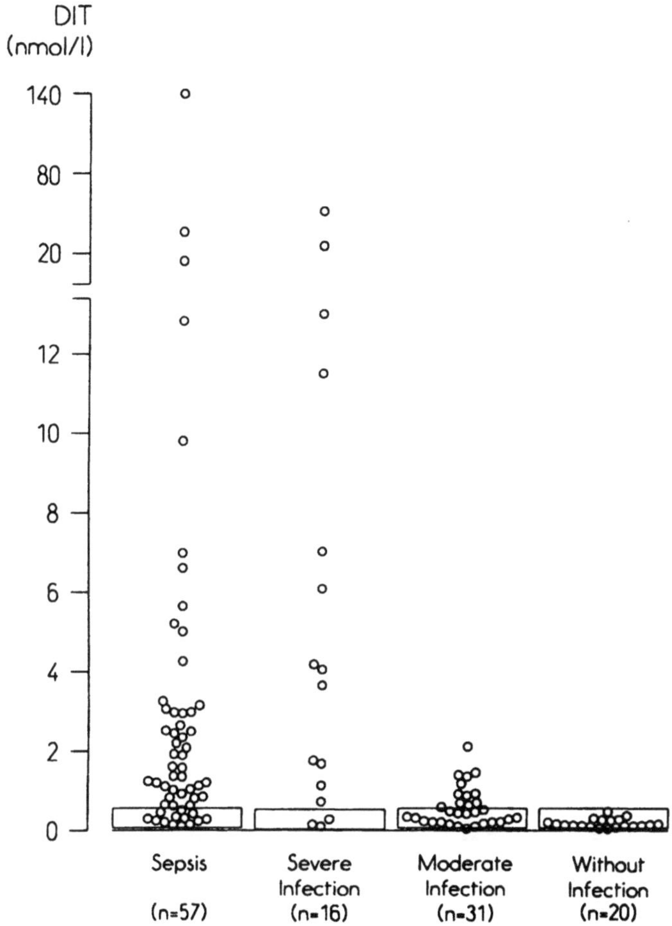

Figure 5
Serum DIT concentrations in critical care patients. The rectangles indicate the normal range (0.02-0.55 nmol/l) (Meinhold et al. 1991a)

Table 5: Prevalence (%) of abnormal thyroidal parameters in critically ill patients (Data from Meinhold et al. 1991a)

		Sepsis	Severe infection	Moderate infection	Without infection
DIT	> 0.55 nmol/l	77	81	39	0
TT_4	< 58 nmol/l	27	12	0	0
FT_4	< 7.7 pmol/l	2	6	0	0
TT_3	< 1.2 nmol/l	84	69	53	58
rT_3	> 0.80 nmol/l	88	53	52	60
TSH	< 0.3 mU/l	36	6	19	21
	> 4.0 mU/l	5	24	0	0

died. Serum DIT was elevated in most of the patients with sepsis and severe local infections such as peritonitis or abscesses. There were only slight elevations in moderate infections like pneumonia and tracheobronchitis. DIT was normal in the control group of critically ill patients without infections. The percentage prevalence of abnormal thyroidal parameters (table 5) clearly demonstrates that DIT is abnormally high only in critical care patients with infections, while the low-T_3 syndrome accompanied by high rT_3 values was seen in all patient groups. FT_4 was normal in almost all patients studied. Thus, in contrast to low T_3 and high rT_3 as general markers for critical illnesses, serum DIT appears to be a specific infection marker and reflects - at least in part - an increased ether link cleavage of T_4 due to increased leukocyte activity associated with defense reactions against bacterial attack.

After this excursion to the DIT-forming pathway of T_4 ether-link cleavage, the last part of this contribution will again focus on thyroid hormone monodeiodination and shortly review some very recent studies on the biochemical characterization of the type I iodothyronine deiodinase. Beckett et al. (1987) first demonstrated that acute selenium deficiency inhibits thyroxine deiodination in the liver of rats. We reported on the same topic at the International Thyroid Conference at The Hague in 1991 (Meinhold et al. 1991a). Figure 6 shows results of these studies, which were done in close cooperation with Dr. D. Behne, Dept. of "Trace elements in Health and Disease", Hahn-Meitner-Institut Berlin. It is evident that long-term selenium deficiency in rats maintained on a low-Se diet for three generations strongly inhibits hepatic T_3 production from its substrate T_4, and that type I deiodinase activity in the liver could be completely restored by Se-replenishment. Similar results were found for the inner-ring deiodination of T_4 to rT_3 in both the liver and the kidney.

These results suggested an association of the trace element selenium with the T_4-deiodinating type I enzyme. There was, however, no clear proof of this assumption without further biochemical investigations. The low stability and abundance of the deiodinase isoenzymes have thus far prevented them from being isolated or purified. Affinity labelling of the enzyme with I-125-labelled bromoacetyl-T_4 (I-125-BrAcT_4) by Köhrle et al (1990) had revealed the substrate-binding subunit of type I deiodinase to be a polypeptide with a molecular weight of 27 kDa. At almost the same time, Behne et al. (1990a) detected a 27.8 kDa selenium-containing protein in the thyroid, liver and kidney after in vivo labelling of rats with the selenium isotope Se-75. The combination of both labelling techniques in a cooperative study finally led to the identification of type I iodothyronine 5'-deiodinase as a selenoenzyme (Behne et al. 1990b).

As shown in figure 6, SDS-PAGE electrophoresis of Se-75-labelled or I-125-BrAcT_4 affinity-labelled microsomal proteins of the rat liver suggested the identity of the selenium-containing and the T_4binding 27 kDa protein. Subsequent trypsin

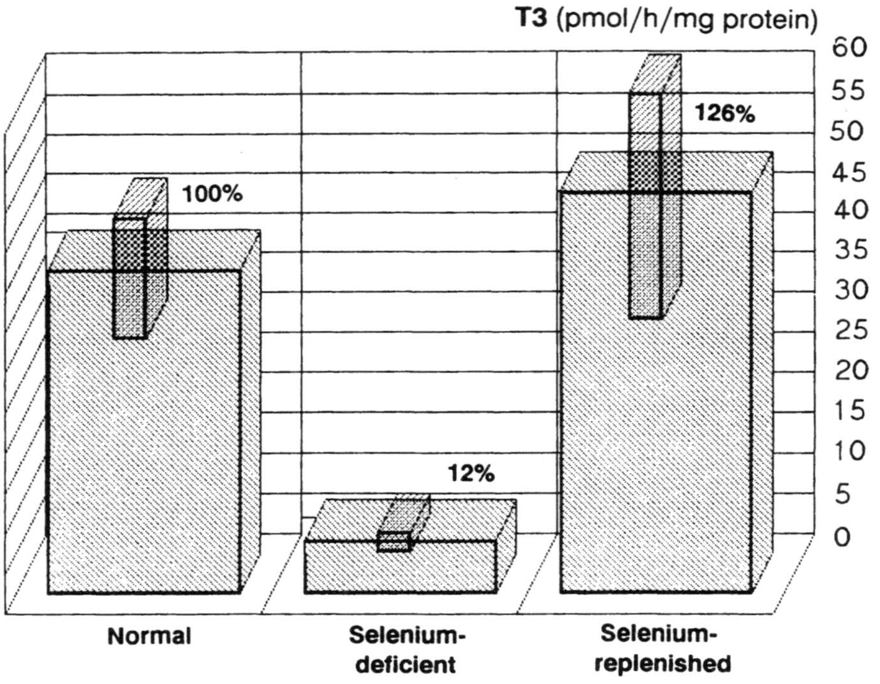

Figure 6

Hepatic T_3 production by 5'-deiodination of T_4 in normal, selenium-deficient and selenium-replenished rats (Meinhold et al. 1991b)

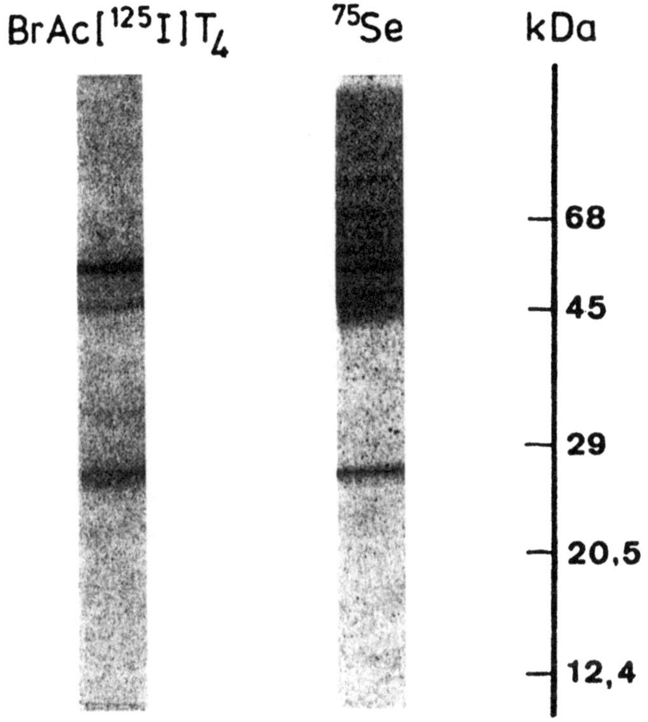

Figure 7

Autoradiogram of Se-75-labelled or BrAc (I-125) T_4 affinity-labelled rat liver microsomal proteins (Behne et al. 1990b)

digestion and cyanobromide cleavage of the double-labelled 27 kDa protein yielded identical distribution patterns and a constant activity ratio of the two radionuclides in each of the protein fragments. The results of these and additional experiments comparing the type I deiodinase and selenium content of the 27-kDa protein gave clear evidence that the active subunit of the type I enzyme contains selenium which might be chemically bound as a selenocystein. Our results were supported and extended by a very recent study (Berry et al. 1991) which demonstrated that selenium is indeed present at the active site of the type I deiodinase in the form of a selenocystenine.

After glutathione peroxidase, a second selenoenzyme with important regulatory functions has been identified by these findings. The fact that type I iodothyronine 5'-deiodinase is responsible for most of the conversion of the prohormone thyroxine to the bioactive T_3 in the body make evident the essential role of the trace element selenium in thyroid hormone metabolism and action.

References

1. Beckett, G.J., S.E. Beddows, P.C. Morrice, F. Nicol, J.R. Arthur: Biochem J. **248** (1987), 443. - 2. Behne, D., S. Scheid, A. Kyriakopoulos, H. Hilmert: Biochem. Biophys. Acta **1033** (1990a), 219. - 3. Behne, D., A. Kyriakopoulos, H. Meinhold, J. Köhrle: Biochem. Biophys. Res. Comm. **173** (1990b), 1143. - 4. Berry, M.J., L. Banu, P.R. Larsen: Nature **349** (1991), 438. - 5. Braverman, L.E., S.H. Ingbar, K. Sterling: J. Clin. Invest. **49** (1970), 855. - 6. Brown, B.L., R.P. Ekins, S.M. Ellis, W.S. Reith: In: In vitro procedures with radioisotopes in medicine, International Atomic Energy Agency, Vienna, 1970, p. 560. - 7. Burger, A.G., D. Engler, U. Buergi et al.: J. Clin. Invest. **71** (1983), 935. - 8. Chopra, I.J.: J. Clin. Invest. **54** (1974), 583. - 9. Chopra, I.J., U. Chopra, S.R.

Smith, M. Reza, D.H. Solomon: J. Clin. Endocrinol. Metab. **41** (1975), 1043. - 10. Chopra, I.J., J.M. Hershman, W.M. Partridge, J.T. Nicoloff: Ann. Intern. Med. **98** (1983), 946. - 11. Gharib, H., W.E. Mayberry, R.J. Ryan: J. Clin. Endocrinol. Metab. **31** (1970), 707. - 12. Gross, J., R. Pitt-Rivers: Lancet **I** (1952), 439. - 13. Hesch, R.D., G. Brunner, H.D. Sölling: Clin. Chim. Acta **59** (1975), 209. - 14. Köhrle, J., R.D. Hesch: In: Endokrinologie, R.D. Hesch (Hrsg.), Urban & Schwarenberg, München, 1989, S. 172. - 15. Köhrle, J., U.B. Rasmussen, D.M. Ekenbarger et al.: J. Biol. Chem. 265 (1990), 6155. - 16. Meinhold, H., J.W. Dudenhausen, K.W. Wenzel, E. Saling: Clin. Endocrinol. **10** (1979), 355. - 17. Meinhold, H., A. Beckert, K.W. Wenzel: J. Clin. Endocrinol. Metab. **53** (1981), 1171. - 18. Meinhold, H., H.J. Gramm, W. Meissner et al.: J. Clin. Endocrinol. Metab. **72** (1991a), 945. - 19. Meinhold, H., G. Böhm, U. Haselbach, R. Giencke, H. Gessner, D. Behne: Effects of selenium deficiency on thyroid hormone synthesis and metabolism. Abstractbook, 10th International Thyroid Conference, The Hague, 1991b, p. 187. - 20. Schwander, J., H. Meinhold: Acta Endocrinol. **114** (Suppl. 283) (1987), 11. - 21. Silva, J.E., P.R. Larsen: J. Clin. Invest. **61** (1978), 1247. - 22. Visser, T.J., i. Van der Does-Tobé, R. Docter, G. Hennemann: Biochem. J. **150** (1975), 489.- 23. Visser, T.J., J.A. Mol, M.H. Otten: Endocrinology **112** (1983), 1547. - 24. Vagenakis, A.G., A. Burger, G.I. Portnay et al.: J. Clin. Endocrinol. Metab. **41** (1975), 191. - 25. Wenzel, K.W., H. Meinhold: Lancet **II** (1975), 413.

Discussion

Leövey: We found with my coworker Dr. Biro in 1983 that the human leukocytes are able in cell culture to produce monoiodine - thyrosine (MIT) and DIT too. We also found that cultured human leukocytes have TSH,they produce MIT and DIT. We do not know the exact explanation of this phenomenon.
Meinhold: Before we came to the clinical studies we performed

for one ore two years in vitro studies with leukocytes. But we were not able to found DIT in resting leukocytes. We had to stimulate them to phagocytosis, and it's essential for the uptake of T_4 to the cell and also essential that the leukocytes make the metabolic worst reaction with oxidizing to establish this oxidizing system.

Leövey: In our investigations the normal leukocytes were stimulated by TSH and after stimulation they produced DIT.

Benker: At the Hague, the group of Prof. van der Heide from Leiden reported on a new class of drugs which differentially inhibit various kinds of deiodinases. Would you speculate about possible clinical applications of such substances?

Meinhold: As I showed in that small table the brain and pituitary deiodinase type-2 enzyme is especially used for local T_3 production from circulating T_4. And in a situation of beginning hypothyroidism, when the T_4 level in the circulation decrease whereas T_3 levels are quite normal, than the pituitary is able to produce its own T_3 by using this T_4 from the plasma whithin the pituitary cells by type-2 deiodination. So it is possible to maintain a euthyroid status whithin the cells with that central function, but I can't say anything about the possibilities that are given with the new drug.

Value of the estimation of peripheral serum T_3 and rT_3 for prognosis assessment in patients with liver cirrhosis - a prospective study

Chr. Rink[1], U. Siersleben[2], J. Haerting[3], T. Mende[2], R. Nilius[1]
Department of Internal Medicine[1], Department of Radiology[2] and Institute for Biostatistics and Medical Informatics[3] of the Martin-Luther-Universität Halle-Wittenberg, Germany

In the last decade it was established that serum triiodothyronine (T_3) level reflects the severity both of acute and chronic liver diseases /3,4,8,14,19/. In particular, in patients with liver cirrhosis the so-called low-T_3-syndrome /3,12-14/.
Therefore, it has been suggested that the estimation of peripheral serum thyroid hormone levels may provide an early prediction of the prognosis of patients with liver cirrhosis /6,19/.

In view of modern therapeutic possibilities available also in hepatology, e.g. immunosuppression and liver transplantation, it is a very important task for hepatologists to predict more precisely the prognosis of patients with liver cirrhosis.

So the search for new and more reliable prognostic parameters is being continued.
It is the aim of our study to prove whether the development of low T_3 serum levels is associated with a poor prognosis and whether the T_3 serum concentration can be used as a predictive parameter regarding the fate of patients with liver cirrhosis.

For this purpose we used a Prognostic Index (PI) reliable for prognosis assessment in cirrhotics which was recently developed by us /15,16/.
By means of this statistical model it is possible to prove other parameters than that used in the index with regard to their predictive value.

Material and methods

To achieve our objectives we determined the peripheral thyroid hormone levels in 28 patients with liver cirrhosis. The diagnosis was established by laparoscopy and/or liver histology. The mean follow-up time of the 22 survivals was 13 months, the mean survival time of the 6 decreased patients was 4.3 months (control on April 30, 1991).

Seventeen of the patients were males and 11 were females. for prognosis assessment of the liver disease we calculated the Prognostic Index (PI) in all of the patients on the basis of the COX regression model /22/: $PI_{(zo)} = \beta' zo = \beta_1 z_1$ 4 ... + $\beta_p z_{op}$, where ß is the coefficient of the variable z in the COX model. Calculating this index for each patient we used 11 parameters as recently described /16/ (table 1).

Table 1: Variables and their coefficients necessary for calculation the Prognostic Index

variables	coefficients ß		covariables z
diagnosis	- 0.9699		1 (micromodular)
			2 (other types)
encephalopathy	- 0.5572		0 (no PSE)
			1 (PSE)
spider naevi	+ 0.9635		0 (no spiders)
			1 (spiders)
PCV	+ 4.8837	)	
platelets	- 0.0158	)	
Quick's value	- 0.0206	)	absolute
albumin	- 0.1164	)	values
cholesterol	- 0.4183	)	of variables
γ-GT	+ 0.0001	)	
IgA	+ 0.0948	)	
potassium	+ 1.2792	)	

The index calculated by these variables permits a precise prediction of the prognosis of cirrhosis /15,16/.
According to the value of the PI we classified all of the patients into three risk groups:

risk group A: index > -2 to +2 = poor prognosis
risk group B: index > -4 to -2 = mean prognosis
risk group C: index -6 to -4 = good prognosis.

We measured tri-iodothyronine (T_3-RIA)[1)], reverse T_3 (RIA)[2)], thyroxine (T_4-RIA)[1)] and basal thyroid-stimulating hormone (TSH-RIA)[1)] as well as the laboratory parameters of the PI as routine determinations in peripheral venous blood.

Statistical analysis was performed on the computer ES 1040 of the Centre of Organization and Calculation of the Martin-Luther-Universität Halle-Wittenberg with statistical software both by the Karl-Weierstraß-Institut of the Academy of Sciences Berlin and by using BMDP in the versions of 1979 an 1985 /2,15/.

1) RIA of Henning Berlin GmbH, FRG
2) RIA of the Academy of Sciences Berlin, FRG

Results

Out of the total of the 28 patients examined 7 patients were classified into risk group A, 12 into risk group B, and 9 into risk group C. The differences between the risk groups with respect to the mean serum T_3 concentrations resulted in a tendency of significance (A/B: $p = 0.06$; A/C: $p = 0.04$; B/C: $p = 0.54$) (figure 1). The regression of the prognostic index values on T_3 demonstrated an inverse correlation ($y = -1.8 -0.7x$; $r = 0.4$; $p = 0.03$) (figure 2).
On the other hand, the slope of the regression of PI on basal TSH was also negative ($y = -2.01 -0.72x$; $r = 0.54$; $p = 0.0028$), although a positive one was expected (figure 3).
The differences between the risk groups A and B or C regarding basal TSH were highly significant (A/B: $p = 0.004$; A/C: $p = 0.0025$; B/C: $p = 0.43$) (figure 4). It is noteworthy that the serum T_3 concentration correlates well with such synthesis parameters of the liver, e.g. serum albumin, cholesterol,

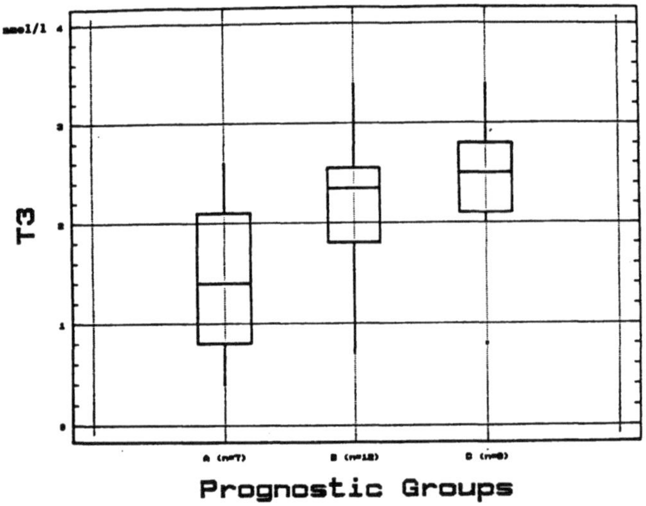

Figure 1

Serum concentrations of T_3 in the three risk groups of the PI (multiple box and whisker plot).

(Wilcoxon: A/B: $p = 0.06$, A/C: $p = 0.04$, B/C: $p = 0.54$)

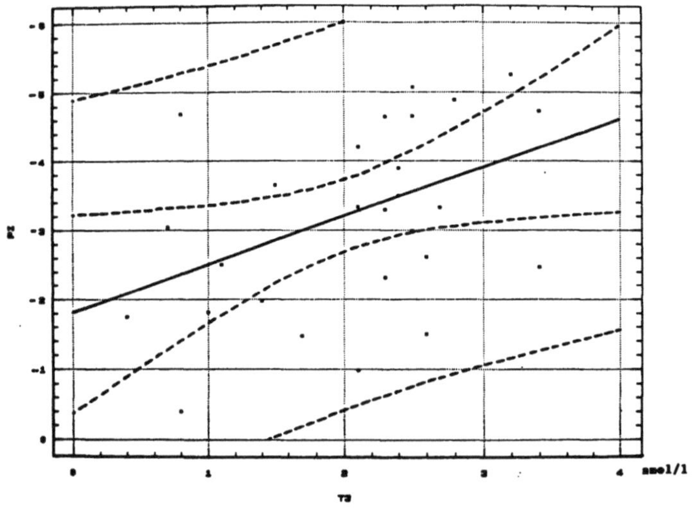

Figure 2

Regression of PI on T_3 (with 95 % confidence interval).

($y = -1.8 -0.7x$; $r = 0.4$, $p = 0.03$)

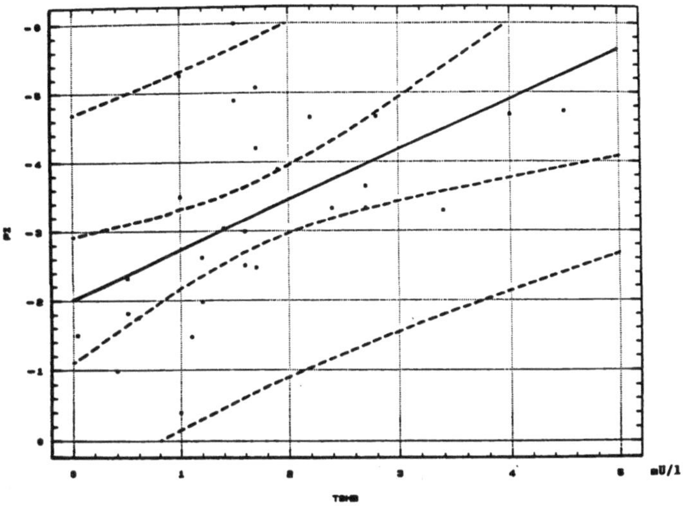

Figure 3

Regression of PI on basal TSH (with 95 % confidence interval).

(y = -2.01 -0.72x; r = 0.54, p = 0.0028)

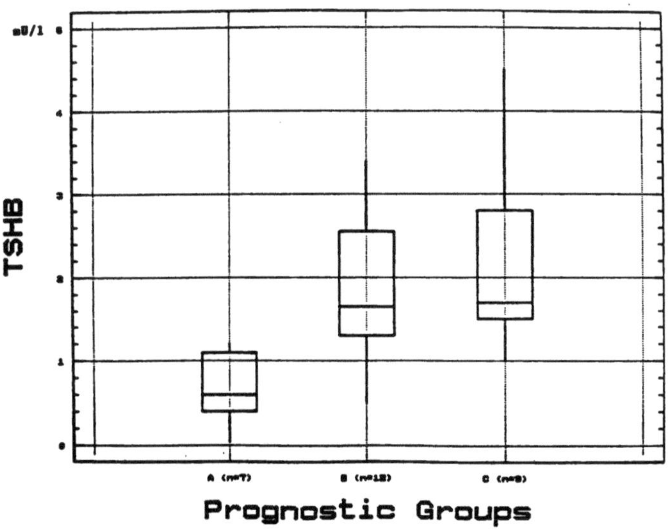

Figure 4

Serum concentrations of basal TSH in the three risk groups of the PI (multiple box and whisker plot).

(Wilcoxon: A/B: p = 0.004, A/C: p = 0.0025,
B/C: p = 0.43)

Quick's value, and IgA, whereas no other thyroid hormone did so (table 2).

Table 2: Correlation matrix (extract of significant correlations, $p < 0.05$) of thyroid hormone and laboratory liver parameters

	TSHb	T_3	T_4	rT_3	PCV	thrombo	chol.	alb.	Quick	K	PI
TSHb	1	-	-	-	-	-	-	-	-	+	+
T_3	-	1	+	-	+	-	+	+	+	-	+
T_4	-	+	1	+	-	-	-	-	-	-	-
rT_3	-	-	+	1	-	+	-	-	-	-	-
PCV	-	+	-	-	1	-	+	+	-	-	
thrombo	-	-	-	+	-	1	-	-	-	-	
chol.	-	+	-	-	+	-	1	-	-	-	
alb.	-	+	-	-	+	-	+	1	+	-	
Quick	-	+	-	-	-	-	-	+	1	-	
K	+	-	-	-	-	-	-	-	-	1	
PI	+	+	-	-							

Moreover, the mean serum T_3 concentration differed significantly between surviving and deceased patients (Wilcoxon-Test, $p = 0.00076$) (figure 5).

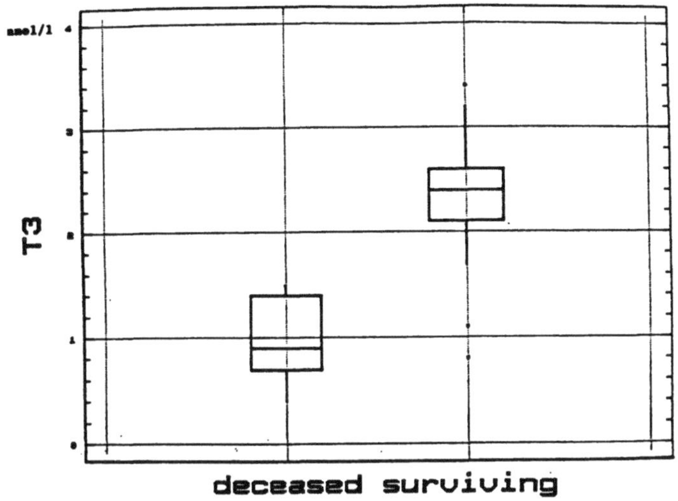

Figure 5

Serum concentrations of T_3 in deceased and surviving patients with liver cirrhosis (multiple box and whisker plot)

(Wilcoxon: $p = 0.00076$)

Discussion and conclusions

The liver is the most important site of the peripheral conversion of T_4 to T_3 /5,6,17/. Therefore, it is not surprising that in chronic liver diseases, in particular in cirrhosis, the T_3 serum concentrations decrease and the low T_3-syndrome develops /3,12, 13,14/. The reason for it is assumed to be an enzymatic shift from phenolic to nonphenolic deiodination of T_4 yielding reserve T_3 (rT_3) /7,10,12,17/. But it could be demonstrated that this switch over to the rT_3 production cannot be the only reason for the deviation of the peripheral hormone metabolism /14/. As earlier observed /14/, we could not find any correlation between T_3 and rT_3 in our cirrhotic patients. But there is a strong inverse correlation between the prognosis of cirrhotic patients, expressed as Prognostic Index /15,16/, and serum T_3 (figure 2). Interestingly, the low T_3 serum concentrations do not induce an increase in the basal TSH. On the contrary, in the risk group A the basal TSH levels are significantly lower than in groups B and C. Since there is no correlation between basal TSH and rT_3 it seems to be more improbable that rT_3 compensate the lacking T_3 and will block up the tri-iodothyronine receptors of the pituitary gland /18/. Instead of this hypothesis there are arguments that give cause for the assumption that in patients with liver cirrhosis toxic substances from the gut reach the brain by-passing the liver by hepatofugal collaterals and may be responsible for a derangement in neurotransmitter metabolism associated with alterations of the pituitary receptors for TRH on TSH secretion /11/ so as to prevent increases of TSH secretion in response to decreased serum T_3 concentration /20/.

Nevertheless, the development of low T_3 serum concentrations in patients with liver cirrhosis indicates poor prognosis for them. If the T_3 values do not increase to normal ranges by means of therapy, the course of the disease will turn out to be fatal (see figure 5).
It seems to be true that low serum T_3 levels are a very sensitive parameter for prognosis prediction in patients with liver cirrhosis.

References

1. Cox, D.R.: J. R. Statist. Soc. (B) **34** (1972), 187. - 2. Dixon, W.J., M.B. Brown, L. Engelman, J.W. Frane, M.A. Hill, R.I. Jennrich, J.D. Toporek: Berkely, University of California Press, 1983. - 3. Hampel, R., W. Meng, A. Weber, R. Michael: Dt. Gesundh.-Wesen **37** (1982), 1563. - 4. Hampel, R., A. Weber, B. Jäger, W. Meng: Dt. Gesundh.-Wesen **39** (1984), 1755. - 5. Hellthaler, G., S. Appelt: Dt. Gesundh.-Wesen **36** (1981), 425. -6. Hepner, G.W., I.J. Chopra: Arch. Intern. Med. **139** (1979), 1117. - 7. Hesch,R.D.: Dt. med. Wochenschr. **106** (1981), 971. -8. Itoh, S., Y. Yamata, T. Oda, K. Kawagoe: Am. J. Gastroenterol. **81** (1986), 444. - 9. Kano, T., T. Kojima, T. Takahashi, Y. Muto: Gastroenterol. Japan. **22** (1987), 344. - 10. L'Age, M., H. Weinhold, K.W. Wenzel, H. Schleusener: J. Endocrinol. Invest. **4** (1980), 379. - 11. Langer, M., P.P. Rovasio, A. Masala, S. Alagna, S. Rassu, A. Solinas, A. Deplano, G. Madeddu, L. Chiandussi: Ital. J. Gastroenterol. **17** (1985), 69. - 12. Rink, Chr., U. Siersleben, J. Haerting, M.

Klaua, E. Mertens: Radiol. diagn. **23**(1982), 88. - 13. Rink, Chr., U. Siersleben, H. Haerting, M. Klaua, E. Mertens: Z. ges. inn. Med. **37** (1982), 532. - 14. Rink, Chr., U. Siersleben, E. Meyer, Th. Zeisler, E. Mertens, M. Klaua, J. Haerting, W. Teichmann, R. Nilius: Radiol. Iugosl. **23** (1989), 45. - 15. Rink, Chr., J. Haerting: Martin-Luther-Universität Halle-Wittenberg, Wissenschaftliche Beiträge 1990/21 (R 118), Halle (Saale) 1990. - 16. Rink, Chr., J. Haerting, R. Nilius: Z. Gastroenterol. (Suppl. 2) **29** (1991), 163. -17. Salata, R., J. Klein, G.S. Levey: Sem. Liver Dis. **5** (1985), 29. -18. Schlienger, J.L.: Z. Gastroenterol. **17** (1979), 452. - 19. Seitz, H.K., P. Czygan, F. Weber, R. Götz, B. Kommerell: L. Chiandussi, I.J. Chopra, I. Martini (eds.): Academic press London and New York 1982, p. 471. - 20. Utiger, R.D.: The thyroid. In: Felig, Ph., J.D. Baxter, A.E. Broadus, L.A. Frohman (eds.): Endocrinology and metabolism 2nd edition. McGraw - Hill Book Comp. New York, 1987, p. 389.

Discussion

Peschel: Did you find some differences of your results concerning the different etiology of your cases of liver cirrhosis whether they are of alcoholic, viral or autoimmune origin, because these various kinds have a different prognosis per se?

Rink: No, we could not demonstrate such differences because the sequels of a cirrhosis are the same, nevertheless the etiology. You can find a collateralisation and we have arguments for such hypothesis that the collateralisation in the liver is a very important reason for the development ot low-T_3 syndrome. These collaterals develop in every cirrhosis in a final state of the disease. We could not demonstrate differences in etiology statistically.

Limanova: We did some examination in myocardial infarction with T_3-low syndroma. We found the same as you, that patients with very low T_3 level died and that patients that had T_3 lower and after seven days the T_3 improved survived.

I would like to ask, did you examine T_3 total or T_3 free? Additionally, I remember a paper, seven or eight years old, the author tried to treat patients with liver cirrhosis, with PTU (Propylthiouracil). They had very good results, but since that we never red those articles - the other authors did not have

success.

Rink: We determined total T_3 and our study is going on and we will also measure the free T_3-fraction.

We know the papers from the Toronto-group and as I know they are the only group that described such a positive effect of PTU-treatment in cirrhotic patients. We did not use such a treatment in our patients because we are not sure that there results a benefit for our patients.

Meinhold: May I make a short comment to your findings regarding rT_3 - this was not a parameter which could be used as a survival parameter. I think it is not surprising. In a paper this year they found that the rT_3-production is not changed in all of that situations with the low T_3 syndrome. One can't speak from a swich to higher rT_3-production and so it's not surprising regarding the T_3 that's a clear decrease. rT_3 remains in it's production stable or constant and its elimination is inhibited. And so rT_3 is not a good parameter in your system.

Thyroid hormones and TSH in acute myocardial infarction

Pechán, J., I. Vereš, J. Murín
Department of Nuclear Medicine of 1st Medical Clinic, Faculty of Medicine, Comenius University, Bratislava, CSFR

The acute and chronic nonthyroidal diseases are often accompanied with abnormal changes of thyroid hormones (TH) metabolism and functional defects of axis hypothalamus-hypophysis-thyroid gland /1/. The acute myocardial infarction (AMI) occupies among these diseases an important place for the well-known influence of TH on myocardial oxygen consumption and thereby for the possibility to influence the course of the disease. Therefore, the serum level changes of TH and thyroid-stimulating hormone (TSH) are in the **foreground** of the interest of many authors. However, conflicting reports have been published /2-4/.

The aim of our study was to investigate the dynamics of TH and TSH changes during AMI on bigger set of patients and to try to find the differences in the behaviour of TH in patients who died within 96 hours from the onset of illness in comparison with patients who survived longer than 3 weeks. Second aspect was to determine the diagnostic value of serum TH and TSH levels on thyroid function evaluation during the course of AMI.

Patients and methods

The study was performed in 88 patients with AMI. No patient showed clinical symptoms of functional changes of thyroid gland. Patients treated with corticosteroids or anticoagulants were exclude.

The parameters were evaluated on the 1st day in 72 patients who survived more than 21 days and in 16 patients who died 96 hours from admission.

In 58 patients the blood samples were taken in addition to the 1st day on the 3rd and the 7th day.

The following commercial kits were used: total serum thyroxine (T4) was evaluated by RIA-T_4, total serum triiodothyronine (T_3)

by RIA-T_3 (both from Košice, ČSFR), effective thyroxine ratio (ETR) by Thyro-KT (Feinchemie Sebnitz) and TSH by Riamat TSH (Byk **Mallinckrodt**). The measurements were always made according to recommendations of the producer.

The medians and 95 % confidence intervals were established. In the statistical analyses non parametrical methods were used: Friedman two way analysis of variance, Wilcoxon's paired signed-ranks test and Mann-Whitney U test.

Results

The values of investigated parameters in survived patients and in those who died are compared in figure 1.

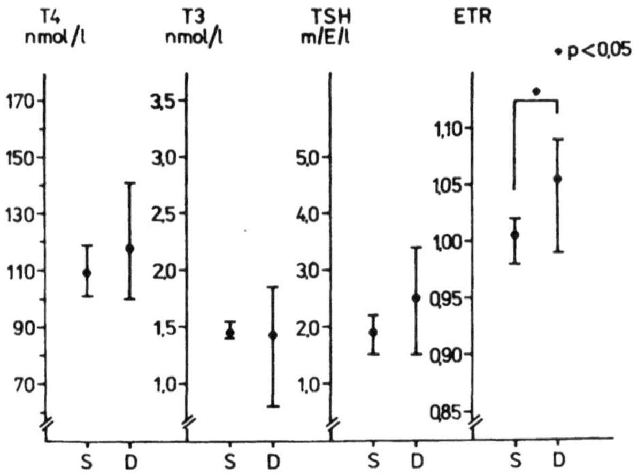

Figure 1

Total serum thyroxine (T_4), total serum triiodothyronine (T_3), basal serum TSH and ETR on the 1st day in patients with acute myocardial infarction. S = patients who have survived, D = patients who have died. Medians, 95 % confidence intervals and statistical significance are shown.

Patients who have died have significantly higher value of ETR on the 1st day in the comparison with the patients who survived AMI. The results of other parameters were not significantly different in survived and died patients but the medians of T_4 and TSH were higher in patients who died.

The level dynamics of TH, TSH and ETR on the 1st, 3rd and 7th day of hospitalization represent figure 2 and 3. The values of T_4, T_3 and ETR decreased on the 3 rd day in comparison with the 1st day. Whereas T_4 and T_3 returned to starting values, ETR remained significantly lower also on the 7th day. The values of TSH did not significantly change, however they tended to increase on the 7th day of hospitalization.

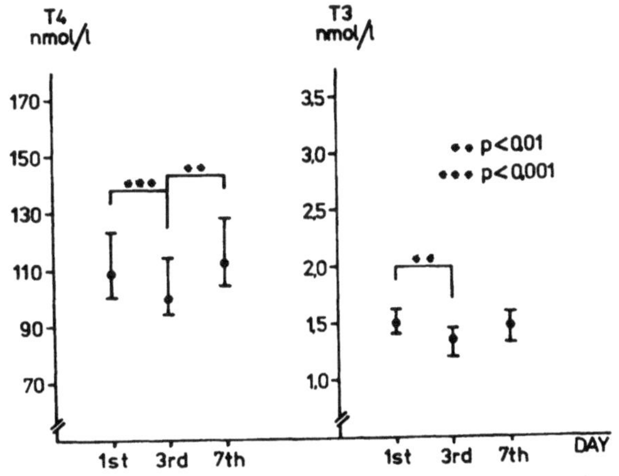

Figure 2

Total serum thyroxine (T_4 and total serum triiodothyronine (T_3) on the 1st, 3rd and 7th day in Surviving patients with acute myocardial infarction. Medians, 95 % confidence intervals and statistical significance are shown.

The frequency of abnormal values of investigated parameters in all patients on the 1st day is shown in table 1. More than one abnormal result was not found in any patient. From the point of view of thyroid function evaluation the most suitable parameter was ETR with the lowest frequency of abnormal values. The most frequent occurence of abnormal values was found in TSH levels.

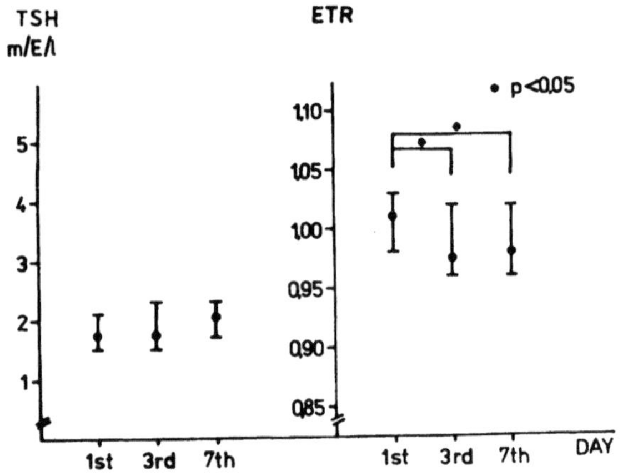

Figure 3

Basal serum TSH and ETR on the 1st, 3rd and 7th day in patients as on figure 2

Table 1: The frequency of abnormal values of thyroid hormones and TSH in 88 patients with acute myocardial infarction

Parameter	Increased	Decreased	Total abnormal
T_4	13.6 %	0	13.6 %
T_3	0	15.9 %	15.9 %
TSH	17.0 %	1.1 %	18.1 %
ETR	9.1 %	0	9.1 %

Discussion

In the difference of many authors we did not find lower levels of T_3 in patients who died, so we cannot explain the relatively higher levels of T_4 and ETR only by disordered peripheral deiodination of T_4 to T_3. However, the uptake of T_4 by tissue may be also diminished, further, it can be caused by relatively increased production of TH by thyroid gland.

The significant decrease of T_4, T_3 and ETR on the 3rd day in survived patients might be explained by several mechanisms. The decrease of TH secretion is probably the most important mechanism, that can be conditioned by the increase of circulating cortisol level /5/. Other mechanism can be the presence of an inhibitor of TH to binding proteins /1/. The decrease of T_3 can be also explained by the defect in T_4 to T_3 deiodination /1/. Decreased T_3 production could result in decreases in the rates of oxygen consumption, substrate utilisation and various catabolic processes. So the decreased secretion of TH in AMI can present the mechanism protecting the myocardium to more extensive breakdown.

The increase of ETR in the group of died patients (in comparison with survivors) is very interesting finding that shows a participation of relative elevated free thyroxine fraction on the course of fatal AMI. However, it is not clear from our work whether this result can be of therapeutic importance (for example thyroid inhibition by iodine) and other works - partly experimental - are necessary.

Conclusion

In 88 patients with AMI the changes in T_4, T_3, TSH levels and ETR were investigated. The T_4 and T_3 values significantly decreased on the 3rd day of hospitalization with the return to starting values on the 7th day. Similarly, ETR values were significantly decreased on the 3 rd day and remained lower on the 7th day. The serum TSH values were nonsignificantly increased on the 7th day of hospitalization in comparison with starting values.

The ETR values were significantly increased on the 1st day of hospitalization in the subgroup of 16 patients who died within 96 hours in comparison with the subgroup of AMI surviving patients.

With respect on thyroid function evaluation, the most suitable parameter was ETR with the lowest per cent of abnormal values.

The finding indicate some thyroid hormones metabolism changes during acute myocardial infarction that could be of importance for the pathogenesis and adjuvante therapy of AMI as well as for thyroid function evaluation during AMI.

References

1. Hennemann, G., E.P. Kreuning: Horm. Res. **26** (1987), 100. - 2. Nabiulin, M.S., A.D. Kuimov: Kardiologija **22** (1982), No. 7, 72. - 3. Vanhaelst, L. et al.: Horm. metab. res. **8** (1976), 42. - 4. Wiersinga, W.M., K.I. Lie, J.L. Tauber: Clin. Endocrinol. **14** (1981), 367. - 5. Marek, H. et al.: Abstracts: XVI. International congress of internal medicine, 1982, 337.

Discussion

Leövey: The changes in thyroid hormone levels in stroke and AMI are different aspects of "sicken thyroid syndrome". These changes may serve as prognostic values of patients with very severe diseases. No threat by thyroid hormones of patients with low-T_3 or T_4 syndrome! Because presumably they are the consequences of the adaptation of human organism.

Meinhold: I would support this comment on the difficulties to use T_3 or T_4 as therapeutic agents in this diseases. There is no definite prove and it is suggested that the low T_3-syndrome is a mechanism which protects the body against energy-providing T_3. So it is very difficult to decide a therapeutic application of T_4 and T_3.

Pechan: The only unexpectable finding of our work was the relative increase of ETR (free thyroxine fraction) in patients who died in the acute phase of myocardial infarction. I think that the usual oxygen consumption may be critical in acute period of myocardial infarction for the survive of myocardial cells. The results of other authors with beneficial effect of beta-blockers on myocardial metabolism during acute myocardial infarction could support this idea.

Deiodination of thyroxine and reverse triiodothyronine in cells of human adipose tissue

Ch.-F. Wolf, J. Wieberneit, L. Duntas, F.S. Keck
Abteilung für Innere Medizin I, Klinik und Poliklinik der Universität Ulm, Ulm/Donau, Germany

The generation of the metabolically most active iodothyronine 3,5,3'-triiodothyronine (T_3) does not direktly derive from thyroidal secretion but from extrathyroidal phenolic deiodination (5'DA) out of thyroxine (T_4) in man /1,2/. Different types of deiodination have been classified by anatomical localization, biochemical patterns, substratum specificity and pathophysiological reactivity etc. /3/. It has been reported, that about 80 % of circulating T_3 are produced by 5'DA whereas 20 % of circulating T_3 derive from direct thyroidal secretion. These figures refer to the plasma pool of T_3 distribution /3/. Focussing the T_3 distribution in man it appears to be noteworthy, that only 5 % of total body's T_3 are found in the plasma. It has been circulated that the distribution of total T_3 in man covers by 76 % the "slow pool" (predominantly adipose tissue, muscle) by 19 % the "fast pool" (e.g. liver, kidney) and by 5 % the plasma /4/. The slow pool has been defined by a plasma exchange time of T_3 of about 17 h, the fast pool has a plasma exchange time of about 30 min. Since the plasma half life of T_3 is about 19 h, we assume a intracellular state of T_3, which is separated from plasma T_3-concentrations in the slow pool. In order to study the intracellular ability of 5'deiodination in the slow pool we investigated adipose tissue, which is White Adipose Tissue (WAT) in adult man. It is a form of connective tissue that constitutes approximately 20 % of the weight of an individual on average nutrition. The morphological compounds of WAT are adipocytes and "stromalvascular cells" (SVC). SVC are defined as fibroblasts, endothelial cells and adipocyte precursors. About 50 % of subcutaneous human SVC are reported to be able to develop the enzymatic patterns of adipocyte-differentiation in vitro /5/.

Materials and methods

Adipose tissue samples has been fractioned in order to isolate the cells using the methods of Petterson et al. /6/ in slight modification. In short: Subcutaneous adipose tissue specimen were immediately cut into small fragments and incubated for 50 min at 37 °C in a solution containing collagenase (2 mg/ml phosphate buffered saline; 6 mg per g adipose tissue). The probes were washed twice. Final centrifugation at 400 yielded a separation of adipocytes and stromalvascular cells and erythrocytes (pellet). As erythrocytes do disturb the cultivation of SVC the pellet was rehomogenized and incubated in a solution containing 8.3 g/l NH_4Cl, 1.0 g/l $KHCO_3$, and 0.0371 g/l EDTA (15 min) at room temperature in order to eliminate red blood cells. Isolated SVC were washed in PBS and resuspended in the final medium for cell cultivation consisting of EMEM / Ham's F-12 (1:1 / v:v) + 10 % fetal bovine serum in order to enhance the amount of specimen: About 10,000,000 SVC are required for the 5'DA assay. As the cultivation of differentiated adipocytes does not lead to a substantial increase of specimen, liberated adipocytes were directly employed for the assay. In order to exclude a possible effect of the proteolytic enzyme collagenase on 5'DA, we also studied intact adipose tissue fragments.

Cells or tissue were mechanically minced and sonified in a buffer containing 250 mM sucrose, 20 mM TRIS, 5 mM EDTA, 1 mM $MgCl_2$ and 10 mM Dithioerythritol as described previously /7/. Differential centrifugation yielded in the subcellular fraction which contains the microsomes. We incubated 400 ug microsomal protein (0.5 ml/ sample) in the buffer system as mentioned above together with T_4 (concentrations as indicated) or rT_3 at 4 °C and 37 °C for 2 or 25 hrs. In order to identify the type of 5'DA, Propylthiouracil (PTU, 1 mM) and Aopodate (IOP, 0.5 mM) were coincubated as indicated. The chemical stability of rT_3 was proven by the simultaneous incubation of an equivalent in the buffer without cellular protein. Incubations were stopped by addition of ice-cold ethanol. The iodothyronine content of ethanol-extracts was determined radioimmunologically. 5'DA was calculated out of the amount of newly generated T_3 or decomposed rT_3 and presented as pg iodothyronine /mg microsomal protein * min of incubation. Chemicals were purchased from Biochrom/Berlin, Henning/Berlin and Serva/Heidelberg. Radioimmuno-assays were obtained from Henning/Berlin and Serono/ Freiburg. Cultivation dishes were purchased from Nunc/Wiesbaden.

We employed truncal subcutaneous adipose tissue from surgical patients. Since a high vascularisation is described for omental specimen we avoided the study of endothelial cells by excluding the greater omentum from our experimental design. The experiments with human adipose tissue samples have been approved by the local authorities for ethics. The study included patients of both sex (n = 5), the age was ranging between 43 and 67 years.

Results

Concerning intact adipose tissue differential centrifugation yielded an amount of 150-200 /ug microsomal protein / g w.w.; so was the protein content of isolated cells. IOP did, PTU did not inhibit 5'DA. There were no substantial differences regarding inhibitory effects on 5'DA between isolated stromalvascular cells, adipocytes and intact adipose tissue (cf. figure 1). T_4 to T_3-deiodination by isolated microsomes was continuously detected over 25 hours at body temperature. Generation of T_3 out of T_4 was not detectable at 4 °C (cf. figure 2). The degration of the substratum rT_3 at nM concentrations resulted in an almost linear decomposition over 25 hours both at 37 °C and at 4 °C from 410 ng/dl rT_3 to 180 ng/dl rT_3. IOP did (data not shown) and PTU didnot inhibit decomposition of rT_3. When rT_3 was incubated without microsomal protein the substratum of 5'DA remained stable over 25 hrs. (cf figure 3). Regarding the enzyme kinetics of 5'DA in human adipose tissue we found an apparent k_M of about 1 /uM for the substratum T_4 and of about 3 nM for the substratum rT_3 (cf. figure 4).

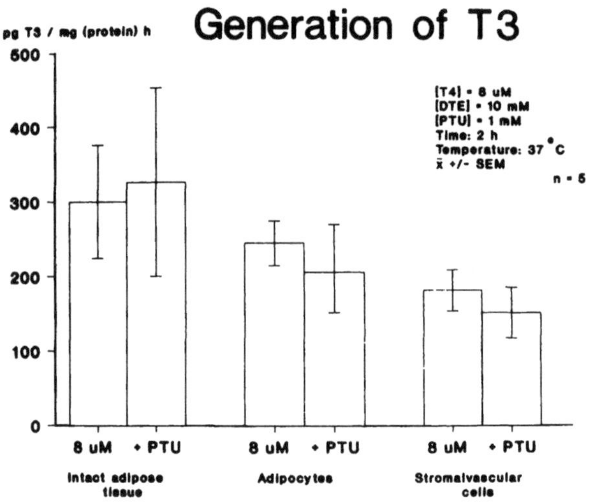

Figure 1

5'-deiodinating activity in intact adipose tissue (IAT), stromalvascular cells (SVC) and adipocytes (ADI)

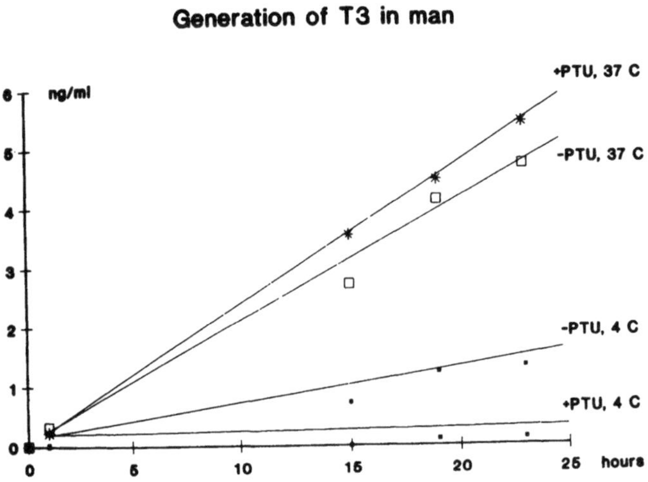

Figure 2

T_3-production out of T_4 at 37 ^oC and at 4 ^oC over 25 hrs. with and without PTU

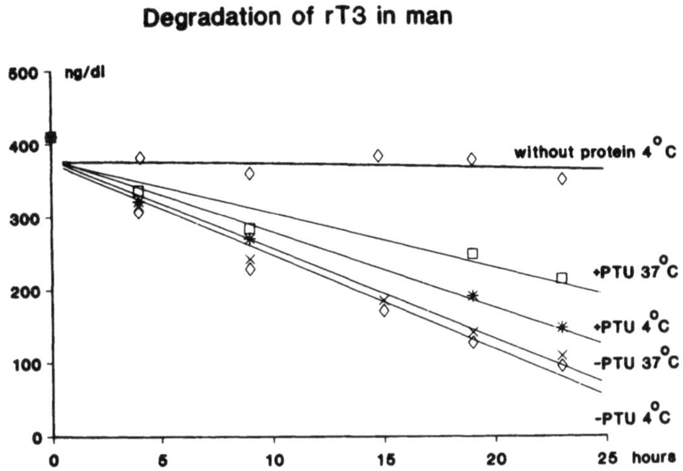

Figure 3

rT_3-decompensation at 37 °C and at 4 °C over 25 hrs. with and without PTU

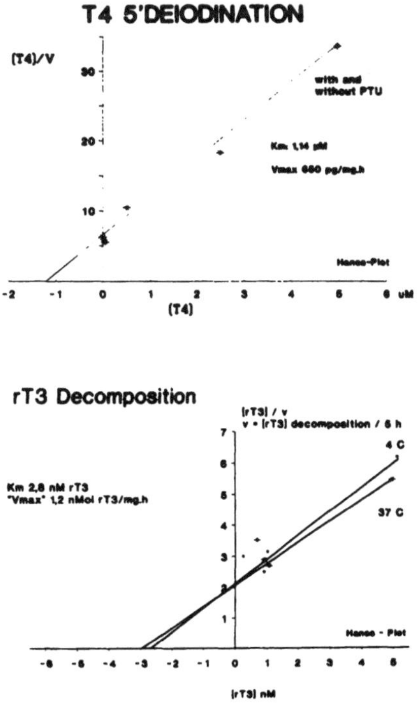

Figure 4

Enzyme kinetics of human adipose tissues 5'DA for the substrata T_4 and rT_3

Discussion

Few studies have employed human tissue for the investigation of thyroid hormone metabolism /8-11/. Our data suggest a PTU insensible 5'DA, which degradates nanomolar concentrations of the substratum rT_3 at body temperature as well as at 4 ^{o}C. Since the general physiological purpose of rT_3 is uncertain (i.e. possible inhibitory effects on 5'DA via actinmediated mobilization /12/, etc.) or none, the meaning of a decomposition of rT_3 at lower temperatures than body temperature remains to be speculative. Regarding the biochemical classification of 5'DA in adipose tissue we have found the typical pattern of type II deiodination apart from the k_M of 1 /uM for T_4. The inhibitory effects of IOP, the lacking effects of PTU and the k_M for the substratum rT_3 do fit into the characteristics of a type II 5'DA. This conclusion is supported by the findings of Naumann et al. /11/, although these data referred to omental specimen. In rat adipose tissues type II 5'DA has been exclusively described for brown adipose tissue, whereas the 5'DA in rat epididymal fat pads is reported to be inhibited by PTU /13/. In contrast to the type II 5'DA of human keratinocytes, which is capable to generate up to 20 % of circulating T_3 in hypothyroid beings /14/, the function of 5'DA in human adipose tissue is probably strictly intracellular. According to DiStefano III /4/ total body's T_3 is exchanged between the plasma and the slow pool by only 10 %, 62 % of the T_3 in the slow pool are generated locally. Since the plasma pool is basically served by the type I 5'DA, we want to emphasize that we can demonstrate a generation of T_3 in about 20 % of body weight, which is almost separated from the plasma.

We demonstrate a PTU-insensitive 5'DA in adipocyte precursors and in differentiated adipocytes. Therefore the activity of 5'-deiodination is not related to the state of differentiation, as reported for other endocrinologically activating enzymes (e.g. aromatase; /15/).

References

1. Hesch, R.D., J. Köhrle: In: Ingbar, S.H., L.E. Braverman (eds.) The Thyroid J.B. Lippincott Company, Philadelphia (1986).-
2. Cavalieri, R.R., B. Rappaport: Ann. Rev. Med. **57** (1977), 57.-

3. Kaplan, M.M.: Neuroendecrinology (1984), 254. - 4. DiStefano III, J.J.: in: Georg Hennemann (ed.): Thyroid Hormone Metabolism (1986). - 5. Hauner, H., G. Entenmann, M. Wabitsch, D. Gaillard, G. Ailhaud, R. Negrel, E.F. Pfeiffer: J. Clin Invest. **84** (1989), 1663. - 6. Petterson, P., R. Van, M. Karlsson, P. Björntorp: Metabolism **34** (1985), 808. - 7. Grau, R., F.S. Keck, U. Loos, E.F. Pfeiffer: Horm. Metabol. Res. Suppl. (1984), 62. - 8. Kaplan, M.M., E.A. Shaw: J. Clin. Endocrinol. Metab. **59** (1984), 253. - 9. Hardy, J.J., C.L. Thomas, R.D. Utiger: Am. J. Med. Sci. (1987), 193. - 10. Visser, T.J., E. Kaptein, O.T. Terstra, E.P. Krenning: J. Clin. Endocrinol. Metab. **67** (1988), 17. - 11. Naumann, A., J. Naumann, G. Sypniewska, K. Fiedorowicz, K. Bielecki, D. Pastuszko: In: Björntorp, P., S. Rössner (edts.): Obesity in Europe **88** (1988). - 12. Farwell, A., R. Lynch, W. Oculicz, A. Comi, J. Neonard: J. Biol. Chem. **265** (1990), 18546. - 13. Leonard, J.L., S.A. Mellen, P.R. Larsen: Endocrinology **112** (1983), 1153. - 14. Kaplan, M.M., C.Y. Pan, P.R. Gordon, J.K. Lee, B.A. Gilchrest: J. Clin. Endocrinol. Metab. **66** (1989), 815. - 15. Mendelson,C.R., E.R. Simpson: Molecul. Cell. Endocrinol. **52** (1987), 169.

Comparison of natural killer activity with thyroid function in Graves' disease

A. Sztankay, Gy. Bakó, E. Fórizs, E. Mezösi, A. Leövey
I. Department of Internal Medicine, University Medical School, Debrecen, Hungary

Growing number of data have been accumulated for some time supposing that the immune system is under hormonal regulation. In some pathological conditions, alteration in hormone levels is accompanied by abnormal immunological findings. Several studies have indicated that thyroid hormones may exert an influence on the immune system. However, the effect of thyroid hormones on the immune system has not been yet well established.

The activity of natural killer (NK) cells is of great importance in autoimmune diseases. NK activity is decreased in patients with autoimmune diseases such as systemic lupus erythematosus and Sjögren's syndrome. Hashimoto thyroiditis and Graves' disease are also considered to be autoimmune diseases. However, results of studies dealing with NK activity of peripheral blood mononuclear cells obtained from patients with autoimmune thyroid disease are conflicting. The cytotoxic activity of NK cells in hyperthyroidism has been reported as normal /1/, higher than normal /2/, or decreased /3/. The lack of uniformity is perhaps in part due to the variety of techniques used.

The aim of our study was to determin in which direction and extent is changing the NK activity in patients suffering from Graves' disease, comparing the spontaneous cytotoxic activity with the actual thyroid hormone levels (T_4, rT_3, TSH). We tried to find inherence between different hormone levels and NK activity.

Patients and methods

Peripheral blood samples were taken from 26 patients with Graves' disease (6 hypothyroid, 7 had normofunction, 16 hyperthyroxinemic at the time of the study).

Mononuclear cells were separated by centrifugation through Ficoll/Hypaque density gradient, followed by washing in Hank's balanced salt solution (HBSSF) and suspended in RPMI 1640 supplemented with 10 % fetal bovine serum.

Mononuclear cells were assayed for NK activity against the NK-sensitive cell line K 562, as described by White et al. /4/. Cytotoxicity was expressed as described by Pross and Maroun /5/.

Hormone (T_4, rT_3, TSH) and antibody (TRAK) determinations were carried out in our clinical laboratory by radioimmunoassay kits.

Results

Compared with the normo-, and hyperthyroxinemic group, cytotoxic activity was diminished in all of the hypothyroid patients. On the other hand no significant difference of NK activity has been detected in the normo-, and hyperthyroxinemic group compared to each other (figure 1). There has not been found correlation in the latter two groups regarding the actual thyroid hormone levels (T_4, T_3, TSH) and the NK activity.

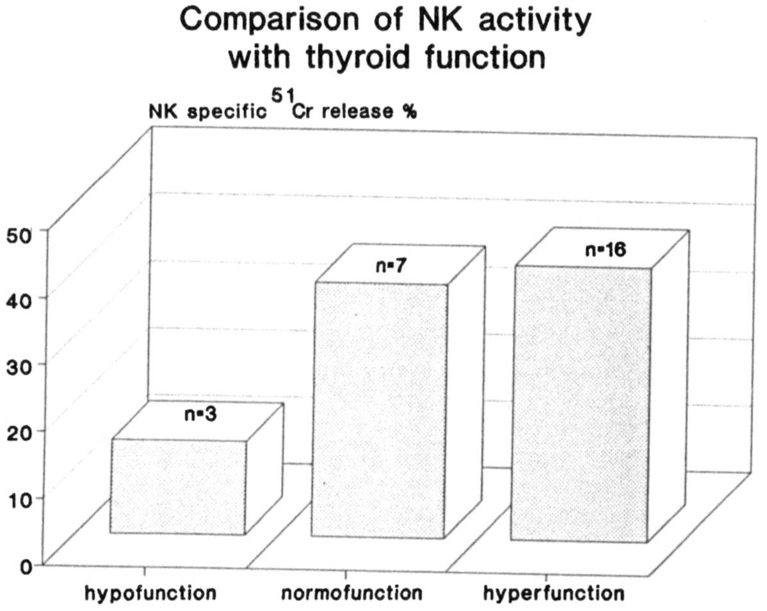

Figure 1

In the hyperthyroxinemic group rT_3 was in the normal range in 4 patients, and was elevated in 12 patients. We have not found significant alteration of NK activity when compared to the different rT_3 levels (figure 2).

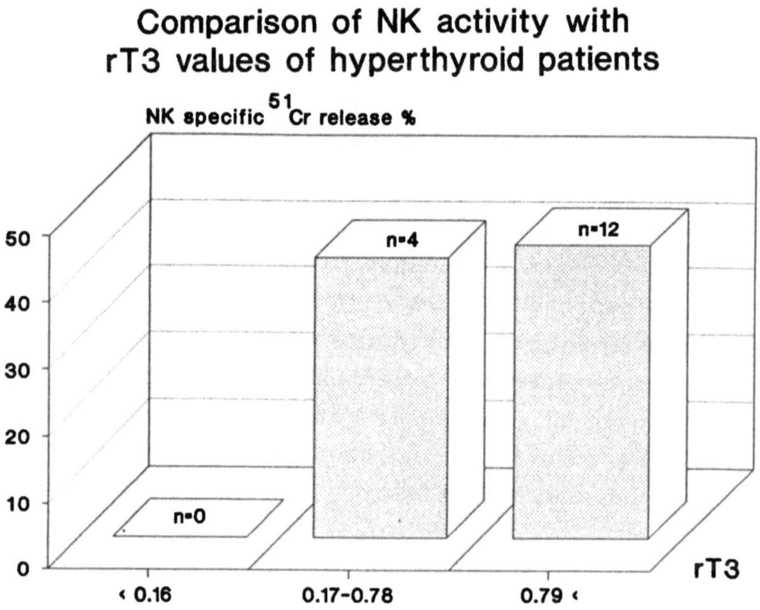

Figure 2

We tried to find inherence between cytotoxic activity and the presence of the pathological anti TSH receptor antibodies that are usually present in the sera of patients suffering from Graves' disease. Assessing the anti TSH receptor antibody levels by TRAK assay, it was elevated in 10, and normal in 6 patients.There was no difference of NK activity between the two groups (figure 3).

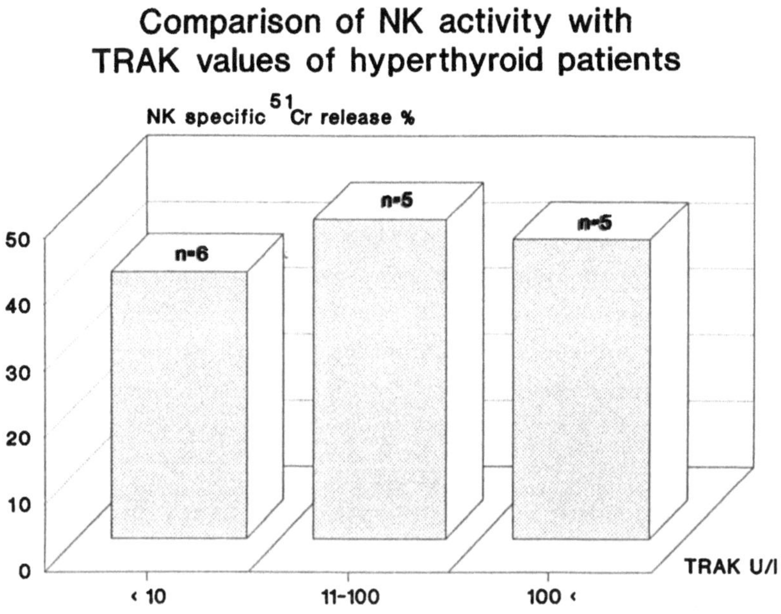

Figure 3

Discussion

The possible role of NK cells in autoimmune thyroid diseases is well known from the works of Papic /6/, Tezuka /7/, and others. NK cells are capable of inhibiting in vitro antibody production by antibody induced lymphoblastoid B cells /8/. With respect to peripheral blood 2- or 3-fold increase of B cell lineage expressing surface markers of in vivo activation has been found among mononuclear cells separated from thyroid glands of patients with Graves' disease /9/. It is also known that NK activity is not only by hormones influenced but by lymphokines too /10/.

In our study we tried to find inherence between the actual thyroid hormone levels and NK activity of peripheral mononuclear cells. Summarizing our findings: we found that the NK activity was diminished in hypothyroid patients, but no significant difference has been noticed between patients with normal thyroid function and with hyperthyroxinemia. We could not have found correlation in the latter two groups regarding the actual thyroid hormone levels, anti TSH receptor antibody values and the NK activity.

We plan to extent our further work on patients with different types of thyroiditis for - according to our opinion - cytotoxic activity may play an important role in these disease. The use of lymphokines (gamma-IFN and IL-2) for in vitro experiments may help us to get closer to the understanding of the role of NK cells in autoimmune thyroid diseases.

References

1. Wall, J.R., R. Baur, H. Schleusener, P. Bandy Dafoe: J. Clin. Endocrinol. Metab. **56** (1983), 164. - 2. Calder, E.A., W.J. Irvine, N.M. Davidson, F.Wu: Clin. Exp. Immunol. **25** (1976), 17. - 3. Iwatani, Y., N. Amino,, H. Mori, H. Tamaki, M. Aozasa, O. Kabutomori, M. Mori, O. Taniazawa, K. Miyai: J. Steroid Biochem. **20** (1984), 1641. - 4. White, D., D.B. Jones, , T. Cooke, N. Kirham: Br. J. Cancer **46** (1982), 611. - 5. Pross, H.F., J.A. Maroun: J. Immunol. Methods **68** (1984), 235. - 6. Milivoj Papic, Joan Stein-Streilein, Margita Zakarija, J. Maxwell McKenzie, Judy Guffee, Mary Ann Fletcher: J. Clin. Invest. **79** (1987), 404. - 7. Hiroshi Tezuka, Katsumi Eguchi, Takaaki Fukuda et al.: J. Clin. Endocrinol. Metab. **66** (1988), 702. - 8. Brieva, J.A., S. Targan, R.H. Stevens: J. Immunol. **132** (1984), 611. - 9. McLahlan, S.M., C.A.S. Pegg, M.C. Antherton et al.: Clin. Exp. Immunol. **65** (1986), 319. - 10. Joan Stein-Streilein, Margita Zakarija, Milivoj Papic, J. Maxwell McKenzie: J. Immunol. **139** (1987), 2502.

The influence of the calcium antagonist nitrendipine on thyroid hormone status in the baboon

J. Wieberneit, F.S. Keck, U. Loos, Ch.-F. Wolf
Department of Internal Medicine I, University of Ulm, Germany

Since 1963, when Douglas and Rubin /1/ developed the hypothesis of "stimulus-secretion coupling", which links an increase in intracellular free calcium concentration (Ca^{++}) with the endocrine secretion of some hormones, interest has focused on the mechanism of calcium-induced hormone release. The introduction of organic calcium antagonists (blockers of the slow Ca^{++}-channel) exerted a new tool for the evaluation of this process. In recent years there has been much interest in interactions between calcium antagonists and thyroid hormone homeostasis on both pituitary and thyroid level.

Several investigations using verapamil revealed an inhibitory effect on pituitary basal or TRH-stimulated TSH-release when given intravenously /2,3/, whereas oral administration was without any effect /4/. On the other hand, dihydropyridine-type calcium antagonists like nifedipine failed to show any changes in pituitary TSH-secretion /5,6/. Serum thyroid hormone concentrations were also unaltered by dihydropyridines /7/.

Beside the two regulatory levels in thyroid state homeostasis (pituitary and thyroid gland) it is well established, that the peripheral conversion of T_4 produces 70 % to 90 % of triiodothyronine (T_3), the metabolically active thyroid hormone. The liver is known to be the organ which contributes to a large extent to circulating T_3 (approx. 40 %) by outer ring deiodination (5'-DA) of the "prohormone" T_4 /8/. The aim of this study was to evaluate the influence of the calcium antagonist nitrendipine upon thyroid hormone serum levels and to compare these parameters with the simulataneously determined hepatic deiodination of thyroxine.

The lack of effect of dihydropyridines in therapeutical doses on thyroid hormone status in previous studies led us to speculate on physiological regulatory mechanisms, which could have overcome possible changes induced by these calcium antagonists. We therefore used the specific high affinity calcium antagonist nitrendipine in doses exceeding the usual therapeutical range in man considerably. The investigation was done in a primate model in order to keep species differences in thyroid hormone regulation to humans low.

Materials and methods

Serum concentrations of T_4, free T_4 (FT_4), T_3, free T_3 (FT_3), thyroxine binding globulin (TBG) and TSH as well as T_3-uptake were measured by luminescence immunoassays (Amersham Buchler Ltd., Braunschweig, Germany), serum concentration of rT_3 by radioimmunoassay (reverse T_3, Serono, Freiburg, Germany). For the evaluation of TBG and TSH conventional kits were used for reasons of convenience; our interest focused primarily on relative changes of these parameters due to the treatment rather than on absolute values.

Baboons (papio sp.) weighting 4.8 to 5.7 kg were allowed to get acquainted to experimental conditions for three weeks before the onset of the study. Nitrendipine in oral preparation was then administered daily for 3 months at the doses 24, 48 and 320 mg/kg bodyweight (N24; N48; N320) respectively. Experimental groups as well as the placebo treated control group (Control) consisted of 8 animals each (4 male and 4 female). In order to control for the integrity of 5'-DA regulation under calcium antagonists an additional group (N320+T_3) was treated simultaneously with high nitrendipine doses (320 mg/kg bodyweight) and T_3 (7.5 μg T_3/kg bodyweight i.m.). Blood samples as well as samples of bile were drawn at the end of the in vivo experiments and livers were rapidly excised on ice. Activity of hepatic 5'-deiodination was measured in the microsomal fraction in the presence of dithioerythritol 10 mM (DTE) as cofactor. Incubation was started by the addition of T_4 and terminated with ice-cold ethanol. Newly generated T_3 of rT_3 were detected radioimmunologically. Endogenous cofactors of 5'-DA represented by non protein-bound sulfhydryl groups (NP-SH) were measured according to the method of Sedlák and Lindsay /9/. Total iodide content of bile was determined with the catalytic-reaction method. Statistical evaluation was done using one-way-analysis of variance followed by Duncan's procedure. Linear regression analysis was done by the method of least squares. Results are given as mean ± SEM. The level of significance was put to a = 0.05.

Results

Serum concentrations of T_4 were lowered after three months of oral nitrendipine administration in the group with highest doses only (figure 1), whereas no change occurred in T_3 at all dosages investigated. Decreased T_4 levels were accompanied by an elevated basal TSH (figure 2). The determination of free thyroid hormone concentrations in serum (FT_4 and FT_3) as a term with closer relationship to the actual thyroid state revealed similar results as total iodothyronines (see table 1) with linear correlations to total iodothyronines ($r = 0.97$, $p < 0.001$ for T_4; $r = 0.80$, $p < 0.001$ for T_3). Parameters of iodothyronine binding in serum as TBG and T_3-uptake showed dose dependent reciprocal changes ($r = - 0.71$, $p < 0.001$) with an increase of TBG and a fall of T_3-uptake (see table 1). Commonly used free hormone equivalents as FT_4- or FT_3-index and T_4/TBG ratio gave comparable results (data not shown). Serum rT_3 dropped in group N320 exhibiting a parallelism to T_4 levels ($r = 0.80$, p ; 0.001). Total iodide content of bile was reduced dose dependently.

The highest nitrendipine dose applied revealed a stimulatory effect upon the activity of hepatic deiodination concerning newly generated T_3 out of T_4 (see figure 3); there was no newly synthesized rT_3 detectable in the ethanol-extracts (data not shown). The additional treatment with triiodothyronine (N320+T_3) resulted in a further increase of 5'-DA, which was significantly higher than both the control group and the exclusively nitrendipine treated group. Cytosolic NP-SH content increased vs. control in the N320 and in the N320+T_3 group, respectively, with the additional T_3 (N320+T_3) being significantly lowered ($p < 0.05$) vs. N320 (see table 1). Serum T_3/T_4 ratio in the nitrendipine treated animals showed a similar rise as 5'-DA, but gave poor correlation between both parameters ($r = 0.35$, p ; 0.05).

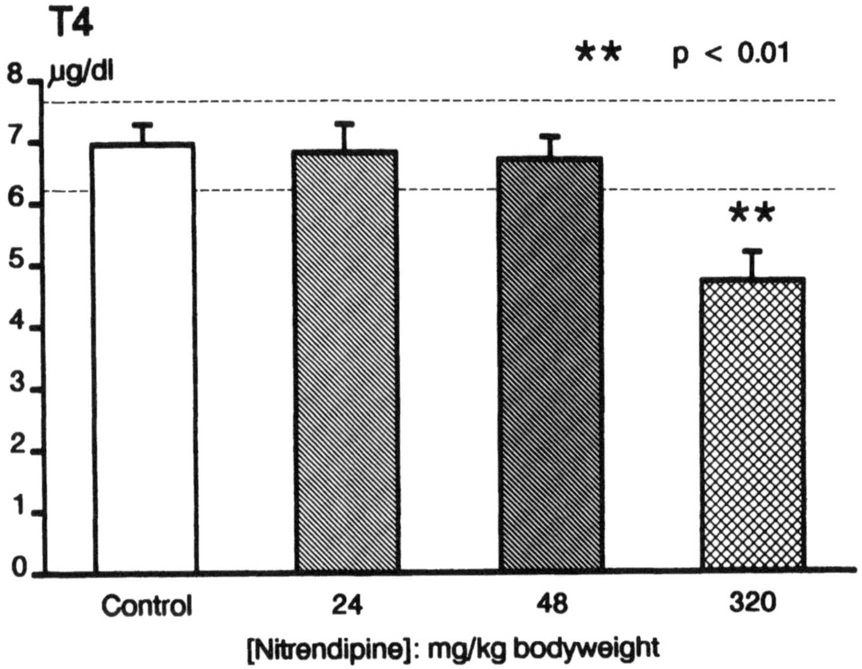

Figure 1

Serum levels of total T_4 under different doses of nitrendipine (for details see text); area between dashed lines: 95 % confidence interval of control group

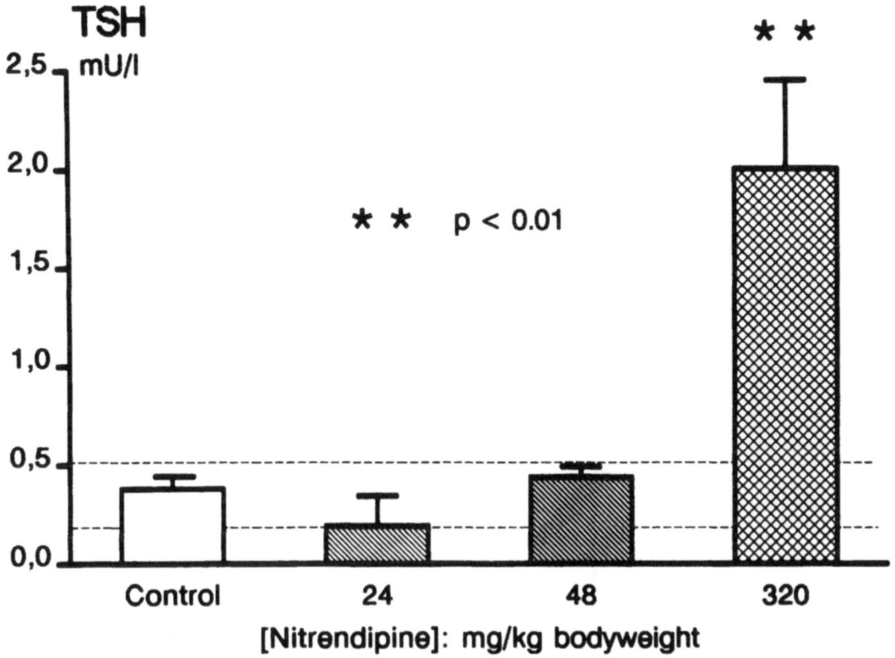

Figure 2

Serum levels of TSH under different doses of nitrendipine; area between dashed lines: 95 % confidence interval of control group

Table: Serum levels of thyroid-related parameters and cytosolic NP-SH content of liver under treatment with nitrendipine; $*p < 0.05$, $** p < 0.01$

	Control	N24	N48	N320
TT_3 (ng/dl)	149.3 $\pm$ 7.4	145.8 $\pm$ 5.8	141.5 $\pm$ 3.4	153.6 $\pm$ 5.8
FT_3 (pg/ml)	6.32 $\pm$ 0.42	6.05 $\pm$ 0.19	5.92 $\pm$ 0.93	5.94 $\pm$ 0.27
TT_4 (/ug/dl)	6.96 $\pm$ 0.34	6.83 $\pm$ 0.45	6.71 $\pm$ 0.38	4.74 $\pm$ 0.48**
FT_4 (ng/dl)	1.05 $\pm$ 0.05	0.91 $\pm$ 0.04	0.90 $\pm$ 0.06	0.57 $\pm$ 0.08**
rT_3 (ng/dl)	26.1 $\pm$ 1.2	26.4 $\pm$ 1.3	26.6 $\pm$ 1.4	21.2 $\pm$ 1.4 **
TSH (mU/l)	0.38 $\pm$ 0.05	0.35 $\pm$ 0.05	0.44 $\pm$ 0.05	2.01 $\pm$ 0.43**
T_3-Up (%)	31.9 $\pm$ 0.6	30.0 $\pm$ 0.8 *	29.3 $\pm$ 0.7 *	27.1 $\pm$ 0.5 **
TBG (mg/l)	1.12 $\pm$ 0.02	1.14 $\pm$ 0.02	1.20 $\pm$ 0.03*	1.30 $\pm$ 0.03**
NP-SH (/uM/g)	4.13 $\pm$ 0.29	4.54 $\pm$ 0.22	4.98 $\pm$ 0.32	6.38 $\pm$ 0.29**

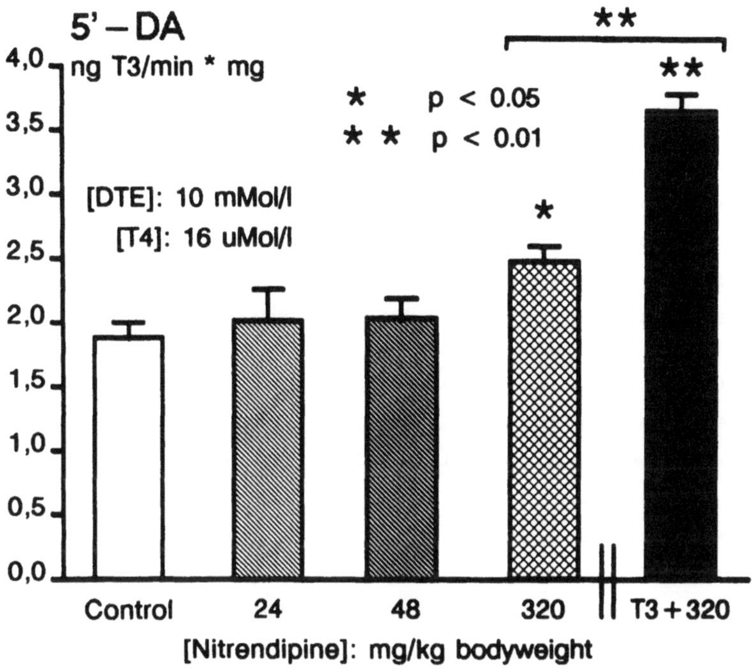

Figure 3

Activity of hepatic 5'-deiodinating activity (5'-DA) in vitro under increasing doses of nitrendipine and after high dose nitrendipine simultaneously given with T_3

Discussion

The results of this study demonstrate considerable alterations on several levels of thyroid hormone homeostasis mechanism under high doses of nitrendipide. The principle finding is a reduction of serum T_4 and rT_3 concentrations below normal control values (< 95 % confid. interval of controls) with unaltered T_3-, but elevated TSH levels, indicating a hypothyroid state. These results are in contradiction to earlier investigations with calcium antagonists, which lacked to show any effect on iodothyronines in serum /2-7/. In these studies much lower doses were employed, however. In addition our study revealed a stimulatory effect on hepatic 5'-deiodinating activity by nitrendipine.

The high correlation of free hormones with total hormone concentrations makes binding abnormalities of iodothyronines due to the nitrendipine treatment highly unlikely. However, an influence of nitrendipine on thyroid hormone binding proteins (TBG, T_3-uptake) can not be excluded. One possible explanation could be a unspecific stimulatory effect of nitrendipine on liver protein synthesis, that could have lead to the increase in 5'-DA as well. The rise in TSH is considered to be not directly induced by nitrendipine, but rather secondarily due to low serum T_4, since calcium antagonists are known to have an inhibitory impact on TSH secretion /2,3/. The decreased T_4 values point at an impairment of thyroid hormone secretion and/or synthesis under high doses of nitrendipine. Our data do not allow to exclude a concommittantly increased clearance rate of iodothyronines.

Normal T_3 serum levels in a state of reduced T_4 serum concentrations might reflect increased peripheral 5'-deiodination. Low rT_3 serum values fit well into this hypothesis since rT_3 derives by more than 95 % from peripheral deiodination and is at the same time the prefered substratum of type I deiodinase with a 500-fold higher affinity to the enzyme than T_4 /10/. From a teleological point of view it is tempting to speculate that the stimulation in 5'-DA counteracts the decreased T_4 secretion in order to maintain T_3 values normal. Previous studies on the influence of thyroid hormones upon hepatic deiodination revealed an opposite effect with decreased 5'-DA in hypothyroidism and a rise in hyperthyroidism /11,12/, however. Therefore the rise in 5'-DA must be ascribed to a direct effect of nitrendipine. The parallel course of NP-SH levels with 5'-DA reflects a sufficient amount of natural cofactor for increased in vivo deiodination.

The low correlation of serum T_4/T_4 ratio with hepatic 5'-DA gives evidence for possible other factors than peripheral deiodination in keeping T_3 levels in a normal range. T_3 levels might therefore reflect a relative increase in thyroidal T_3-secretion as compared to T_4, which is known to occur in hypothyroidism or due to enhanced TSH-levels /13/. This effect is partly ascribed to a stimulatory effect of TSH on 5'-DA (type I) in the thyroid itself and might have been further increased by the nitrendipine treatment.

In conclusion, these results demonstrate an inhibitory effect of high nitrendipine doses on serum T_4 levels, which can be assigned to an impairment of hormone release from the thyroid. While serum T_4 levels were low, T_3 levels were kept normal, which might be ascribed in part to an enhanced peripheral 5'-DA.

References

1. Douglas, W.W., R.P. Rubin: J. Physiol. (London) **167** (1963), 288. - 2. Geras, E., M.J. Rebecchi, M.C. Gershengorn: Endocrinology **110** (1982), 901. - 3. De Marinis, L., A. Mancini, S. Miniel-li, C. D'Amico, M.L. Di Pietro, C. Albini, M. Passeri, I. Liberale, E. Menini, A. Barbarino: Hormone Res. **25** (1987), 5. - 4. Semple, C.G., J.A. Thomson, G.H. Beastall, A.R. Lorimer: Brit. J. Clin. Pharmac. **17** (1984), 179. -5. Haitas, B., B.I. Joffe, D. Edelstein, V. Panz, J.M. Laprey, H.C. Seftel: J. Cardiovasc. Pharm. **8** (1986), 1284. - 6. Struthers, A.D., J.A. Millar, G.H. Beastall, W.B. Mcintosh, J.L. Reid: J. Clin. Endocrin. Metab. **56** (1983), 401. - 7. Lalau, J.D., E. Miteljan, S. Arlot, J.Quichaud: Horm. Metabol. Res. **19** (1987), 40. - 8. Distefano III,J.J. in: Georg Hennemann: Thyroid Hormone Metabolism (1986). - 9. Sedlak, J., R.H. Lindsay: Analyt. Biochem. **25** (1968), 192. - 10. Visser, T.J., D. Pekkes, R. Docter, G. Hennemann: Biochem. J. **179** (1979), 1740. - 11. Grussendorf, M., M. Hüfner: Clin. Chim. Acta **80** (1977), 61. -12. Keck, F.S., Chr.-F. Wolf,

E.F. Pfeiffer: Exp. Clin. Endocrinol. **96** (1990), 269. -
13. Laurberg, P.: Metabolism **33** (1984), 379.

Effect of thyroid hormones on lipoprotein (a) level in hypothyroidism

S. Oravec
Department of Internal Medicine, University Hospital, Bratislava, CSFR

Hypothyroidism belongs to the frequent causes of secondary hyperlipoproteinemia. The most significant alteration is the increase of Low Density Lipoprotein (LDL) in the lipoprotein spectrum accompanied at the same time by increased value of apolipoprotein B (Apo B) in serum.

An elevated concentration of lipoprotein (a) (Lp(a)), called also a sinking pre beta lipoprotein, seems to be a risk factor for coronary heart disease being independent from other risk factors of premature atherosclerosis development.

For the time being the role of Lp(a) in the development of coronary heart disease in hypothyroidism is not obvious, although it is known, that the patients with high LDL-concentration in serum can also have increased serum concentration of Lp(a) /1/.

The aim of my study was to analyse the effect of thyroid hormones substitution therapy on Lp(a) in the longitudinal study at the group of hypothyroid patients and to look for the answer to the question, whether thyroid hormones (thyroxine (T_4) and triiodothyronine (T_3)) decrease the Lp(a) concentration in serum and so by this mechanism brake the development of coronary heart disease, especially in hypothyroid patients.

Material and methods

Author has been observing a group including 12 hypothyroid patients (11 women and 1 man) at the average age of 48 years. This group embraced patients with spontaneous primary hypothyroidism, hypothyroidism after strumectomy and after radiotherapy of the toxical thyroid gland.

The diagnosis of hypothyroidism was determined on the basis of clinical features and laboratory examinations including T_4 and thyrotropin (TSH) analysis in serum.

These patients have been receiving the clinically optimal dosis of thyroid hormones (Thyreotom VEB Berlin-Chemie FRG, each tables contains levothyroxine 40 /ug and triiodothyronine 10 /ug).

After 12 hour fasting period blood before and every 2 months during hormones substitution was collected by puncture of the cubital vein, the serum was obtained and stored at -20° Celsius, up to the time of lipoproteins and hormones analysis.

The serum concentration of total cholesterol (TC), triglycerides (TG) (both Fa. Lachema, CSFR), Apo B / EIA method as reported in 1965 by Laurell /2/, Lp(a) (ELISA method Fa. Immuno AG, Austria), T_4 and TSH (both Fa. Imuna, CSFR), before and during substitution therapy has been observed.

For reference values of biochemical parameters, as a control group a group of 40 healthy volunteers at the age between 21 and 30 years without clinically manifested and biochemically demonstrable parameters of thyroid gland dysfunction was employed. The obtained results were statistically evaulated by Student t-test; by method of linear regression the equation of line in individual patients and in every observed parameters was calculated and 95 % confidence interval was stated /3/.

Results

"Do the observed parameters, especially Lp(a) show during the hormonal substitution therapy of hypothyroid patients the tendency of changing their serum concentration in time t?"

To answer this question we have been testing two hypotheses:
1. There are no changes in patient's condition after the hormones application with respect to the level of T_4 in serum.
2. Test of the 2nd hypothesis: Slope is zero; i.e. observed parameters show no tendency of increase or decrease of the concentration in serum ($b_1 = 0$) in time.

By testing the hypotheses it has been found:
1. The 1st and 2 nd hypothesis cannot be refused in group of 7 patients. In these so called non-responders, the concentration of T_4 remains unchanged, even after the substitution therapy

($Y_o = Y_t$), it varies around the regression line within the 95 % confidence interval and didn't show any alteration depending on time t, i.e $b_1 = 0$ (figure 1).

The same trend is being found with Lp(a) as well with other observed parameters TC, TG, Apo B. Their serum concentration doesn't change in the time t, but varies around the regression line, its $b_1 = 0$ (table 1).

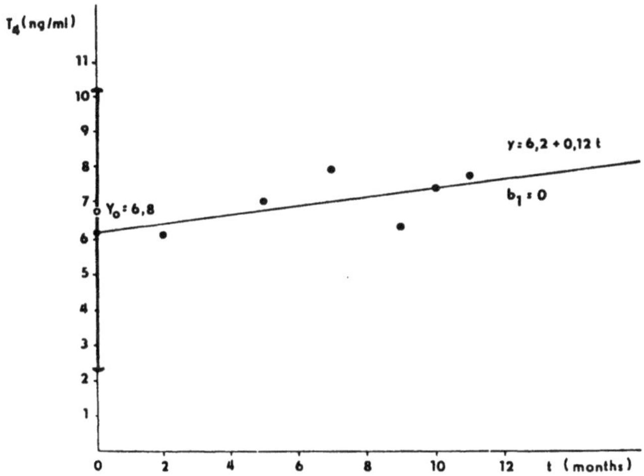

Figure 1
Regression line of T_4 at the "responder" group

Table 1: Biochemical parameters at the "non responder" group n = 7

	T_4 (ng/ml)	TSH (µU/ml)	TC (mmol/l)	TG (mmol/l)
0.M.	13,2±11,4	106,4±45,7	8,2±2,7	2,8±1,6
4.M.	12,8±7,5	76,1±53,7	7,7±2,8	2,4±1,1
8.M.	22,1±13,5	63,9±55,9	6,2±1,1	2,0±1,0

	Apo B (mg/dl)	Lp(a) (mg/dl)
0.M.	100,8±29,8	6,3±6,1
4 M.	107,1±29,4	6,4±4,6
8.M.	93,7±25,0	7,0±4,0

Legend

T_4	Thyroxine
TSH	Thyreotropin
TC	Total cholesterol
TG	Triglyceride
Apo B	Apolipoprotein B
Lp(a)	Lipoprotein (a)

2. In another group of patients with hypothyroidism ($n = 5$) in so called responders, during hormonal substitution the concentration of T_4 - compared with its value in time $t = 0$ - increase significantly ($p < 0.01$). The value of T_4 before the hormonal treatment (Y_o) appears outside of the confidence interval and acquires its new steady state ($Y_o = Y_t$) (figure 2).

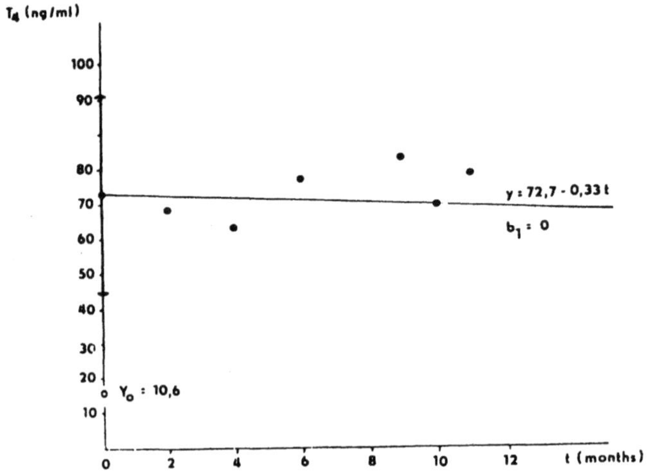

Figure 2
Regression line of T_4 at the "responder" group

Lp(a) being analysed, one cannot refuse the hypothesis 1st and 2nd. The concentration of Lp(a) during the therapy remains unchanged ($Y_o = Y_t$) and varies around the regression line with $b_1 = 0$. The behaviour of some further parameters Tc, TG, Apo B can be valuated in a similar way, although the tendency of decrease of TC and Apo B concentration in time can be observed. However, testing did not prove significance of this decrease ($p > 0.05$) (table 2).

3. In the group of non responders the low Lp(a) concentration before starting the substitution therapy were found 15 mg/dl. On the other hand, in the group of responders the value of Lp(a) in serum have been varying and reached about 30 mg/dl.

Table 2: Biochemical parameters at the "responders" group n = 5

	T_4 (ng/ml)	TSH (µU/ml)	TC (mmol/l)	TG (mmol/l)
0.M.	8,18 ± 1,7	102,2 ± 31,1	8,3 ± 3,1	1,7 ± 1,1
	p < 0,01			
4.M.	62,9 ± 5,2	50,0 ± 22,4	6,2 ± 0,8	1,8 ± 1,0
		p < 0,05		
8.M.	95,4 ± 40,3	2,6 ± 2,9	5,3 ± 1,1	2,2 ± 1,8

	Apo B (mg/dl)	Lp(a) (mg/dl)
0.M.	109,0 ± 29,4	28,4 ± 10,8
4.M.	100,3 ± 14,8	28,3 ± 15,8
8.M.	84,3 ± 26,1	37,9 ± 19,9

Legend

T_4	Thyroxine
TSH	Thyreotropin
TC	Total cholesterol
TG	Triglyceride
Apo B	Apolipoprotein B
Lp(a)	Lipoprotein (a)

Discussion

Lp(a) is one of the risk factor of coronary sclerosis development, independent from other risk factors /1,4-7/. In hypothyroidism increased values of TC, Apo B and LDL were observed /8/, all of them being risk factors connected with the development of serious coronary sclerosis. Up to day the role of T_4 deficiency in Lp(a) metabolism in hypothyroidism is not explained, although it is known, that the patients with the increased LDL concentration, especially in hypothyroidism can at the same time have the increased concentration of Lp(a) in serum /1/. The treatment with thyroid hormones decreases the TC, Apo B and LDL level and their decrease in serum is one of the signs of the succesful therapy /9/. The question: does the therapy with thyroid hormones influence or decrease the concentration of Lp(a) in serum becomes a topical one. Because of physical and chemical characteristics shared equally by Lp(a) and LDL, Lp(a) was supposed to be eventually the genetic variation of LDL /10/. An positive answer would mean the possibility to influence the concentration of Lp(a) in serum as the risk factor, which especially when combined with higher Apo B concentration increases the risk factor of coronary attack up to 5 times /11/.

From this study it follows, that the concentration of Lp(a) doesn't change during the treatment with thyroid hormones and T_4 doesn't influence the serum level of Lp(a) in patients with hypothyroidism. We did not succeed in proving the significance of TC and Apo B decrease in serum, although this tendency in time t can be stated.

But rather interesting is the low Lp(a) concentration in non responders and increased values of Lp(a) in responders already before the treatment. Thus Lp(a) could fulfil the function of an index whether the substitution therapy with thyroid hormones will bring a long a real therapeutic effect in patients with hypothyroidism and will positively influence the level of coronary sclerosis risk factors, such as LDL, Apo B and TC.

Reference values

Total cholesterol	(mmol/l)	(TC)	5.8 ± 1.0
Triglyceride	(mmol/l)	(TG)	1.4 ± 0.6
Apolipoprotein B	(mg/dl)	(Apo B)	74.0 ± 20.0
Lipoprotein (a)	(mg/dl)	(Lp(a))	20.0 ± 5.5
Thyroxine	(μg/ml)	(T_4)	106.0 ± 42.0
Thyreotropin	(μU/ml)	(TSH)	2.75 ± 2.25

Acknowledgement

I would like to express my gratitude for the generous help in my study to Dr. Langer Dr.Sc., Dr. Štrbák Dr.Sc., Dr. Wimmer CSc. from Slovak Academy of Sciences CSFR, as well as to Dr. Dieplinger OhD from Institute of Biology and Human Genetic Innsbruck, Austria.

References

1. Kostner, G.M., P. Avogaro, G. Cazzolate, E. Marth, G. Ben Bittolo, G.B. Qunici: Atherosclerosis **38** (1981), 51. - 2. Laurell, C.B.: Analyt. Biochem. **15** (1965), 45. - 3. Snedecer, G.W.: Statistical methods 5th ed., Iowa State college Press, Ames Iowa, 1965. -4. Armstrong, V.W., P. Cremer, P. Eberle, A. Manke, F. Schulze, H. Wieland, H. Kreuzer, D. Seidel: Atherosclerosis **62** (1986), 249. -5. Dahlen, G., J.R. Guyton,

M. Attar, J.A. Faemer, J.A. Kautz, A.M. Gotto Jr.: Circulation **74** (1986), 758. - 6. Rhoads, G.G., G. Dahlen, K. Berg, N.E. Horten, A.L. Danneberg: JAMA **256** (1986), 2540. - 7. Krempler, F.: Berichte der OGKC **10** (1987), 17. - 8. Dori, L., P.S. Roheim: J. Lipid Res. **22** (1981), 287. - 9. Schwandt, P., P. Weisweiler: Atherosclerosis **35** (1980), 301. - 10. Kostner, G.M.: In: Low Density Lipoproteins eds.: Ch.E. Day and R.S. Levy, Plenum Press (1976), 229. - 11. Molinari, E., P. Pichler, A. Philapitsch, H. Aicher, S. Pfeiler, J. Schuster: Die Ellipse 1989, **18** (1989), 229.

Discussion

Leövey: How does thyroid hormones (T_4) act on the serum cholesterol level, especially in hyperthyroidism?

Oravec: T_4 accelerates the synthesis of cholesterol and its degradation by BE-receptors in liver and in the peripheral tissues too as well. As the degradation ratio of cholesterol is higher than in its synthesis, the endeffect of T_4 on cholesterol is lowering its concentration in serum.

The main part of serum cholesterol is localized in LDL (transport of endogenous cholesterol), which degradation is performed by BE-receptors, predominantly in liver. As the T_4 increases the synthesis of BD-receptors, under T_4-deficiency condition (hypothyroidism) the amount of BE-receptors is significantly reduced, the LDL degradation by this way damaged and higher LDL-cholesterol concentration in serum persists.

THYROIDITIS

Thyrotoxicosis due to thyroiditis

A. Leövey
1st Department of Internal Medicine, University Medical School, Debrecen, Hungary

Thyrotoxicosis associated with an inflammatory, destructive process in the gland has become recognized in recent years as an important entity. This category of thyrotoxicosis includes subacute thyroiditis, silent (or painless) thyroiditis, postpartum and Hashimoto's thyroiditis. The features that are common to all four types are a transient, spontaneously resolving phase of thyrotoxicosis. The pathophysiologic mechanism of the thyrotoxicosis is the release of preformed hormone from an inflamed thyroid gland.

Subacute thyroiditis, also termed granulomatous thyroiditis or de Quervain's disease, presents typically with abrupt onset of severe pain in the thyroid region (often referred to the jaws), fever, and malaise (figure 1).

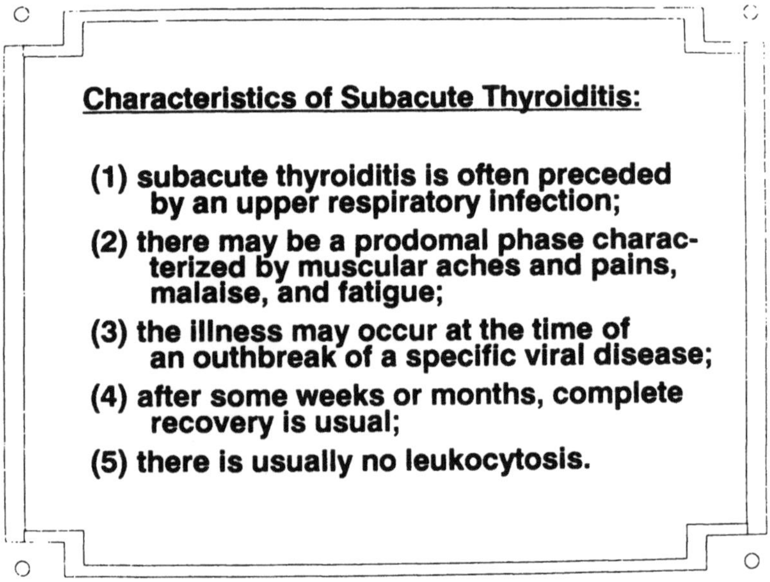

Figure 1

Examination shows exquisite tenderness of the gland, which may be only slightly enlarged or normal in size. Most of the patients also have signs and symptoms of mild thyrotoxicosis. The erythrocyte sedimentation rate (ESR) is elevated in nearly all cases, often to very high values, but the leukocyte count is usually normal. The serum T_4 and T_3 concentrations are elevated as is the serum thyroglobulin level, and the TSH level is suppressed. The RAI uptake is invariably low, usually near zero, during the thyrotoxic phase, and this finding is very helpful in making the diagnosis. Antithyroid antibodies are usually not detectable or, if present, are low in titer. Biopsy of the gland shows extensive follicular destruction and a granulomatous infiltrate with characteristic giant cells ingesting colloid /14/.

The disorder is self-limited, running its course over a period of 2 to 5 months. The initial thyrotoxic phase may be followed by a period of hypothyroidism, but eventual recovery is complete and recurrences are unusual.

Management in the initial phase is directed at the local inflammation and pain, using salicylates or nonsteroidal anti-inflammatory drugs and a betablocking agent to ameliorate the thyrotoxicosis. In severe cases unresponsive to salicylates, corticosteroids may be neccessary to control the local inflammatory process. The RAI uptake may be used to monitor recovery of glandular function during such therapy, so as to avoid relapse due to inadequate duration of treatment.

There is indirect evidence that subacute thyroiditis is caused by a viral infection of the thyroid /14/, but an underlying genetic susceptibility is suggested by a female-male ratio as high as 6:1 and in association with HLA-Bw35 /6/.

<u>Silent (Painless) Thyroiditis:</u> More properly termed subacute lymphocytic thyroiditis /6/, this is characterized by clinical manifestations of thyrotoxicosis, usually mild in degree, which goes on to spontaneous recovery (sometimes with a temporary hypothyroid phase). The gland may be enlarged or normal in size, but as the name implies it is not painful or tender. The diagnosis rests on finding laboratory evidence of thyrotoxicosis and a

low RAI uptake that is not accounted for by excess iodine intake or thyroid hormone administration. In contrast to subacute granulomatous thyroiditis, the ESR is normal or only slightly elevated. Antithyroid antibodies (antimicrosomal) are positive in 10 % to 50 %, but antibody titers are only mildly to moderately elevated. Thyroid stimulating immunoglobulin is not present. Thyroid biopsy shows follicular disruption and dense infiltration with lymphocytes, but no giant cells (as in subacute thyroiditis). Most patients recover without sequelae, but a minority show evidence of a chronic thyroiditis with goiter, rising antibody levels, and even hypothyroidism /18/. The continued presence of antimicrosomal antibodies in the serum during recovery from the thyrotoxic phase of this disease appears to predict eventual hypothyroidism /19/.

Postpartum Thyroiditis: Soon after the original descriptions of atypical or silent thyroiditis /4,5,12,17/, it became apparent that many of these patients were postpartum (figure 2). Since then, surveys of women in the postpartum period have revealed a high incidence of thyroid dysfunction /1,9,11,15/. The manifestation run the variation from frank thyrotoxicosis to hypothyroidism; often both occur at different times in the same patient. From 2 % to 3 % of all postpartum women show clinical and biochemical evidence of thyrotoxicosis during the first 2 to 3 months following delivery. Typically, the thyrotoxic period is short and resolves spontaneously within 2 to 3 months, being followed by hypothyroidism and then recovery and euthyroidism. A goiter may persist, and recurrences are not unusual following subsequent pregnancies.

The diagnosis may be missed entirely if not suspected; the thyroid is minimally enlarged or normal to palpation, and symptoms of mild thyrotoxicosis or hypothyroidism may be dismissed as the "tired mother syndrome".

The laboratory findings are the same as those of silent thyroiditis, except that antithyroid antibodies are positive more often in the postpartum cases. The differential diagnosis includes Graves' disease (presumably triggered by the immunologic reactivation following pregnancy), thyrotoxicosis factitia, and iodine-

Characteristics of transient postpartum thyrotoxicosis due to painless thyroiditis

(1) Thyrotoxicosis (often abrupt onset and short duration)

(2) Low thyroid uptake of iodine

(3) Thyroidal pain and tenderness absent

(4) Lymphocytic thyroiditis in fine-needle biopsy

(5) Thyroid microsomal autoantibodies often present (and may persist after recovery)

(6) Subsequent hypothyroid phase develops in less than 50%

Figure 2

induced thyrotoxicosis. Management is symptomatic, using beta-blocking agents for the thyrotoxic phase, if necessary, and thyroid hormone for the hypothyroid phase.

An autoimmune pathogenesis is strongly suggested by the presence of antithyroid antibodies in more than half the cases, the histologic picture in the gland, a strong family history of thyroid disease, and an association with HLA-B8 and B-35 in whites of North America. An association with other HLA haplotypes has been found in other ethnic groups /15/.

It is reasonable to postulate that an underlying defect in immunity may predispose some individuals to one or another form of thyroiditis. In fact patients have been described in whom subacute or silent thyroiditis and Graves' disease occurred sequentially /16/. In another instance, a patient with a history of Graves' hyperthyroidism had an episode of typical postpartum thyroiditis /2/.

Hyperthyroidism in Chronic Lymphocytic Thyroiditis: Hashimoto' thyroiditis is a common thyroid problem that may affect up to 2 per cent of the population, 95 per cent of whom are women. It can present with hyperthyroidism, or as a euthyroid goiter. There is universal agreement that it is an autoimmune disorder and that it is associated with a high incidence of other autoimmune diseases. There is an increased prevalence of HLA-D5, and although uncommon there is an increased predilection for the development of a primary thyroid lymphoma. The thyroid gland is universally enlarged and usually quite firm. Occasionally it is rock-hard, suggestive of a thyroid neoplasm. Although the enlargement is generally diffuse, it can be asymmetric or nodular. Thyroidal pain is distinctly uncommon, but symptoms of pressure and dysphagia may be present. The hallmark of the disease is the presence of antithyroglobulin and antimicrosomal antibodies, which if present in high titers are pathognomonic. Thyroid hormone levels may be normal, low, or high, depending upon the degree of thyroid destruction. Despite normal T_4 and T_3 levels, TSH may be mildly elevated or the TSH response to TSH exaggerated, indicating the presence of compensated hypothyroidism. In patients who are euthyroid at the time of presentation, the development of overt hypothyroidism is uncommon. Only 3 of 52 patients became hypothyroid over 14 years in one series /7/, while there was an incidence of 2 per cent per year in another among patients who had both thyroid antibodies and an elevated TSH /13/. An abnormal response to perchlorate in some patients indicates the presence of an underlying organification defect. The thyroid scan classically shows as "salt and pepper" pattern. Histologic examination of the thyroid reveals destruction of the follicles, infiltration of the gland with lymphocytes which may form germinal centers, epithelial enlargement with oxyphilic cytoplasmic changes (Hurthle-Ashkanazy cells) and dense fibrosis. There is no effective, safe treatment for the chronic inflammation.

Whereas most patients with Hashimoto's disease are either euthyroid or hypothyroid, occasionally mild hyperthyroidism may be encountered early in the course of the disease /6/. In such patients the disorder may be indistinguishable from Graves' disease, with ophthalmopathy and positive TSab in some cases (figure 3). Indeed, the two conditions are probably expressions of the same underlying autoimmune disorder. In contrast to destructive types of thyroiditis with thyrotoxicosis, however, the thyrotoxicosis of Hashimoto's disease ("Hashitoxicosis") is characterized by an elevated or high-normal RAI uptake. This finding, the clinical picture, and very high titers of antimicrosomal and/or antithyroglobulin antibodies usually point to the diagnosis.

Hashimoto's thyroiditis may be associated with unusual manifestations:

1. A transient phase of hyperthyroidism (Hashitoxicosis), which rapidly evolves into permanent hypothyroidism.
2. Infiltrative ophthalmopathy identical to that seen with Graves' disease.
3. Focal thyroiditis resulting in a palpable nodule that appears cold on scan.
4. The fibrous variant, which may present as a firm or hard thyroid lump.

Figure 3

According to present knowledge, both B-G disease and Hashimoto's thyroiditis are attributed to an autoimmune process /8,10/. It seemed, therefore, of interest for us to examine the incidence of the association of the two processes. The behaviour of the thyroid membran-receptor antibodies (MRab) in this association was regarded as a question of particular importance. For this reason fine needle biopsy of the thyroid gland was performed in such 170 patients with B-G disease in which the clinical features or laboratory findings (microsomal, thyroglobulin antibodies, ESR) were compatible with the possibility of CLT. The microscopic findings proved positive for CLT in 93 (54.7 %) of 170 patients subjected to biopsy.

Typical microscopic features, as well as antibody-positivity were found in a total of 48 cases. These patients were corresponded to Hashimoto's thyroiditis, and from these 39 were in a period of activity at the time of study, showing the criteria of Hashitoxicosis (figure 4). In the latter cases the membrane-receptor assay (MRA) was in 77.1 % and the cAMP assay in 56.2 % positive. This seems to suggest that Hashitoxicosis may well be associated, in addition to the traditional antibodies, with thyroid-receptor antibodies, which implies that "blocking" (TBII), and 'stimulating", i.e. functional, mechanisms may operate side by side in the same patient and at the same time (figure 5). This might be one of the immunopathogenetic features of Hashitoxicosis.

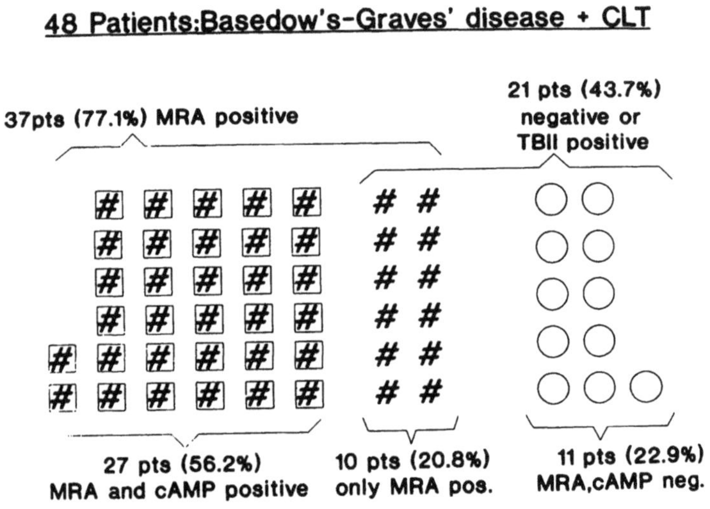

Figure 4

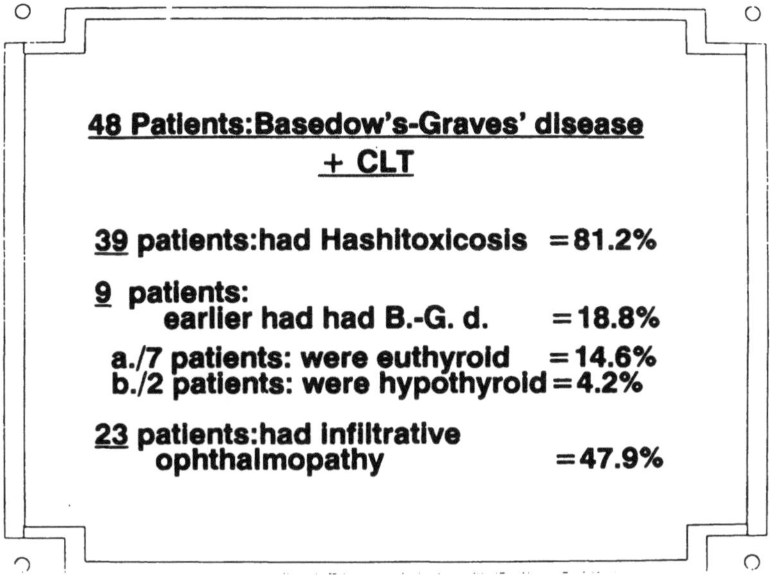

Figure 5

Infiltrative ophthalmopathy was present in 23 patients so that its frequency was higher in our study than in B-G disease (47.9 % vs. 38 %).

The features of CLT showed a considerably higher incidence in females than in males. The typical prevalance of B-G disease was even more marked when the condition was associated with CLT. The female-to male ratio, 3.6:1 for the total patient material, was 15:1 for CLT. Such increase in the female-male ratio presumably is a result of a genetic linkage to the chromosome X or a connection with the endocrine environment.

On the basis of our observations we may suppose that Hashimoto's thyroiditis joins B-G disease far more often than any other disease. Multiple associations of different immune processes are frequent but the association of CLT with B-G disease is of particular interest as in this instance a single organ would provide the site for two different clinical conditions. It is presumed that Hashitoxicosis represents an unique instance in which B-G disease and Hashimoto's cohabit the same gland, but the eventual dominance of the latter results in permanent hypothyroidism.

The pathogenetic background of this constellation is obscure.

References

1. Amino, N.: N. Engl. J. Med. **306** (1982), 849. - 2. Eckel, R.H.: JAMA **243** (1980), 1454. - 3. Fischer, D.A. In: The Thyroid. Eds.: Hershman, JM., Bray, GA, pp. 487-500, Pergamon Press, Oxford - New York - Frankfurt (1979). - 4. Gluck, F.B.: N. Engl. J. Med. **293** (1975), 624. - 5. Hamburger J.L.: J. Nucl. Med. **15** (1974), 81. - 6. Hay, I.D.: Mayo Clin. Proc. **60** (1985), 836. - 7.Khangure, M.S.: Clin. Endocrinol. **6** (1977), 41. - 8. Kidd, A.: Metabolism **29** (1980), 80. - 9. Lervang, H.H.: Acta Med. Scand. **222** (1987), 368. - 10. Mori, T.: J. Clin. Endocr. **33** (1971), 688. - 11. Nikolai, T.F.: Arch. Intern. Med. **147** (1987), 221. - 12. Pappetrou, P.D.: Lancet **1** (1975), 361. - 13. Turnbridge, W.M.G.: Clin. Endocrinol. Metab. **8** (1979), 21. - 14. Volpe, R.: Pharmacol. Ther. C. **1** (1976), 171. - 15. Walfish, P.G.: Clin. Endocrinol. Metab. **14** (1985), 417. - 16. Wartofsky, L.: Am. J. Med. **83** (1987), 761. - 17. Woolf, P.D.: Am. J. Med. **60** (1976), 73. - 18. Woolf, P.D.: Endocrine Rev. **1** (1980), 411. - 19. Yamamato, M.: Endocrinol. Jpn. **34** (1986), 357.

Discussion

Knappe: May I ask you, whether you see post partum thyroiditis very often or can you say anything about the incidence of post partum thyroiditis?

Leövey: The incidence of post partum thyroiditis varies from two to three percent. It means, that every post partum woman can get this. But in the majority of the cases this transient form of thyrotoxicosis is very mild; therefore they generally missed the diagnosis. I suppose that they diagnose that thyrotoxicosis only if the patients have clinical symptoms of thyrotoxicosis. It is necessary to screen all post partum women by antithyroglobulin antibodies to examine the exact incidence of this disease.

Thyroiditis - a histopathological review

H.G. Peschel
I. Institute of Pathology, Klinikum Berlin-Buch, Berlin, Germany

Inflammatory changes and diseases of the thyroid gland are acute, subacute or chronic. They are caused by infectious organisms, represent accompanying reactions of other lesions or are of immunological origin. The organ is involved diffuse or focally.

1. Acute thyroiditis, usually of infectious nature, is often associated with infections of the upper respiratory tract. The most common organisms are Streptococcus hemolyticus, Staphylococcus aureus and Pneumococcus. Other forms are caused by traumas, radiation or tumour necrosis. They don't play any role in biopsy investigations.

2. Subacute granulomatous thyroiditis, described by de Quervain in 1936 /12/, is thought to be of viral origin. The process involves the whole organ in different intensity so that the enlargement is often asymmetric. Usually there is no adherence to the surrounding tissue. Typical cases present pain or marked sensitivity of the gland, about 40 % show a painless course. Histologically granulomatous pseudotubercular arrangements are found consisting of histiocytes and foreign body giant cells around destroyed follicular epithelium and degenerated colloid. In the development of the inflammatory process, initially there is an alteration of the follicular epithelium with desquamation and degeneration, followed by colloid depletion and a cellular response of polymorphonuclear leucocytes. In its progression lymphocytes, plasma cells and histiocytes become the major component of the inflammatory response. Follicular epithelium disappears and is replaced by palisading histiocytes and giant cells, which we usually detect in biopsies. Subsequently fibrosis occurs in interfollicular areas, finally regeneration of the follicles, so that complete histological recovery takes place. Focal fibrosis will still remain (Woolner et al. /14/).

3. <u>Other granulomatous inflammations</u> are caused by tuberculosis via hematogen spread, Mycosis or Syphilis in its tertiary phase. Sarcoidosis may also involve the gland. These lesions seldom occur in biopsies, but in patients who died of miliary tuberculosis, the thyroid gland has to be carefully investigated for its involvement in the specific inflammatory process. Multifocal granulomatous thyroiditis is a histological finding rather than a true lesion of the thyroid. It probably represents a response to minor trauma. It is found in surgically resected thyroids and is believed to be the result of rupture of follicles caused by palpation of the gland. Therefore it is referred to as "palpation thyroiditis". The term was coined by Carney et al. in 1975 /2/. The involved follicles show partial loss of the epithelium and are replaced by inflammatory cells, predominantly macrophages, but also lymphocytes, plasma cells and a few multinucleated giant cells. Only the palpated lobe contains this lesion, as has been disclosed in experiments, so that other factors, which would effect both thyroid lobes, could be eleminated. The histological changes regress spontaneously.

4. The classification schemes of chronic thyroiditis are numerous. <u>Hashimoto's disease</u> /6/, also known as autoimmune thyroiditis and struma lymphomatosa, is a chronic thyroiditis of immunological origin. Both lobes are enlarged symmetrically showing firm consistency, in some cases with a distinct multinodular pattern. There is no extension beyond the gland.
Histologically the stroma contains numerous lymphocytes, arranged in follicles with large germinal centers. Plasma cells and histiocytes are usually present. Occasionally multinucleated giant cells can be seen (Knecht et al. /8/).
The thyroid follicles are small and atrophic. Colloid may be absent or developed focally. Characteristically, oxyphilic metaplasia is found with abundant pink granular cytoplasm. These follicular cells, variously called oxyphils, oncocytes, Askanazy or Hürthle cells, frequently contain large nuclei with prominent nucleoli. Usually connective tissue is scarce, but in the fibrous variant keloid-like fibrosis is more extensive. The architecture of the thyroid is destroyed

displaying severe follicular atrophy. Included islands of epithelium often show squamous metaplasia.
Ultrastructurally, the epithelial cells can be derived into three types (Bastenie and Ermans /1/):

a) Hyperplastic cells with well developed Golgi complex, normal mitochondria, dilatated endoplasmatic reticulum and increased numbers of large mitochondria.

b) Oncocytes (oxyphilic cells) with poorly developed Golgi complex, decreased endoplasmatic reticulum and increased numbers of large mitochondria.

c) Colloid cells with large homogenous areas.

The cellular infiltrates are mainly transformed B lymphocytes, plasma cells and immunoblasts. Follicular basement membrane deposits have been found, which are identified as immunoglobulins and complement (Kalderon et al. /7/). The ratio of B to T lymphocytes is elevated. T lymphocytes are predominantly of suppressor type which demonstrate cytological activity in vitro /3/. The main failure of the disease seems to be an organspecific defect in suppressor T lymphocytes. Circulating antibodies against thyroglobulin and other follicular cell antigen exist in Hashimoto's thyroiditis, in a milder form also in other thyroid diseases with lymphocytic infiltration, especially in Graves' disease and toxic nodular goitre. But plasma cells are rare in toxic goitre, fibrosis is unusual. Oxyphilic metaplasia occurs only of the disorder is of long standing. So there are some histological differences. Nevertheless these lymphocytic infiltrations reveal the relationship between Hashimoto's and Graves' disease as the two ends of the spectrum of autoimmunothyroid lesions (LiVolsi /10/) with a transition stage sharing features of both disorders so-called Hashitoxicosis.
Lymphoma-like thyroiditis is a variant of Hashimoto's disease (Woolner et al /15/) with a dense lymphocytic infiltrate which mimics malignant lymphoma. The presence of thyroid follicles, the pleomorphic cell population with various types of lymphocytes, and the rather frequent plasma cell are helpful in distinguishing this process from true lymphoma of Non Hodgkin's

type, which is usually of B cell origin. The two actually occur side by side. Immunohistochemical investigations elucidate whether the cell population is of polyclonal inflammatory or of monoclonal neoplastic nature. We had to register an over-diagnosis of such a lesion in our biopsies. Further complications are papillary and oncocytic carcinoma. All these disorders evolve from a setting of hyperplasia of the respective cell component in Hashimoto's disease. In our surgical biopsies struma lymphomatosa has been decreasing in the recent years, obviously due to improved diagnostics and nonsurgical therapy (table 1).

Table 1: Hashimoto's thyroiditis in biopsies.
Period 1. 1. 86 to 31. 12. 90.
I. Institute of Pathology Klinikum Berlin-Buch

Years	Biopsies	Hashimoto's thyroiditis	Per cent	with Ca, NHL
1986	885	14	1.6	-
1987	981	16	1.6	1
1988	932	22	2.4	3
1989	856	8	0.9	-
1990	857	7	0.8	-
Total	4511	67	1.5	4

5. The so-called juvenile variant of lymphocytic thyroiditis is a common cause of asymptomatic goitre in children and adolescents. Grossly, there is diffuse enlargement of the gland with increased consistency. Microscopically, an extensive lymphocytic infiltration is obvious, germinal centers often being present. Contrary to the classical Hashimoto's disease, follicular atrophy and oxyphilic metaplasia are usually absent, but the similarity of the histological changes to the so-called Hashitoxicosis or hyperthyroiditis with transient hyperthyroidism is remarkable /4/.

6. Focal nonspecific thyroiditis is seen in older patients without special symptoms, in nodular hyperplasia and adenomatous goitre, in the surrounding tissue of thyroid cancer, especially papillary carcinoma, and in other lesions. Focal aggregates of lymphocytes with a formation of germinal centers are detected. Adenomas are usually spared. The incidence is about 20 percent with a female predominance /9/. The ratio has been increased since the addition of iodide to the water supplies /5/.

7. Riedel's thyroiditis, the so-called iron-hard struma /13/, also known as invasive fibrous thyroiditis, is a very rare disease that can simulate malignant tumour clinically because of the asymmetric firmness and of the tendency to invade both thyroid and perithyroid tissue. The thyroid follicles are destroyed and replaced by a dense fibrosis and an inflammatory infiltrate associated with an occlusive phlebitis /11/. Biopsy is necessary to establish the definitive diagnosis.

References

1. Bastenie, P.A., A.M. Ermans: Oxford, Pergamon Press 1972. - 2. Carney, J.A., S.B. Moore et al.: Am. J. Clin. Pathol. **64** (1975), 639. - 3. DelPrete, G.F., E. Maggi et al.: J. Clin. Endocrinol. Metab. **62** (1986), 52. - 4. Fatourechi, V., W.M. McConahey, L.B. Woolner: Mayo Clin. Proc. **46** (1971), 682. - 5. Harries, M., M.K. Palmer: J. Pathol. **110** (1980), 309. - 6. Hashimoto, H.: Arch. Klin. Chir. **97** (1912), 219. -7. Kalderon, A.E., H.A. Bogaars, I. Diamond: A. J. Med. **55** (1973), 485. - 8. Knecht, H., C.E. Hedinger: Histopathology **6** (1982), 511. - 9. Kurashima, C., k. Hirokawa: Survey Synth. Pathol. Res. **4** (1985), 457. - 10. LiVolsi, V.A.: Volume 22 in the Series Major Problems in Pathology, W.B. Saunders Company 1990. - 11. Mayer, S., R. Hausman: Am. J. Clin. Pathol. **65** (1976), 274. - 12. de Quervain, F., G. Giordanengo: Mitt. Grenzgeb. Med. Chir. **44** (1936), 538. -13. Riedel, H.:Die chronische, zur Bildung eisenharter Tumoren führende Entzündung der Schilddrüse. Verh. Dt. Ges. Chir. **225** (1986), 101. - 14. Woolner, L.B., W.M. McConahey, O.H. Beahrs: J. Clin. Endocrinol. Metab. **17** (1957), 1202. - 15. Woolner, L.B., W.M. McConahey, O.H. Beahrs:

J. Clin. Endocrinol. Metab. **19** (1959), 53.

Discussion

Leövey: In how many cases did you see patients with Hashimoto's thyroiditis together with lymphoma? In earlier times it was written that this association is relatively common. But later they say, it is very rare..

Peschel: I think its a rare incidence, but in former times we had detected more forms of true lymphoma of non-Hodgkin type. But in the last years only one case per year we could detect. And today it is the question: is it a primary thyroid lymphoma or is it an involvement of an organ by a nodular lymphoma of the lymphnodes in the primary development.

Deckart: How many cases do you remember in your institute where Hashimoto's thyroiditis is transverted into malignant lymphoma? I think it is very difficult to observe these situations in the clinical case. We just observe such a case and we have to do a "criminalistic" analysis.

Peschel: Usually we register the malignant lymphoma and we detect in the surrounding non neoplastic infiltrated tissue (the lymphocytic infiltration of probably Hashimoto's thyroiditis). When you find oxyphilic metaplasia you can say, this is a development in such lesion, but on the other hand you must say that you can have focal lymphocytic thyroiditis in the surrounding tissue of a malignant lymphoma. That must not be the classical type of Hashimoto's disease. And if you have follow-up investigations it might be more clear. In the last 15 years we detected 10 to 12 malignant lymphoma which had primary developed in thyroid gland.

Weiss: On the one slide you had the postulation that the Hashimoto's thyroiditis is a prelymphoma, but I see there is a lot of literature mainly in the United States (a study of the Armed Forces Hospital) where was shown that in case of Hashimoto's thyroiditis is no higher rate of lymphoma!

Peschel: Yes, you have to compare it with the other population - in this slide you can see it seems to be a prelymphoma. But this sentence is obtained by a paper of the United States.

Weiss: I think prelymphoma is a hard definition and is precancerous condition and then perhaps the therapeutic strategy should be operate all cases of proven Hashimoto's thyroiditis!

Peschel: I agree with you - this must to be handled in a sufficiant critical way.

Benker: Did you see cases of "anaplastic" thyroid carcinoma, that later turned out to be malignant lymphomas?

Peschel: In the former diagnostics there were difficulties to distinguish between small cell carcinoma of undifferentiated carcinoma and malignant lymphoma. But now with immunological investigations you can detect this. But we had no case with undifferentiated carcinoma in Hashimoto's disease.

Simova: A clinical remark: our clinical experience with several cases of lymphoma developed in thyroid with Hashimoto's thyroiditis was, that in all of them the goitre started to grow although suppressive therapy with thyroid hormone was continously applied.

Clinical and cytological classification of lymphocytic thyroiditis

Z. Limanová
III Medical Clinic Prague, CSFR

Lymphocytic thyroiditis (LT) is considered to be a typical autoimmune disease. The consequences of this disease still are not fully evaluated and elucidated. LT can be iniciated experimentally and testosteron or thymosine fraction prevents its outbreak. There are still doubts concerning etiology, its course and prognosis, and the danger of the disease: even the method of the treatment is still vague and the prevalence in female remains an enigma. There are reports that viruses, iodine and probably fluor influence the outbreak of LT and there are some immune stigmata observed in part of the patients with LT. Holm (1985) /1/ proved the higher incidence of myeloproliferative disease in patients with LT.

As we have the opportunity to diagnose lymphocytic thyroiditis, we tried to correlate the cytological picture, clinical course and the thyroid function of the patients with this disease.

Method

There were 415 patients diagnosed with LT in our outpatient department from 1980 till 1990: it formed 15.9 percent of all of our fine needle biopsies (FNB). The diagnosis of LT was based on FNB, the cytological results were compared to the clinical findings and the level of T_4, TSH. The level of antibodies, the ultrasound and the thyroid scan were the complementary examinations not applied to all patients.

Results

According to different characteristics of cytological smears we divided the patients into five groups: 400♀ and 15♂ (figure 1).

The youngest patient was 6 years old, the oldest 81: see figure 2. The distribution of cytological groups in relation to the age is on the figure 3.

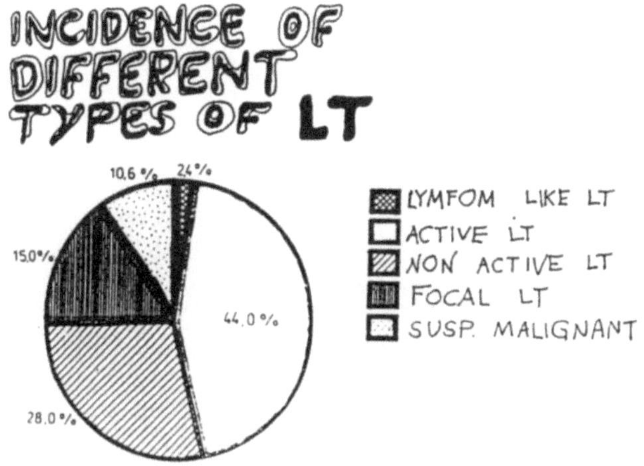

Figure 1

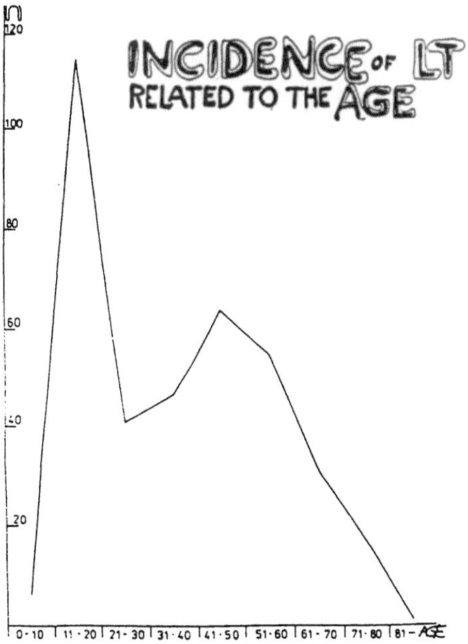

Figure 2

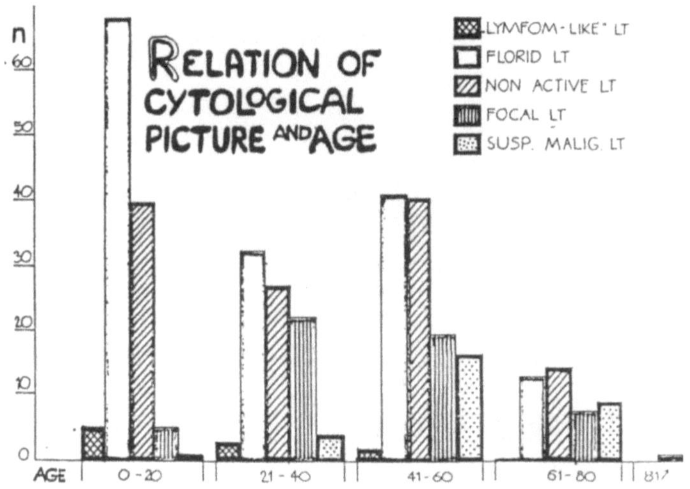

Figure 3

1. "Lymphoma Like" LT - 2.4 %: very cellular smears, represented only by elements of lymphocytic origin, matured and mostly younger forms, including lymphoblasts. Neither thyrocytes, nor plasmocytes.
2. Active LT - 44 %: matured and younger forms of lymphocytes: plasmocytes are present, thyrocytes with marked anisocytosis and anisonucleosis; oncocytes are present, but rarely in children.
3. Non active LT - 28 %: thyrocytes without pronounced atypie: lymphocytes are matured, plasmocytes are present, but not numerous.
4. Focal LT - 14 %: thyrocytes without atypie, matured lymphocytes but not numerous, often elements of monocytomacrophag. system.
5. Thyroid malignancy suspects - 10.6 %: thyrocytes with marked atypie/anisonucleosis, anisocytosis, prominent nucleolus, lymphocytes mostly younger forms, plasmocytes, rarerly.

Thyroid disease appeared in 49 % of patients first degree relatives, especially: LT in twins (one case), LT in sisters (two cases), LT in mothers or fathers (two cases), LT in daughter (two cases), surgery for thyroid carcinoma in mothers (one case) or fathers (one case), in one case a patient's father died of leukemia and patient's daughter had surgery for thyroid papillary carcinoma.

The patient underwent investigation for:

mechanical difficulties	31.0 %
susp. functional disorder	25.0 %
regular check up	29.7 %
difficulties resulting from influenza	5.0 %
remaining reasons	9.3 %

Results of thyroid scan:

multinodular goiter	21.0 %
diffuse goiter	24.3 %
cold nodule	39.3 %
adenoma	1.5 %
normal	3.9 %

After clinical and laboratory evaluation including TRH test when necessary the following groups were diagnosed:

euthyroid	57.0 %
hypothyroid	25.0 %
subclinical hypothyroid	12.0 %
thyrotoxic	5.0 %

In all of cytological different groups thyroid functional disturbance were observed.
The level of T_4 and TSH is on the table 1 and 2. The distribution of different cytological appearance and thyroid function is on the figure 4.

Table 1

T_4 nmol/l

	Euthyroid	Subclinical hypothyroid	Hypothyroid
	108.07 ± 23.10	61.08 ± 23.88	52.82 ± 21.34
1:	99.97 ± 17.11	58.06	42.75
2:	107.16 ± 23.77	55.81 ± 19.36	54.27 ± 16.22
3:	110.03 ± 24.05	66.51 ± 27.07	68.87
4:	110.51 ± 23.56	71.00	--
5:	105.35 ± 22.60	57.86 ± 23.33	40.73 ± 10.16

Table 2

TSH /uU/l mean + 50

	Euthyroid	Subclinical hypothyroid
	2.14 ± 1.30	12.85 ± 7.30
1:	2.00	12.00
2:	2.47 ± 1.44	11.84 ± 6.82
3:	1.94 ± 0.98	12.06 ± 7.59
4:	2.01 ± 1.29	10.00 ± 4.81
5:	1.90	17.60 ± 9.29

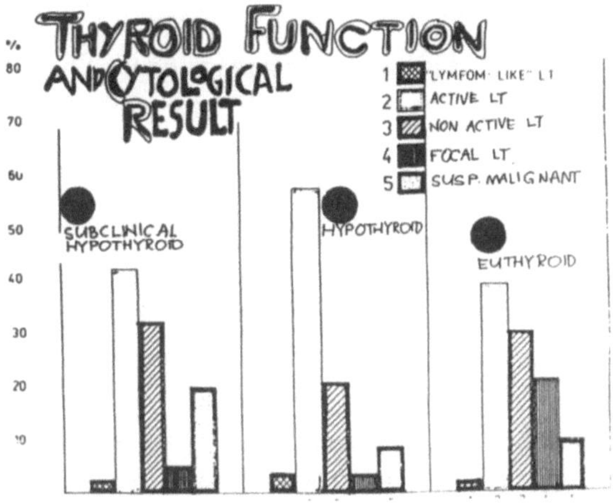

Figure 4

The incidence of myeloproliferative disease in patients with LT was observed in 9 out of 415 patients during follow up in our out-patient department:

age	type of myeloprolif. disease	cytolog. group:
38	acute myeloid leukemia	3
58	chronic myeloid leukemia	3
26	NHL centroblastic. high gr. of malign.	2
56	NHL immunoblastoma B. high gr. of malign.	2
48	NHL centr ocyto-centroblastic	2
73	NHL immunoblastoma typ B	2
73	NHL centrocytoblastic	2
77	NHL typ B	5
68	NHL histiocytic	atrophy

+/ NHL = Non Hodgkin lymphoma

Summary

The highest incidence of LT was observed in teenagers and in fifties, the prevalence in women to men being 26:1.

According to the different cytological results gained from FNB the patients were divided in to five groups, and the cytological findings were correlated to the age and to the thyroid function. The cytological smears from young patients (often lymphoma-like appearance, no oncocytes) differed from those acquired from the older patients (oncocytes, thyroid malignancy suspected).
Fourty three percent of all patients under investigation had thyroid function failure: fifty percent from cytological group 1, 2 and 5, fourty one percent in group 3 and thirty percent in group 4.
The level of T_4 was 108,07 $\pm$ 23.0 nmol/l in euthyroid, 52.82 $\pm$ 21.34 hypothyroid and 61.08 $\pm$ 23.88 nmol/l in subclinical hypothyroid patients.
The level of TSH was 2.14 $\pm$ 1.3 /uU/l in euthyroid and 12.85 $\pm$ 7.30 /uU/l in subclinical hypothyroid patients and in hypothyroid patients was above 25.0 /uU/l in most of cases.
in 9 out of 415 persons, i.e. in 2.17 % the diagnosis of myeloproliferative disease was confirmed during follow-up for LT. The incidence is higher than was published by Holm (1985) /1/.

As the thyroid function fails in almost 50 % of the patients with LT the lipid variable appears in some of the patients with LT (De Maertelaer, V., 1987) /2/, the postpartum thyroiditis occures in some of the women with LT (Othman et al., 1990) /3/, the incidence of myeloproliferative disease is diagnosed more often than in the control group (Holm, 1985, our results), and LT occures in certain families. We suggest the life-long follow-up of all patients with lymphocytic thyroiditis.

References

1. Holm, L., H. Blomgren, T. Lowhagen: New Engl. J. Med. **312** (1985), 601. - 2. De Martelaer, V., R. Calay, P. Neve: Gerontology **33**(1987), 315. - 3. Othman S. et al.: Clin. Endocrinol. **32** (1990), 559.

Discussion

Weiss: What are the cytological criteria for the diagnosis "focal lymphocytic thyroiditis"?

Limanova: It is the group number 4 according our system. We found the normal tissue in some smears and in other smears the infiltration of matured lymphocytes; quite usual we had macrophages and histiocytes around that. But no young types of lymphocytes and no oncocytes and no plasmocytes. It was a small group and I really wonder before I put those patients in the group whether there is really autoimmune etiology. But those patients quite often had higher degree of antibodies. And there we found also a failure of thyroid function.

Weiss: But I think from the cytological point of view, if you perform only one punction in this thyroid, it's not possible to say: this is chronic lymphocytic thyroiditis and this is focal thyroiditis.

Limanova: We never make only one, we usually make most oftenly three punctions in one patient. We don't provide only one.

Weiss: And you just mentioned the autoantibodies. My question is now, how often the autoantibodies in this group were negative?

Limanova: I didn't speak about antibodies in my paper because we tried different types of antibodies - I mean different methods. In all groups we can find antibodies positive and antibody-negative patients sometimes with lymphoma - like, i.e. very high size of lymphocytic infiltration. In the last cases antibodies could be negative. When I had a certain group with certain method, positivity was in 70 % and approximately in 30 % negativity against a mixture of TNM-antibodies.

The role of ultrasound investigation in the diagnosis and treatment of thyroiditis

Z. Novák, V. Zamrazil, J. Němec, P. Vlček
The Institute of Endocrinology, Prague, CSFR

7.5 MHz mechanical sector transducer Hewlett-Packard was used. Two signs were evaluated - the echogenity and the homogenity of tissue in the ultrasound investigation. Three problems were explored: 1. What is the reliability of normal ultrasonographical findings? 2. What changes are visible in subacute and chronic thyroiditis? 3. What changes are recognisible during the longitudinal monitoring?

1. Thirty six patients with thyroid nodule and normal ultrasonographic finding in the rest of the lobe or with normal oposite lobe were operated on. Histological investigations revealed normal findings in 25 patients (69 %), hyperplastic changes in 4 (11 %), focal lymphocytic chronic thyroiditis in 4 (11 %), micrometastases in 1 (3 %), hyperplastic changes combined with chronic lymphocytic thyroiditis in 1 (3 %), mild signs of Graves' hyperthyroidism in 1 (3 %).

2. Sixteen patients suffering from subacute thyroiditis were investigated. The diagnosis in eight of them was approved with a fine-needle aspiration biopsy, eight others of them having obvious symptoms, including pain and tenderness of thyroid gland, highly increased blood sedimentation rate, increased levels of antibodies etc. In seven patients the inflammation began as a focus occupying either a part of a lobe or the whole lobe (44 %) while the other lobe seemed to be normal. In six patients (37 %) the changes, i.e. hypoechogenity of a poorly confined focus, were asymmetrical but afflicting the both lobes. In three patients (19 %) the changes were symmetrically located in the both lobes. The diagnosis of chronic lymphocytic thyroiditis was verified by fine-needle aspiration biopsy in all fifty patients we analyse. In 70 % profound hypoechogenity was seen (thyroid tissue resembling to surrounding muscles), the glands being in addition non-homogenous. Only slight decrease of echogenity and homogenity was

visible in 26 % and in 4 % of patients the echogenity was nearly normal, but the tissue of glands showed numerous slightly hypoechogenic spots. No ultrasound investigation was normal.

3. Eight patients of those with subacute thyroiditis were longitudinally monitored in intervals from two months to three years. In all but one the ultrasonographical finding worsened during the first two months despite the improvement of clinical symptoms. We saw the normalisation of the ultrasound finding in two patients (after five and nine months), partial normalisation in five (in intervals from 2 months to 3 years), persisting changes in one patient (two years). 18 patients with chronic lymphocytic thyroiditis were monitored 1 to 3 years. The partial improvement of changes in ultrasound finding got worse later in one of them. Hypoechogenity and nonhomogenity did not change in 15 (82 %) and got worse in 1 patients (6 %). No entire normalisation was visible.

Conclusions

1. "Normal" ultrasound finding can comprise about 30 % abnormal glands. The most of these are not serious, excluding a micrometastatic spread, that is the most dangerous failure of the method.
2. Non-symmetrical affliction of the gland increase the probability of the presence of subacute thyroiditis. Symmetrical affliction however does not exclude it.
3. Symmetrical affliction of the gland, which is permanent, contributes to the diagnosis of a chronic lymphocytic thyroiditis.
4. The improvement of ultrasonographical changes was delayed after clinical improvement for several months in all investigated cases of subacute thyroiditis. Similar improvement of ultrasound finding is rare in chronic thyroiditis. Its role in the control of the therapy of thyroiditis has remained unclear.

Discussion

Deckart: Only some remarks: We compare now 5.0 MHz transducer and 10.0 MHz transducer and find quite different results if we do this. With 10 MHz we see more. That might be - things you didn't detect with 5.0 MHz. And we had the same observation that the clinical improvement in the subacute thyroiditis runs much quicklier than there is an improvement in the ultrasound picture. But on the other hand it is very important to use this technique especially in the observation of thyroiditis migrans, going from one lobe to the other. And if you always observe new regions with acute inflammation.

Holub: You are perfectly right in the first part of the question. Those ultrasound system differs very much one from the other. So results are oblique from similar type of probe and the frequency of ultrasound. You cannot applay them for another machine. They can differ. To the second part of your question: The improvement that means in our work normalisation of echogenity. That can be caused by normalisation of follicular diameter. But persisting hypoechogenity need not be caused only by inflammatory changes but by increase of fibrotic tissue in gland. This causes hypoechogenity too. One must be very careful if interprete ultrasonographical investigation.

Subacute thyroiditis de Quervain in male subjects

P. Hnilica, J. Podoba, V. Štrbák, Š. Nyulassy
Postgraduate Medical Institute, Inst. Exp. Endocrinology
SAS and Research Inst. of Medical Bionics, Bratislava, CSFR

The association of HLA-B35 antigen /1/ with the subacute thyroiditis de Quervain (deQ) has been generally accepted. Recently we described (as the first to our knowledge) sexual differences in the frequency of this antigen in patients with this disease /2/. The expression of HLA-B35 antigen was found in 74.2 % of female and in 100 % of male patients.

It was aim of our study to see

1. if proportion of male patients changes with age of deQ manifestation,
2. if the frequency of HLA-B35 antigen negative female cases is related to the age.

Material and methods

All cases of deQ diagnosed in the period 1972-1990 were carefully reevaluated and only 204 doubtless cases (172 women and 32 men) were included in this study. The diagnosis of deQ was based on clinical and laboratory examinations including fine needle aspiration biopsy /3/ of goitre in all patients. In 156 cases (76.5 %) HLA typing was also performed; from technical reasons the typing was impossible to perform in 48 patients (41 women and 7 men).

Results

Sex and age at the manifestation of deQ in our series of patients is shown in figure 1. The disease was erupted most frequently at the age period 35 to 54 years (105 patients, 71.1 % of all cases). The highest proportion of female patients was found at the age 40-45 and in men at the age of 55-59 (table 1). The age affects both the sex ratio and rate of cases in different decades but different way (figure 2). The relative proportion of males was the highest in the 55-64 year old patients (F/M 0.6). The maximum of relative occurrence of the disease in female patients was observed at the decade 35-44 years (F/M 13.2). The second peak was

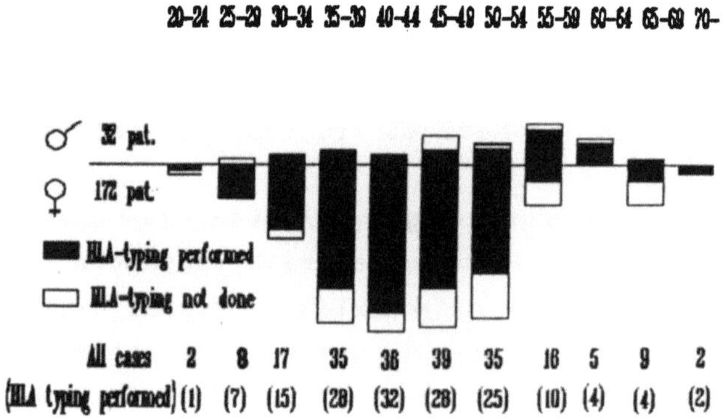

Figure 1

Sex and age distribution of 204 cases

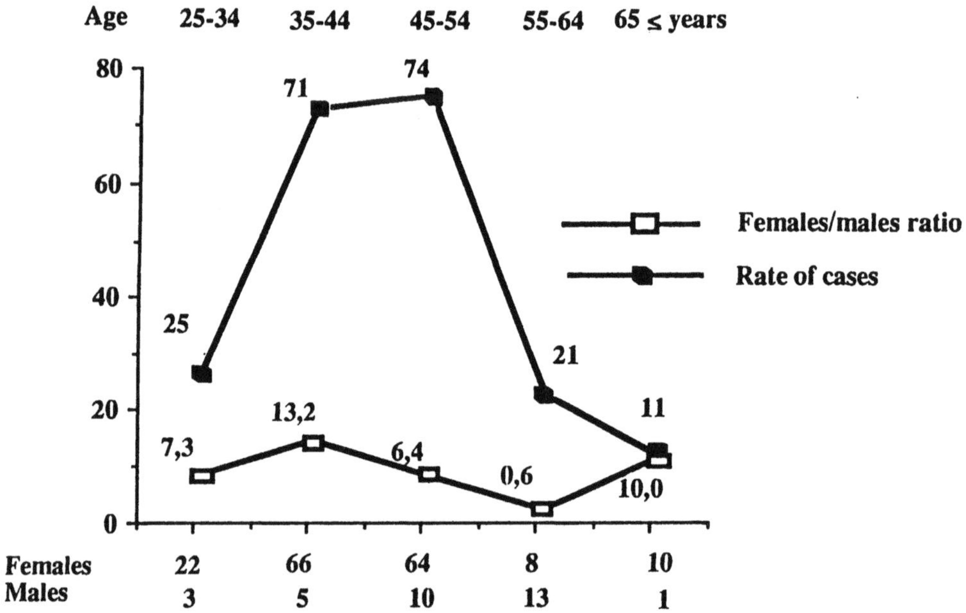

Figure 2

Frequency and sex ratio in age groups

Table 1: Subacute thyroiditis de Quervain in 1972 - 1990
Sex and age distribution

Age (years)	20-24	25-29	30-34	35-39	40-44	45-49	50-54	55-59	60-64	65-69	70 -	All	(%)
Males	-	1	2	3	2	6	4	8	5	1	-	32	(15.7)
Females	2	7	15	32	34	33	31	8	-	8	2	172	(84.3)
All cases	2	8	17	35	36	39	35	16	5	9	2	204	(100)
F/M		7.3		13.2		6.4		0.6		10.0		5.4	

found at the age 65 and older (F/M 10.0).

The results of HLA typing in our patients are shown in figure 3. All men with recognized deQ presented HLA-B35 antigen. The most frequent HLA-B35 antigen negative cases were observed at the age of the most frequent manifestation of deQ i.e. at the age of 35-59 (table 2). In these age groups the ratio positive/negative cases was 3.0; almost one third of patients was HLA-B35 antigen negative. In a group of deQ patients at the age of 20-34 this ratio was 10.5; in patients 60 and over 60 no HLA-B35 antigen negative case was found. The differences in the frequency of HLA-B35 antigen negative female cases are statistically significant (according to chi square test - figure 4).

Conclusion

In a series of 204 (172 women and 32 men) cases of subacute de Quervain's thyroiditis the most frequent manifestation of the disease was found at the age of 40-44 (females) and 55-59(males).

The relative proportion of males in individual age groups (expressed as females/males ratio) was the highest in the 55-64 age group (F/M 0.6). However, the maximum of relative occurence of the disease in female patients was observed at the age of 35-44 (F/M 13.2); the second peak was found at the age of 65 and over 65 (F/M 10.0).

HLA typing was performed in 156 cases (131 women and 25 men). The expression of HLA-B35 antigen was confirmed in all male cases (100 %) but only in 74.8 % female patients.

The occurence of HLA-B35 antigen negative cases was found to be more frequent ($p < 0.01$) in the group with the occurrence of subacute thyroiditis in 35-59 years than in the groups of persons manifesting this disease both at younger and older age.

These data suggest that some factors related to the age of manifestation of the disease influence both sexual distribution and proportion of HLA-B35 negative female cases in series of patients with the subacute de Quervain's thyroiditis.

Table 2: HLA-B35 antigen in patients with subacute thyroiditis de Quervain

Age (years)	20-24	25-29	30-34	35-39	40-44	45-49	50-54	55-59	60-64	65-69	70 -	All
Males	-	-	2	3	2	3	3	7	4	1	-	25
B35-posit.	-	-	2	3	2	3	3	7	4	1	-	25
B35-negat.	-	-	-	-	-	-	-	-	-	-	-	-
Females	1	7	13	25	30	25	22	3	-	3	2	131
B35-posit.	-	7	12	17	21	19	16	1	-	3	2	98
B35-negat.	1	-	1	8	9	6	6	2	-	-	-	33
All cases	1	7	15	28	32	28	25	10	4	4	2	156
B35-posit.	-	7	14	20	23	22	19	8	4	4	2	123
B35-negat.	1	-	1	8	9	6	6	2	-	-	-	33
posit./negat.		10.5				3.0						

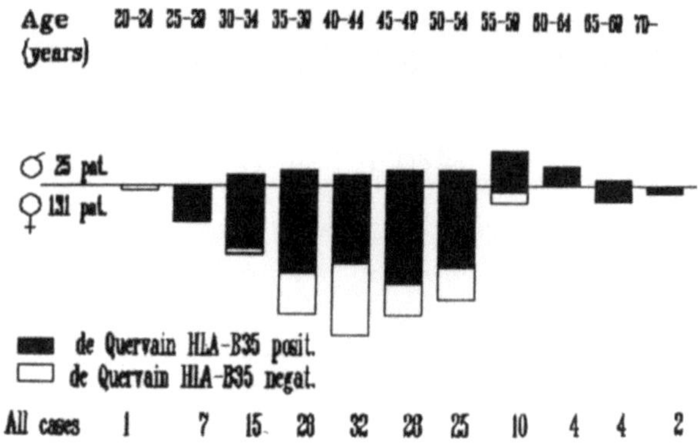

Figure 3

HLA-B35 antigen in 156 examined cases

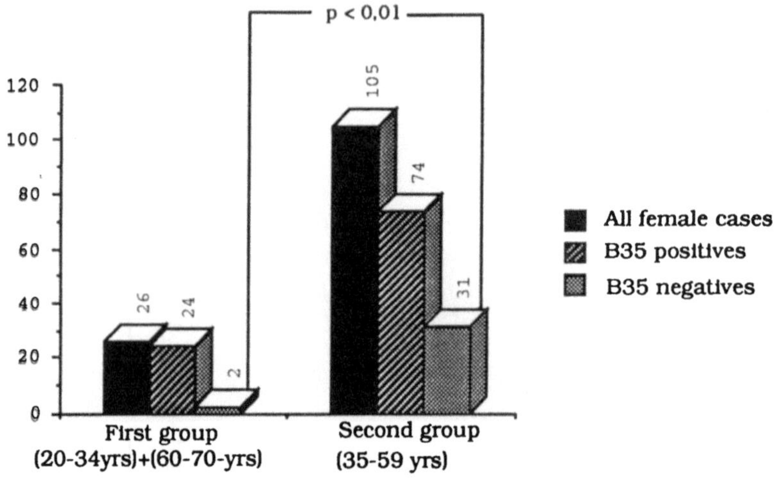

Figure 4
HLA-B35 in 131 female cases of de Quervain' thyroiditis

References

1. Nyulassy, Š. et al.: J. Clin. Endocrinol. Metab. **45** (1977), 270. - 2. Hnilic, P., Š. Nyulassy: J. Endocrinol. Invest. **13** (1990), suppl. 2, 158. - 3. Persson, P.S.: Acta med. Scand., suppl. 483 (1967), 1.

Discussion

Benker: My congratulations for this nice and huge collection of subacute thyroiditis cases - I wonder if you can calculate incidence figures from your data?

Hnilica: The exact incidence of subacute thyroiditis yearly per 100 000 inhibitants in our area is unknown. But our series consists of 204 patients recognized during the period approximately of 22 years.

Leövey: It is interesting, that you find that the patients with de Quervain thyroiditis have HLA-B35 and it predominates. There are interesting findings in the United States that the women with post partum thyroiditis have mostly the HLA-B8 or HLA-B35.

Hnilica: If we meet a male patient with clinical symptoms of subacute inflammation of thyroid without expression of HLA-B35 antigen we must consider a possibility of subacute flare up of chronic diffuse lymphoid thyroiditis.

The finding of HLA-B35 antigen in all our male cases of de Quervain's thyroiditis (100 %) was surprising also for us. We expect the similar reports on this observation from other working teams.

Thyroid function in postpartum thyroiditis and its follow up

Nina Simova
Institute of Pathophysiology and Nuclear Medicine,
Medical Faculty of Skopje, University "Kiril i Metodij",
Skopje, Yugoslavia

The observations of a disordered function of the thyroid in some women during the postpartum period and its relation to autoimmune thyroiditis, have been reported since 1976: Amino et al. /1/, Ginsberg et al. /2/, Hoffbrand and Webb /3/. Nowadays, postpartum thyroiditis (PPT) is considered as a separate clinical entity among the thyroid diseases (Schleusener et al. /4/, Compact Review /5/). Here are presented the results of the evaluation of thyroid function in PPT and during the follow up of a series of patients.

Patients and the methods of evaluation

In the period of 1978 - 1990 in the thyroid department were diagnosed, treated and followed up 56 patients with PPT. The diagnosis was established by these criteria:

- Development of a goitre in postpartum period or enlargement of existing one.
- Abnormal thyroid tests that change in a short time.
- Transience and self-limitation of the thyroid disorder.
- Data for the existence of an immunological involvement (damage) of the thyroid.

Some of the patients seen before the period of observation and followed up as hypothyrotic patients on substitution therapy were added to this series after the correction of the previous diagnosis (by interrupting of the substitution and approval of their euthyroidism.

The patients are 17-36 years old (mean 25.5). In 36 of them (66.1 %) PPT developed after the first delivery, in 15 (26.8 %) after the third and in other 2, it repeated after several pregnancies. Most of them - 50 (94.6 %) are seen after 3-10 months after delivery (m. after 5.6 months), and only 3 (5.4 %) after 10-18 months. The follow up period is 4 months to 15.5 years (m. 5.9 years) in 50 patients (89.3 % of all) and 6 (17.9 %) are seen once or twice (followed up to 3 months). 14 patients (25 %) are followed during and after the next pregnancies.

All patients are examined clinically and laboratory and radioisotope tests are used only for those who have stopped the breast feeding. Therapy with thyroid hormones was given to those with manifested hypothyroidism and also to many others as a suppressive treatment of the goitre.

Results

Most of the women - 30 (53.6 %) when first seen, feeled themselves healthy, apart from the enlarged thyroid, and nervousness and rare heart palpitation in some of them. Weakness, exhaustion, fatigue, headache and other common complaints declared 11 (19.6 %) patients. 10 (17.9 %) complained of coldness, swelling, slowness, and 5 (8.9 %) of weakness, shortness of breath, palpitations, sweating.

The thyroid was of normal size, but firmer, estimated by palpation, in 3 patients (5.4 % of all). In all others, it was enlarged and firm, gummous, often lobulated. The enlargement was diffuse in all, but in 4 (7.1 %) patients, whose glands were nodular. Less than a third of the patients declared a neck discomfort: slight pain, pressure, discomfort with swallowing etc. Scintigraphy of the thyroid in 36 patients revealed on empty scan in 2, who had a high serum thyroxine level, and homogeneous distribution of the activity in the thyroid in almost all-in 30. Not homogeneous scans were seen in 2 nodular thyroids and in 2 others. Ultrasound tomography was done in 20 patients: it was found an echopoor pattern with scarcely hyperechogenic reflects in 18 patients, as it is seen in Hashimoto's thyroiditis. In one patient with reduced thyroid after long suppressive therapy, the finding was normal and in an other, it was not affirmative for a thyroiditis.

Fine needle biopsy was performed in 53 patients (94.6 % of all). The cytologic pattern of Hashimoto's thyroiditis was found in 83 % (44 pat.) of the examined, in 5 of them a marked fibrosis was noticed. 4 findings(7.5 %) were described as an inflammatory process and 3 (5.7 %) as a subacute thyroiditis. One of the latter was with a significant fibrosis and an other, when latter repeated, was described as a Hashimoto's pattern. Two findings (3.8 %) were not affirmative for thyroiditis, although in one of them a high titer of antithyroid was found.

Antithyroid antibodies (ATA) were not detected regularly, but in different phases of the disease, in 34 patients (60.7 % of all). Elevated titers were found in 88.2 % (30 pat.), and low titers or absent ATA in 4 (11 %).

Thyroxine levels (T_4) in serum were determined at every visit of the patients. A disagreement of its value and the clinical state was a frequent finding. The values at first seeing of the 3 patients seen after 10-18 months after the delivery and of an other seen elsewhere and followed up by us are normal. T_4-values of other 50 patients are presented in figure 1 and table 1.

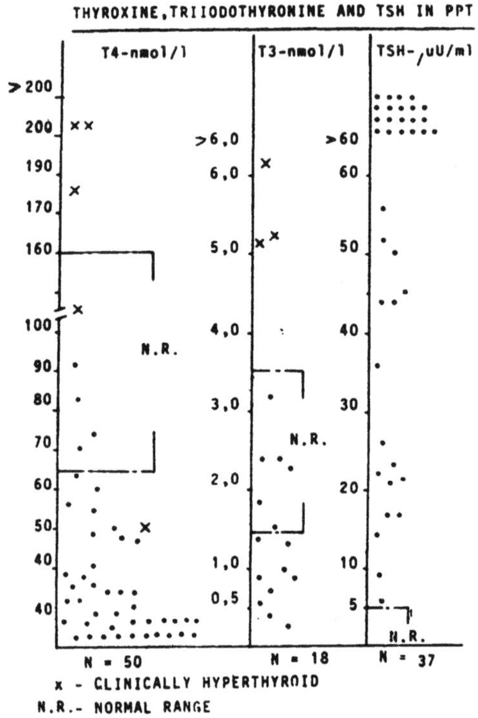

Figure 1

Table 1: T_4 in PPT (at first seeing)

Hyperthyrctic patients (5)

High T_4:	3 patients
Normal:	1 patient (high T_3)
Subnormal:	1 patient (high T_3)

Other patients (50)

$T_4 < 50$ nmol/l:	36 patients (80 %)
$T_4 = 50\text{-}60$ nmol/l:	5 patients (11.1 %)
$T_4 > 50$ nmol/l:	4 patients (8.9 %)
(all with high TSH)	

Triiodothyronine was determined in 18 patients (36 % of all) and values are shown on figure 1. It was high in all 3 tested patients with clinical signs of hyperthyroidism. In the other 15 patients, it was low in 9 (60 %) and with a normal value in 6 (40 %).

TSH was determined in 37 patients (74 % of all), in none of the hyperthyrotics. All values were elevated, ranging from 6 to over 100 μU/ml (figure 1).

The follow up of the patients during the first months is presented on figure 2. It can be seen how quick are the changes of T_4 serum levels. The hyperthyreosis which appear in only 5 patients was mild, without eye's phenomena. In 2 patients the clinical and laboratory signs changed to slight hypothyroidism and in others to euthyroidism in 1-1.5 months. Definitely hypothyroidism developed in 1 patient after a remission of 8 years and a latent hypothyroidism (normal T_4, high TSH) in another, which persisted for 7 years and after that, a therapy was started. The other 3 patients remained euthyrotic.

27 of the patients with low or normal T_4 and high TSH at first seeing could be examined monthly. In 21 of them (77.8 %), T_4 reverted to normal values within 1-10 months (m. 4.5 m.). From the six patients with long standing low thyroxin level, 4 became

definitely hypothyrotic, 1 with latent hypothyroidism and 1 recovered in euthyroidism.

A therapy with thyroid hormones was applied in the most of the followed patients (in about 2/3), either as a substitution in hypothyrotics, or as a suppression of the thyroid enlargement. For an evaluation of the definite status, the therapy has been stopped for several months and the thyroid function was evaluated. It was found that 23 patients out of 37 reevaluated (62.2 %) were euthyroid, with normal thyroid tests, 9 (24.3 %) were clinically euthyroid but with high TSH (latent hypothyrotic) and only 5 (13.5 %) developed definitely hypothyroidism.

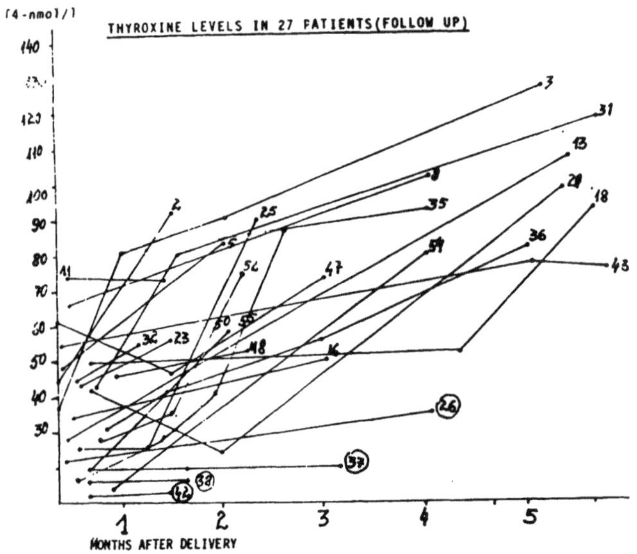

Figure 2
Thyroxine levels in 27 patients (follow up)

Follow up of PPT in 14 patients included the next pregnancies: in 12 the second and in 2 the second and third ones. Relapse of the disorder - a new episode of PPT developed in 6 patients and in 2 of them repeated after the third delivery. Every relapse was associated with low T_4 and high TSH (including that in a patient with hyperthyrosis in the first attack of PPT) and signs of mild hypothyrosis. Ultimate outcome of the relapses is: 4 patients with latent hypothyroidism and 2 euthyrotics. Most of those patients who had no relapses in the consecutive pregnancies had been treated with thyroid hormonal therapy during the pregnancy.

Table 2: Follow up of the hyperthyrotic patients

Patient	time of examin.	Clinical status	T_4 nmol/l	T_3 nmol/l	TSH /uU/ml
	I seeing	hyperthyroid.	187	5.1	-
1.	after 1M	euthyroidism	112	2.6	< 5
	" 2Y.	"	N	N	< 5
	I seeing	hyperthyroid.	202	13.0	-
2.	aft. 1.5M	hypothyr.(mild)	54	-	0.5
	" 3 M	euthyroid	81	-	22.0
	" 6 Y.		N	N	< 5
	I seeing	hyperthyroid.	49	5.2	0.01
3.	aft. 1.5M	hypothyr.(mild)	71	-	20.0
	" 8 Y.	hypothyroidism	low	-	> 6
	I seeing	hyperthyroid.	200	-	-
4.	aft. 1.5M	euthyroidism	90	-	-
	" 10 Y.	"	N	low	> 6
5.	I seeing	hyperthyroid.	109	3.8	-
	after 7Y.	euthyroidism	N		; 5

M - Month; Y - Year; N - Normal value

Discussion

Study of the course of PPT in a relatively large series of patients and over a long period of time, proves the known facts that PPT is a benign, transitory disorder in most of the cases. Even during the acute phase - attacks of the disease, the clinical picture is much milder than could be expected by thy laboratory disorder of the thyroid tests. In more than 60 % of the patients the thyroid function returns to normal after a transitory disorder and in about a quarter of the rest it is normal under augmented pituitary stimulation (latent hypothyroidism). Only in less than 15 % of the cases develops a clinical hypothyroidism. As in other immunologic diseases, the disorder oscilate between episodes of activation-relapses and remissions. The specificity of PPT is that relapses are associated with pregnancies and occur in postpartal period. Very indicative examples are 2 patients with relapses after each of 3 deliveries, when a severe hypothyroidism, even myxoedema developed and then, a full recovery with euthyroidism and reduction of the gland to a normal size followed. In one of them, echographic finding returned to normal pattern, also. Still, PPT may destroy the thyroid to such a degree that its function become insufficient and longlife treatment is necessary. It may happen in the first attack of the disease or after a period of years. By our experience it is not possible to predict the course of this disease, neither the ultimate outcome of it.

An interesting aspect of PPT is its relation to Hashimoto's thyroiditis. Almost in all patients with PPT it was found lymphocytic infiltration of the thyroid and high titers of ATA, by which it is undistinguishable from the former. There are other types of thyroiditis published by Gluck et al. /6/, Nikolai et al. /7/ and cases with a transitory hypothyrosis by Yamamoto et al. /8/, that resemble PPT in some features. By most of its characteristics PPT is identical to Hashimoto's thyroiditis, but the main difference is the reversibility of the thyroid impairment and the change of the thyroid disorder in short intervals, dislike Hashimoto's Thyroiditis which is an irreversible thyroid damage. So, it is an autoimmune thyroiditis occuring in a young woman, with on activation in postpartum period.

What is the incidence of PPT, there are no data for our country. Amino /9/ estimate it to be about 5.5 % of the women in Japan. If the incidence is so high everywhere, and because the clinical disorder is mild and transitory and possibly it passes inapperently in many patients, it may be presumed that it is the cause of many hypothyroidism in mediaeval women. i.e. these women very probably had PPT in their young years.

Concerning the therapy of PPT, it is symptomatic as in other immunological diseases: substitution of the thyroid hormones where they are deficient. Hyperthyroidism usually has not be treated. There are no data for eventualy preventing of the relapses by any treatment. But, by our experience, once started therapy with thyroid hormones, should be revised in every patient, for avoidance of unnecessary, longlife treatment, at least in some patients.

Conclusions

1. Clinical manifestations of PPT are mostly mild and shortlasting. Hyperthyroidism appear in less than 10 % and hypothyroidism in about 20 % of the cases. Less than 20 % of the patients need a substitution therapy during the first attack of PPT.
2. Thyroid tests in PPT are disordered in much greater degree than clinical state.
3. For the diagnosis of PPT very often it is necessary to monitor the thyroid function many times, in the beginning monthly and later 1-2 times in the year.
4. At the end of follow up period of 37 patients of our series, clinical hypothyroidism was found in 13.5 % and latent hypothyroidism in 24.3 % of the patients.
5. Hypothyreosis may develop in the patients who recovered from PPT after many years and that's why longlife controls are recommended.

References

1. Amino, N., K. Miyai, T. Onishi et al.: J. Clin. Endocrinol. Metab. **42** (1976), 296. - 2. Ginsberg, J., P.G. Walfish: Lancet **1** (1977), 1125. - 3. Hoffbrand, B.I., S.C. Webb: Postgrad. Med. J. **54** (1978), 793. - 4. Schleusener, H. et al.: J. Clin. Endocrinol. Metab. **56** (1983), 791. -5. Compact Review, New Compact **16** (1985), 107. - 6. Gluck, F.B. et al.: N. Engl. J. Med. **293** (1975), 624. - 7. Nikolai, T.F. et al.: Arch. Intern. Med. **140** (1980), 478. - 8. Yamamoto, T., H. Sakamoto: Ann. Intern. Med. **88** (1978), 808. - 9. Amino, N. et al.: N. Engl. J. Med. **306** (1982), 849. -

Discussion

Hehrmann: Did you see any linkage or connection to the breast feeding of the mothers? Last year we had a number of young patients who had subacute thyroiditis after they stopped breast feeding.

Simova: No, we have no results. But I have to sum other data, that about 12 % of our patients had goiter or some other thyroid disease in the family.

Limanova: You mentioned, that thyroids were enlarged. May I ask you if the organs in ultrasound were really enlarged? We have the experience that in young women that are really slim, we thought that the thyroid is enlarged, after ultrasound the size is quite normal.

Simova: At first we made palpation and recently a investigation was made by ultrasound also.

Hnilica: We didn't observe any case of subacute thyroiditis in post partal period.

Simova: We had not clinical diagnosed the three cases as subacute thyroiditis, it was only cytological finding. There was no pain, no temperature, no sedimentation rate. But in cytology it was typical Hashimoto when we repeated it in one case. The other had high titers of antibodies.

Riedel's thyroiditis - positive therapeutic response to glucocorticoids

M. Ventz, G. Knappe. D. Zieglitz
I Internal Clinic of University Hospital, Charité Berlin, Germany

Riedel's thyroiditis (struma) is a very rare chronic inflammatory disease of the thyroid gland. Bernhard Riedel first described a chronic sclerosing thyroiditis in 1896. Synonyms of the disease are: invasive fibrous thyroiditis or invasive sclerosing thyroiditis. Woolner et al. reported an operative incidence of 0.04 % that means 1 per 2000 thyroidectomies. The overall incidence of outpatients in this series of the Mayo Clinic was 1.06 per 100000 /2,6/.

Although the condition is rare, benign and in most cases self-limiting, its importance lies in its ability to clinically mimic carcinoma almost completely.

In this paper we report on a case of Riedel's thyroiditis recently seen in our clinic and discuss our experience with steroid treatment.

Case report

A 45 years old female patient first noticed a nonpainful swelling on the left side of the neck. This nodule grew in size progressively to the middle and right of the thyroid. She complained of pressure and dyspnea. Physical examination revealed a non-tender, firm, stonyhard mass on the left side of the thyroid and in the region of the isthmus. Lymphnodes were not palpable. The circumference of the neck was 43 cm.

Thyroid scan with Tc-99 showed no uptake in the left lobe, isthmus and lower part of the right lobe. Normal uptake was seen in the upper region of the right lobe.

Thyroid sonography revealed an enlargement of the whole thyroid gland. Hypoechoic areas were observed in the left region, isthmus and lower part of the right lobe.

FNB and Cytology: Cytology was suspect for malignant cells. Fibrous tissue and inflammation cells were also found.

Laboratory findings:

The first estimation of thyroid hormones showed an euthyroid situation and later a hypothyroid stage.
ESR was high.Gamma-globulins were also elevated.

Wedge resection of the isthmus was performed. Histology revealed a fibrous invasive thyroiditis. Despite surgery patient continued to complain of dyspnea, and pressure in the neck. Therefore we started with the administration of 50 mg prednisolone. The dose was subsequently tapered down and discontinued after 4 months. At the same time we substituted L-thyroxine 100-150 /ug/day.

The circumference of the neck decreased from 43 cm to 39 cm. The thyroid volume fell also from 45 ml to 13 ml in 1 year. Radiologically the trachea is no more stenosed.

Discussion

The etiology of Riedel's thyroiditis remains unknown, although several theories have been advanced. Two theories should be mentioned. It has been suggested that Riedel's thyroiditis may be a collagen vascular disorder because of the presence of vasculitis on pathologic examination. Vasculitis may be prominent, particularly in the extracervical manifestations of this disorder. However, the focal nature of the vasculitis argues against a primary pathogenetic role in this disease /3,4/. The second theory is based on the finding of antithyroid antibodies in a significant percentage of patients suggesting the possibility of an autoimmune disorder, although these antibodies could also be secondary to antigen release by destruction of thyroid tissue. The pathologic feature of cellular infiltration with lymphocytes, plasma cells, and histocytes, while not specific, is typical of an autoimmune response. Cross-reactive antigens in several tissues could explain similar pathologic process in multiple anatomic sites. However, normal serum complement levels and normal lymphocyte subpopulations speak against a immunologic mechanism /3/. The association of Riedel's thyroiditis with other fibrosclerotic

lesions was first suggested in 1958 by Barrett /1/.
He noted a similarity in the pathologic appearance of Riedel's thyroiditis and other fibrosing lesions. Subsequently, examples of Riedel's thyroiditis were reported in association with a variety of other fibrosclerosing lesions, including sclerosing cholangitis, retroperitoneal fibrosis, mediastinal fibrosis, orbital pseudotumor, localized pulmonary fibrosis and fibrous parotitis.

The clinical feature of Riedel's struma is nonspecific and the process is frequently mistaken for neoplasm. The average patient presents in the fourth to fifth decade, and women are effected three to five times more commonly than are men. Most patients present with nonpainful thyroid mass that may produce pressure symptoms such as dyspnea and dysphagia. Growth of the mass may be rapid or gradual over several years. Hoarsness of voice with vocal cord paralysis has been reported to occur in this condition and creats confusion with carcinoma. Cervical lymphadenopathy is not present. The majority of patients are euthyroid, while some are hypothyroid. The status of thyroid function appears to depend on the extent of replacement of the gland by nonfunctioning fibrous tissue.

Laboratory findings in Riedel's thyroiditis are also nonspecific. ESR is frequently elevated. Antithyroid antibodies may or may not be present. Sonography reveales a hypocheoic structure. Scintigraphy shows no uptake in the involved region.
Surgical treatment of Riedel's Thyroiditis is necessary to establish an accurate diagnosis. In addition it may be needed to relieve from significant tracheal compression.
The only medical treatment advocated is steroid therapy. According to literature and our own experience steroid treatment may be successful. However the dose must be high and the duration of treatment long (about 3 months) /3-5/. The prognosis for patients with Riedel's thyroiditis is good, and it is generally considered to be a self-limiting disease. Some investigators have noted slow disease progression. However, spontaneous regression has also been reported.
Extracervical manifestation of the fibrosis may alter the prognosis.

Conclusions

- Riedel's thyroiditis is a very rare disease.
- The origin remains unknown.
- Diagnosis should be histologically proved.
- In the differential diagnosis thyroid cancer, fibrosing variants of Hashimoto's disease and subacute granulomatous thyroiditis should be considered.
- Wedge resection of isthmus is necessary. Steroid administration can be successful.

In general the prognosis is good. In some cases the prognosis depends on the presence of associated diseases such as fibrous retroperitonitis, sclerosing cholangitis, fibrous mediastinitis and so on.

References

1. Barrett, N.R.: Brit. J. Sury **46** (1958), 207. -2. Hay, J.D.: Mayo Clin. Proc. **60** (1985), 836. - 3. Malatte, M.J., G.D. Chintich, C.W. Zuppan: Arch. Otolaryngol. Head Neck Surg. **117** (1991), 214. - 4. Schwaegerle, S.M., T.W. Bauer, C.B. Esselstyn: Am. J. Clin. Pathol. W (1988), 715. - 5. Westhoff, M: Dt. med. Wochenschr. **113** (1988), 337. - Woolner, L.B., W.M. McConahey, O.H. Beahrs: J. Clin. Endocrinol. **17** (1957), 201.

Discussion

Zamrazil: I agree with conclusions about good effect of prednisone treatment. We have observed satisfactory effect of prednisone in our patients too. Unfortunately we lost one patient eight years later for renal failure due to retroperitoneal fibrosis. So prognosis of the disease is not good in all cases.
Ventz: It is discussed also in the literature, but I think sometimes the dose was to low and it was administered in a to short period. But you know the origin, the course is unknown and therefore we don't have a very good treatment.
Bergant: Did you perform frozen section histology?
Ventz: I can't say anything about it.

Management of chronic lymphocytic thyroiditis in children and adolescents

O. Hniková, J. Zikmund and M. Finková
Clinic of Children and Adolescents, 3rd Medical Faculty of Charles University, Prague, Czechoslovakia

Juvenile autoimmune thyroiditis (chronic lymphocytic goitrous thyroiditis, Hashimoto's disease) has been reported in the last decade as quite a common cause of nonendemic goiter also in children and adolescents /2-5/.
In our outpatient ward of the Pediatric Clinic in Prague 10, we have been following 28 patients with lymphocytic thyroiditis for 1-4 years.

Material and methods

There were 27 girls and only one boy with this diagnosis. Twenty of them were referred to our endocrinological ambulance by district physicians for evaluation of enlarged thyroid gland not responding to thyroglobulin therapy and only two for a small firm thyroid gland. The remaining six girls were found during an epidemiological study of goiter prevalence among school children in Prague 10 in 1988. 6020 school children aged 7-14 years were examined by palpation according to WHO goiter criteria (this means grade 0, IA - B, II, III) by school pediatricians. The children who had goiter grade IB and more were sent to endocrinological examination, including hormonal levels (total T_4, TSH) and ultrasound of the thyroid gland. For RIA determination of total T_4 Košice (Slovakia) kits and for RIA TSH Henning's kits were used. In those who had irregular echotexture findings antimicrosomal antibodies by RIA kits from Henning (positive result from 500 IU/ml) and antithyroglobulin antibodies by RIA kits from Serono (positive results more than 50 IU/ml) were performed.

Results

Out of 22 patients who were sent to us by district physicians, as was mentioned above, subclinical hypothyroidism in 4 girls was revealed and in two girls with small firm thyroid glands overt hypothyroidism was diagnosed. One girl had slight hyperfunction by laboratory tests. Adequate TSH-TRH response in subclinical hypothyroidism and hyperthyroidism was present. Ultrasound findings were typical for the diagnosis, which was confirmed with cytological observations from fine-needle aspiration. Eighteen out of 22 cases, i.e. 82 %, had a positive elevation of antimicrosomal antibodies and 13 cases, i.e. 60 %, also antithyroglobulin antibodies. In the group of 6020 schoolchildren in Prague 10, goiter was revealed in 286 children, i.e. in 4.1 % (figure 1). Out of these cases (figure 2) 221 children had goitres of grade IA, i.e. 77.3 %, grade IB was found in 52 children, i.e. in 18.2 % and grade II in 13 children, i.e. in 4.5 %.

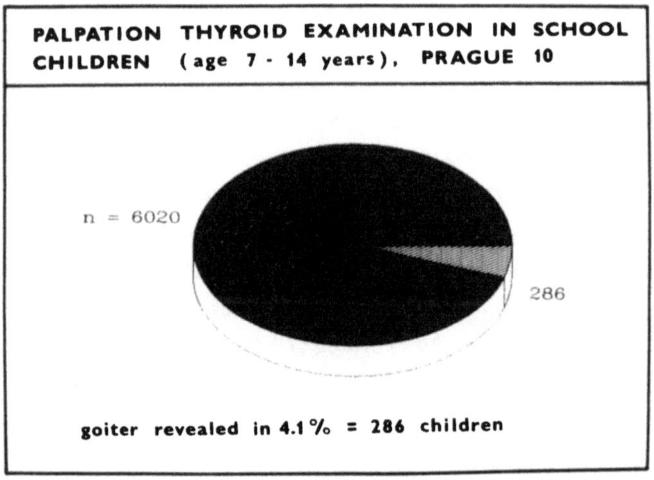

Figure 1

Palpation thyroid examination (epidemiological study from Prague 10)

The sex ratio (girls:boys) in goiter IA was 4:1, in grade IB 3:1 and 10:1 in grade II. Grade III was not encountered. Most cases (figure 3) were between the age of 10-14 years in both sexes. Euthyroidism was diagnosed on the basis of normal serum total T_4 and TSH values in all children with goiter grade IB - II. Echostructure in 55 patients was normal, but in 6 girls was irregular with hypoechogenic and unechogenic loci. Fine-needle aspiration

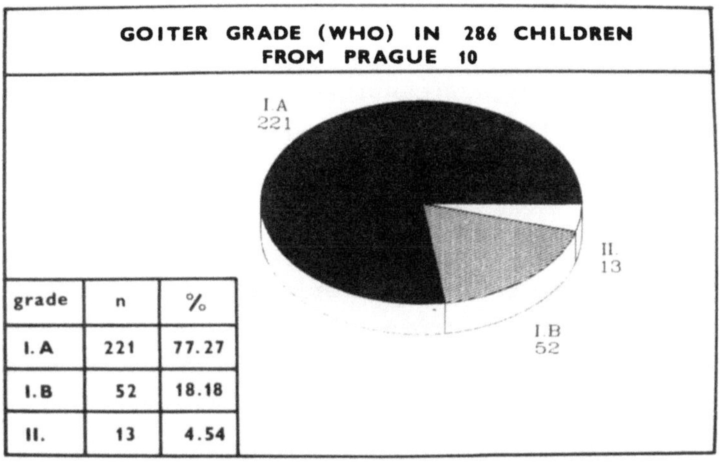

grade	n	%
I.A	221	77.27
I.B	52	18.18
II.	13	4.54

Figure 2

Goiter grade in 286 school children (epidemiological study from Prague 10)

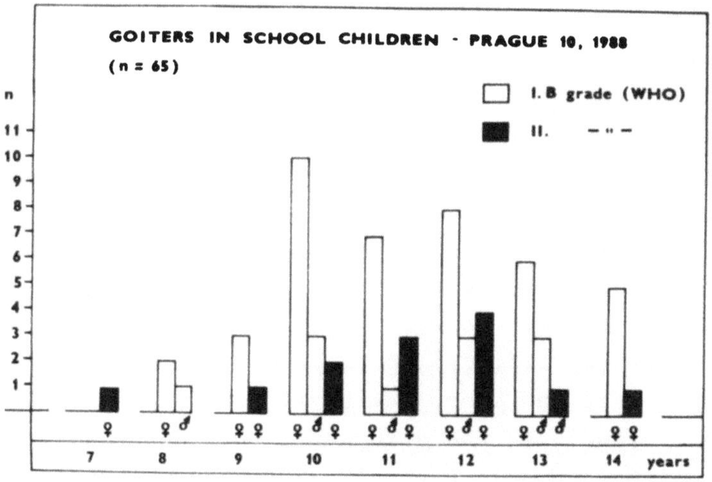

Figure 3

Goiters in school children
(according to sex and age)

in these six patients exhibited a typical cytological picture of lymphocytic thyroiditis. All of them were girls 12.8 years old on the average. All had significantly elevated antimicrosomal antibody titers and 4 of them also antithyroglobulin antibody titers.

Discussion

In children and adolescents, chronic autoimmune thyroiditis may result in either goitrous Hashimoto's thyroiditis, which is very often reported or atrophic thyroiditis, which is quite rare in children. In our group of juvenile lymphocytic thyroiditis it was present only in two girls out of 28 patients. Goiter in juvenile lymphocytic thyroiditis in most cases does not differ at the beginning from simple juvenile goiter by palpation and is often asymptomatic. Ultrasound of the thyroid gland as a screening method should be recommended in enlargements of the thyroid gland (grade IB and more). In our epidemiological goiter study, four girls had tender goiter of grade IB and two of grade II at the time of the diagnosis. All six girls were treated with L-thyroxine 0.05 mg/day because of thyroid enlargement. In these 6 girls, alternate day prednison treatment was also introduced with a 5 mg dose/every other day after initial 5 days' period with 15 mg/day. Alternate day prednison therapy was terminated after 12 months. There were no side effects of this therapy. The evaluation of ultrasound findings, after prednison therapy had been discontinued, showed remarkable improvement in echostructure in 5 girls (figure 4a, b and 5a, b). In one girl the thyroid echostructure did not change at all. Serological findings, hormonal levels and cytological controls in the course of one year's treatment were the same, but thyroid volumes diminished (-6 ml on the average). In the group of 22 patients who were not receiving prednison but only L-thyroxine, the echostructure improved only in 7 cases, while the rest were without change. It can be concluded that the early diagnosis of the juvenile lymphocytic thyroiditis is possible with ultrasound examination as the best screening method with fine-needle aspiration of thyroid tissue under ultrasound control in suspected cases. The patients should be regularly followed and treated with thyroxine in all

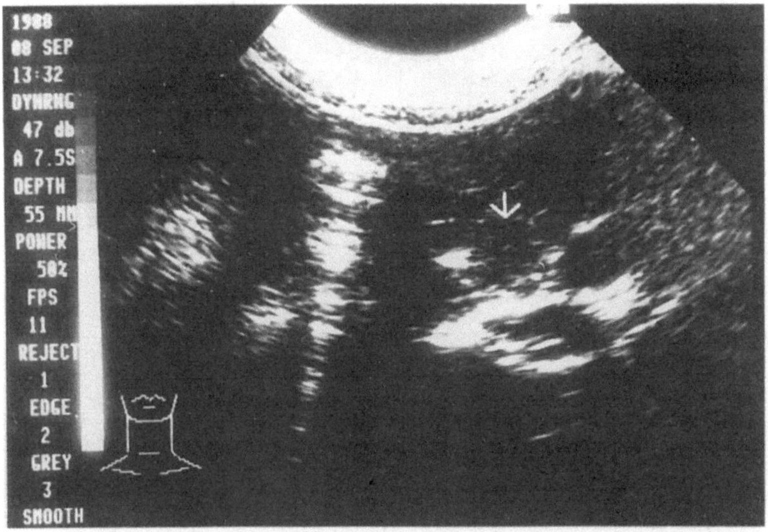

Figure 4a

Hypo- and unechogenic loci of irregular echostructure in a patient with lymphocytic thyroiditis

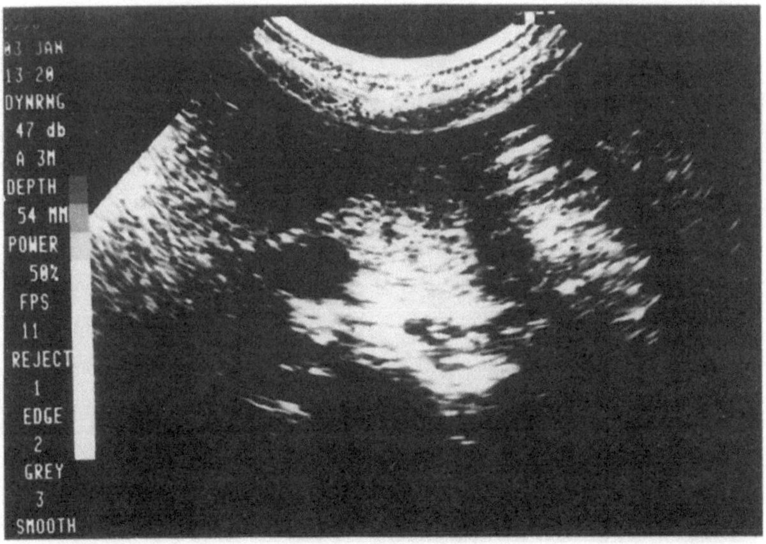

Figure 4b

Mildly hypoechogenic loci and slightly irregular echostructure - same patient as in figure 4a after one year's treatment with L-T_4 and alternate day prednison

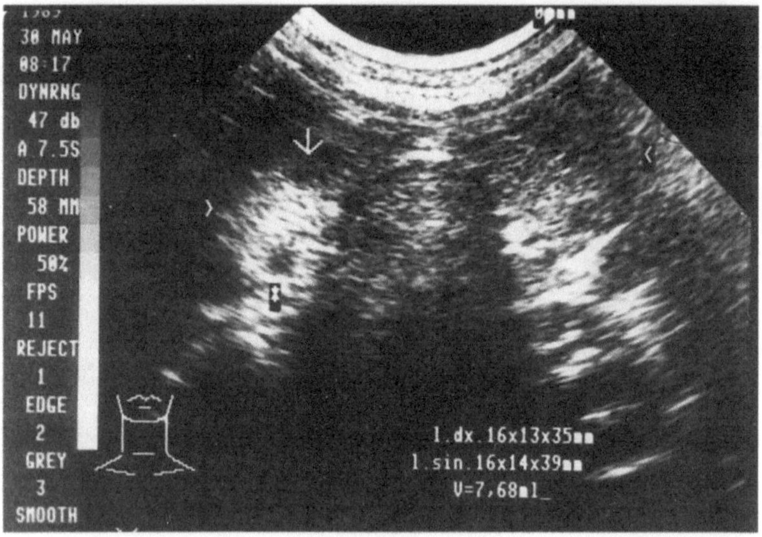

Figure 5a

Unechogenic loci in a patient with lymphocytic thyroiditis

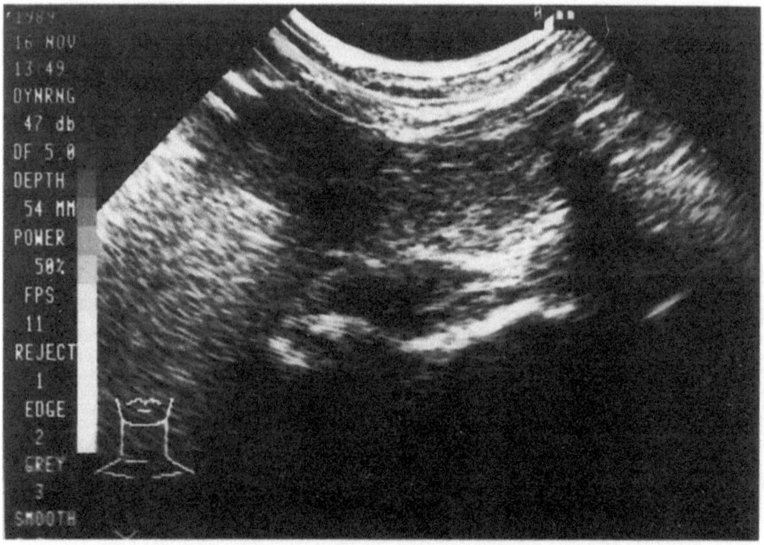

Figure 5b

Unechogenic loci not present, echostructure is regular - same patient as in figure 5a after one year's treatment with L-T_4 and alterate day prednison

cases with overt or subclinical hypothyroidism. Alternate day prednison therapy with small doses is still controversial and would require a long-term follow up. Although it has been reported in the literature /1,4,5,7/ that some cases can recover spontaneously after several years, we only encountered one case in a four-year follow up.

We would like to express our thanks to Dr. Limanová for her participation in the cytological examinations and valuable advice in this matter.

References

1. Frey, H.: Acta Endocrinol. (Copenh.) **98** (1981), 210. - 2. Chiovato, L., P. Vitti, F. Santini, G. Lopez, C. Mammoli, P. Bassi, L. Giusti, M. Tonacchera, G. Fenzi, A. Pinchera: J. Clin. Endocrinol. Metab. **71** (1990), 40. - 3. Inoue, M., N. Taketani, T. Sato, H. Nakajima: Endocrinol. Jpn. **22** (1975), 483. - 4. Maenpaa, J., M. Raatikka, J. Rasanen, E. Taskinen, O. Wager: J. Pediatr. **107** (1985), 898. - 5. Rallison, M.L., B.M. Dobyns, R.R. Kaeting, J.E. Rall, F.H. Tyler: J. Pediatr. **86** (1975), 675. - 6. Yamada, T.: J. Clin. Endocrinol. **46** (1978), 784. - 7. Yamamoto, T., H. Sakamoto: Ann. Intern. Med. **88** (1978), 808.

Thyroiditis and thyroid hyperfunction

V. Zamrazil, J. Němec
Institute of Endocrinology, Prague, Czechoslovakia

Thyroiditis and hyperthyroidism are of particular interest of clinical endocrinologist for several reasons:

1. both diseases are common in population of many countries. In CSFR thyroiditis is the most frequent thyroid disease.
2. clinical picture and some laboratory findings are often similar;
3. interrelationships between thyroiditis and hyperthyroidism are complex and sometimes not yet fully elucidated. From this point of view one should take into account the following fact: both thyroiditis and hyperthyroidism are not defined diseases but complex of several entities with different etiopathogenetic factors, clinical course, laboratory findings and prognosis.

The interrelationships of both diseases can be summarized in simplified form:

1. common autoimmune basis causes both Hashimoto's thyroiditis and Graves'-Basedow a form of hyperthyroidism;
2. hyperthyroidism is a manifestation (sometimes dominant) of thyroiditis (acute and subacute thyroiditis, postpartum thyroiditis, silent thyroiditis);
3. hyperthyroidism and thyroiditis is caused by destruction of the thyroid (actinotherapy, application od I-131);
4. concurrent hyperthyroidism and thyroiditis are sometimes present in thyroid cancer;
5. iatrogenic hyperthyroidism develops during treatment of thyroiditis due to overdosage of thyroid hormones.

Some important combinations are given in figure 1.

From clinician's viewpoint, time relations in manifestations and clinical course of both diseases are important for diagnosis a treatment of patients suffering for thyroiditis and/or hyperthyroidism. For some combinations see figure 2.

INTERRELATION AMONG THYROID INFLAMATION AND FUNCTION

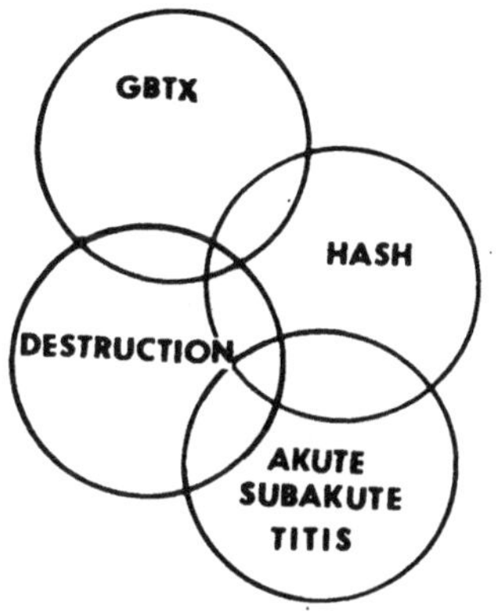

Figure 1

DYNAMICS OF DEVELOPMENT OF THYREOTOXICOSIS AND TITIS

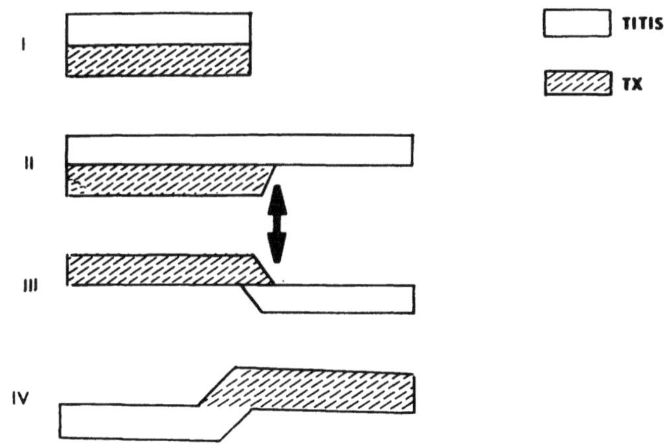

Figure 2

1. The clinical manifestation can be observed in the same time and both diseases ended (are cured) at the same time (figure 2-I).
2. The time of clinical manifestation is identical, but after successful treatment of the first disease, the second one persists (figure 2-II).
3. After hyperthyroidism is cured, thyroiditis occurs (figure 2-III).
4. After thyroiditis is cured, hyperthyroidism occurs (figure 2-IV).

For the illustration of some combinations of thyroiditis and hyperthyroidism allow us to demonstrate three case reports.

Case report I <u>Simultaneous presence of GB TX and Hash</u>

female, 28 years: manifest hyperthyroidism, endocrine orbitopathy painfull goiter
T_4 : 250 nmol/l T_3 6.8 nmol/l ART 240 ms
TRH-TSH test suppressed antithyroglobulin antibodies (TgAtb) pos., antimicrosomal antibodies (MAtb) pos., TRAK pos.

Treatment: carbimazole, prednison, subtotal thyroidectomy (STE)

Present status: therapy with T_4, MATb still pos.

Case report II <u>Occurrence of Hash during treatment of GB TX</u>

female, 24 years: manifest hyperthyroidism, minimal orbitopathy
T_4 232 nmol/l T_3 3.9 nmol/l ART 270 ms
TgAtb neg. MAtb neg.
4 months after STE painfull goiter occured
TgAtb pos. MAtb pos. TSH 7.8 mU/l

Present status: small sometimes painfull goiter, treatment with T_4

Case report III <u>Occurrence of hyperthyroidism during treatment of hypothyroidism caused by thyroiditis</u>

female, 42 years: clinical hypothyroidism, no goiter
TSH > 80.0 mU/l T_4 18.6 nmol/l
ART 465 ms TgAtb pos. MAtb pos.
Treatment: T_4
3 years later manifest hyperthyroidism, no goiter
T_4 > 250 nmol/l T_3 6.0 nmol/l
TSH ; 0.6 mU/l ART 240 ms
2 months after cessation of T_4 treatment:
T_4 > 250 nmol/l T_3 4.9 nmol/l
ART 240 ms
a reactivity of TRH-TSH test, MAtb pos.
TgATB pos. TRAK pos.
Treatment: carbimazole, in preparation for I-131 treatment

As is obvous from presented case reports, combinations of thyroiditis and hyperthyroidism involve various possibilities and at least some of them are of clinical importance. Our knowledge of this problem is still not good. Further studies and systematic evaluation of observed data seems to be necessary. The aim of our presentation is to call attention to this topic. From our material a preliminary conclusions only are possible:

- simultaneous presence of hyperthyroidism and thyroiditis is relatively frequent;
- mechanisms of relationships are various, most important seems to be common autoimmune basis;
- hyperthyroidism is dominant in clinical picture of some types of thyroiditis (silent and postpartum thyroiditis);
- development of thyroiditis during treatment of GB TX is most important combination;
- late occurrence of thyroiditis during and even after successful treatment of GB TX is a strong argument for systematic follow-up of such patients.

References

Hamburger J.I.: Ann. Intern. Med. **104** (1986), 219. - 2. Pinchers, A., S.H. Ingbar, J.M. McKenzie, G.F. Fenzi: Plenum Press (New York, London), 1989. - 3. Zamrazil, V., J. Nemec: Radiobiol. Radiother. **26** (1985), 235.

Clinical and laboratory evaluations of patients with different types of thyroiditis

I. Sztojka, Zs. Karányi, A. Leövey
First Department of Medicine, University Medical School, Debrecen, Hungary

171 patients (164 women (96 %) and 7 men (4 %) aged 14-76 years) with thyroid diseases were studied. We reviewed the clinical data for all cases of thyroid disease in the outpatient clinic.

Methods

Thyroid function was measured with commercial available kits: T_4, TSH by radioimmunoassay, T_3-resin uptake, anti-thyroglobulin antibodies by tanned erythrocyte haemagglutination technique, antimicrosomal antibodies by complement fixation test. Radioactive iodine uptake (RAIU) with scan and fine needle aspiration cytology was performed without local anaesthetic using a 21 gauge needle on a 10 ml disposable syringe mounted in a syringe holder. The smears were stained using the May Grünwald Giemsa technique.

Results

135 patients presented with Hashimoto's thyroiditis (132 women (97.8 %) and 3 men (2.2 %). Diagnosis of Hashimoto's thyroiditis was based on the positive tests for thyroid microsomal and thyroglobulin autoantibodies and cytological features by fine needle aspiration. De Quervain (subacute) thyroiditis was diagnosed in 6 patients (4 women (66.7 %) and 2 men (33.3 %)) by characteristic clinical features and fine needle biopsy. 8 patients (8 women) fit the criteria of "silent" thyroiditis with low RAIU and a nontender thyroid gland with hyperthyroidism, 20 patients presented with a clinically isolated nonneoplastic thyroid swelling (18 women (90 %) and 2 men (10 %)). Of the swellings 18 were solid on aspiration and 2 yielded fluid and were termed cystic. 2 patients with isolated swelling presented carcinoma (2 women) (figure 1).

Average of patients were estimated when the diagnosis was discovered (figure 2). Hashimoto's thyroiditis: 33.5, subacute thyroiditis: 36.5, "silent": 37.1 year. RAIU in Hashimoto's thyroiditis was normal (72 cases (55.4 %) low (41 cases (31 %)) and elevated (17 cases (13 %)). All patients with subacute thyroiditis and "silent" thyroiditis showed very low (2 % or less) RAIU. It returned to normal in all patients in whom we repeated in the recovery.

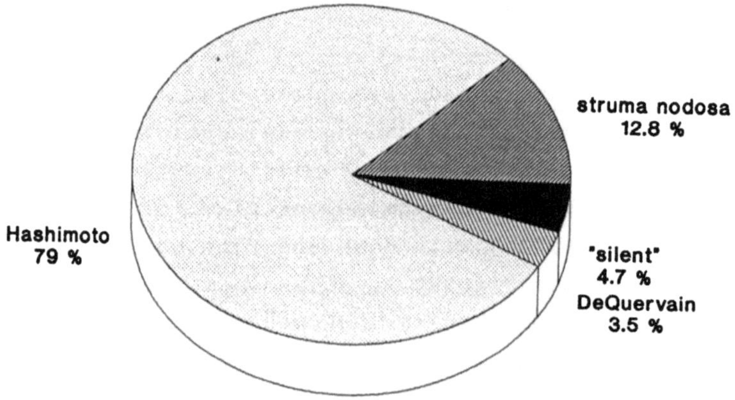

Figure 1
Diagnosis of patients

We investigated the scan in the patients when it was possible (normal or elevated RAIU). Hashimoto's thyroiditis usually showed "scanty" scan (91 cases (69.5 %)) or cold nodule (25 cases (19 %)), but sometimes "warm" nodule (7 cases (5.3 %)), or normal thyroid gland (4 cases (3 %)) can be seen.

Thyroid microsomal and thyroglobulin autoantibodies were estimated at the discovery of disease and after following the patients (figure 3). Hashimoto's thyroiditis is characterized by elevated autoantibody level. Mean value was 98 U at the beginning of disease (normal 16 or less), after the treatment decreased to 15.6 U. Patients with subacute thyroiditis showed normal autoantibody level (12-6 U), and in cases with "silent" thyroiditis the measured were elevated a little, average value was 36 U to 7.7 U. Laboratory findings of thyroid function at the time of

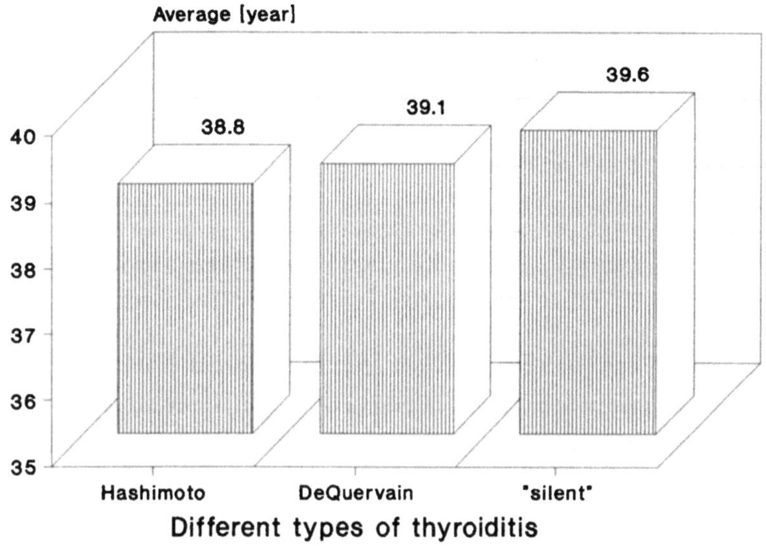

Figure 2

Average of patients with different types of thyroiditis

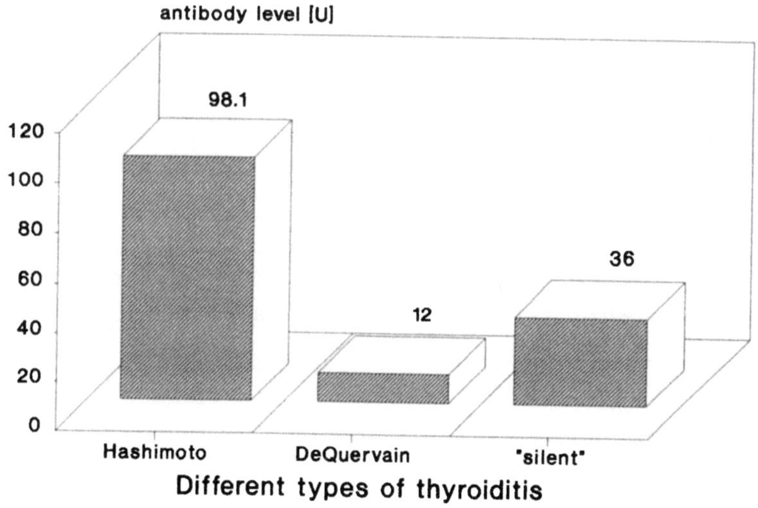

Figure 3

Thyroid microsomal and thyroglobulin autoantibody level in different type of thyroiditis

diagnosis in Hashimoto's thyroiditis: T_3 U was 0.94, T_4 RIA was 105.7 nmol/l. TSH-RIA was 4.1 mU/l. Patients with subacute thyroiditis presented: T_3 U 1.2, T_4 RIA 178 nmol/l, TSH-RIA 3.8 mU/l. Cases with "silent" thyroiditis showed: T_3 U 1.02, T_4 RIA 152 nmol/l, TSH-RIA 1.32 mU/l.

During the following examinations sometimes the patients showed altered thyroid functions both hyperthyroidism and hypothyroidism (table 1).

Fine needle aspiration biopsy was performed in 158 patients from 171. The aspirates were classified into four categories: features of chronic lymphocytic thyroiditis, monolayered sheets with inflammation, "possible neoplastic" increased cellularity and variation in nuclear size, features of inflammation with giant cells (figure 4).

During evaluation of the smears 68 were chronic lymphocytic thyroiditis, 72 showed cytological features of inflammation, 9 were "possible neoplastic" 1 yielded fluid and were termed cystic, and 1 was insufficient. 7 showed features of inflammation with giant cells.

Table 1: Clinical state of thyroid function in different types of thyroiditis

Types of thyroiditis	Thyroid function				
	Transient hyperthyr.	Euthyr.	Transient hypothyr.	Hypothyr.	No of pts
Hashimoto's	21	97	2	15	135
Subacute	5	1	-	-	6
"silent"	8	-	-	-	8

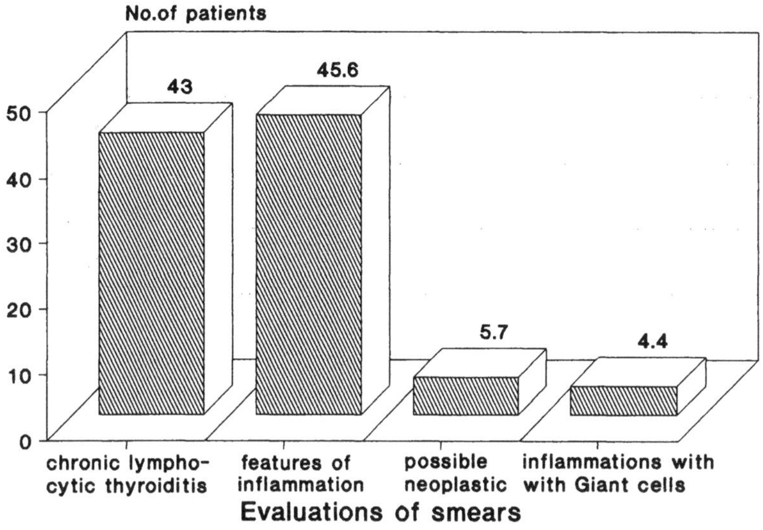

Figure 4
Cytological evaluation of thyroid fine needle biopsy

Discussion

Hashimoto's thyroiditis is the most common cause of hypothyroidism. It is believed to result from a derangement of immune system. Alterations of both cell-mediated immunity and humoral immunity have been proposed /1,13/. The most important characteristics of Hashimoto's thyroiditis are the lymphocytic infiltration of the gland. Fine needle aspiration cytology is used to exclude malignancy without excision and histologies examination. Extensive experience in Sweden /9/ and other centers suggests an accuracy of over 90 %.

Thyroxin therapy is usually recommended for hypothyroid patients with Hashimoto's thyroiditis because the thyroid gland is progressively destroyed, with a permanent defect in thyroid hormonogenesis /2,3/. In our study 97 from 135 patients remained euthyroid and only 15 did not recover thyroid function, and need thyroxin therapy.

The main problem with Hashimoto's thyroiditis is the painful, enlarged thyroid gland. 125 patients from 171 received non-steroid antiinflammatory drugs, and 43 patients need steroid therapy during some weeks to two months. Patients with sub-acute thyroiditis received antibiotic therapy during the febris and two patients were needed short time methimazol therapy against hyperthyroidism. An interesting problem is the "silent" thyroiditis. Several authors have noted the same or a similar disease recently and have suggested a number of names, including silent or atypical subacute thyroiditis /10, 12/, thyrotoxicosis with painless thyroiditis /14/, hyperthyroiditis as a diagnostic pitfall /8/, as well as a post-partum thyroiditis /5/. It need to emphasize that it occurs as a spontane resolving or transient hyperthyroidism with low RAIU and features of thyroiditis by cytological or histological or histologies examinations. It needs to be recognized and differentiated from other forms of hyperthyroidism, and need to be careful receiving definitive, ablative thyrostatic therapy /11/.

The relationship between this form and Hashimoto's thyroiditis is unknown, the low male-to-female ratio /4/, the relatively low family history of thyroid disease /6/, and the normal or a little elevated antithyroid antibody titer suggest differences from Hashimoto's thyroiditis. In our series we could not describe about acute suppurative thyroiditis and Riedel's thyroiditis /7/. Appearance of these is rare, during our investigation there was none of them.

References

1. Brown, J., D.H. Solomon, G.N. Beall: Ann. Intern. Med. **88** (1978), 379. - 2. Buchanan, W.W.: Arch. Intern. Med. **115** (1965), 411. - 3. De Groot, L.J.: The thyroid and its disease. 4th ed. New York; Wiley (1975), 405. - 4. Furszyfer, J.: Metabolism **21** (1972), 197. - 5. Ginsburg, J.: Lancet **1** (1977), 1125. - 6. Heinman, P.: Acta Med. Scand. **179** (1966),

113. - 7. Al-Hilaly, M.A.: Acta Chir. Scand. **156** (1990), 237. - 8. Jackson, I.M.D.: N. Engl. J. Med. **293** (1975), 661. - 9. Lowhagen, T.: Surg. Clin. North Am. **59** (1979), 3. - 10. Morrison, J., R.H. Caplan: Arch. Intern. Med. **138** (1977), 45. - 11. Nikolai, T.F.: Arch. Intern. Med. **140** (1980), 478.- 12. Papapetron, P.D., I.M.D. Jackson: Lancet **1** (1975), 361. - 13. Volpe, R., M. Edmonds: Lamki Mayo Clin. Proc. **47** (1972), 824. - 14. Wool, P.D.: Am. J. Med. **60** (1976), 73.

Hashimoto-Thyroiditis with long-term negative auto-antibody determination: a case report

Marie-Luise Weiss, A. Blottner, H.F.Deckart
Klinik für Nuklearmedizin und Endokrinologie,
Klinikum Berlin-Buch, Germany

Introduction

The incidence of Hashimoto-thyroiditis as a classical autoimmune disease of the thyroid has, as epidemiological studies have shown, considerably increased and it is more frequently diagnosed /8/. Pathogenetically the primary disturbance is based on a defect of the suppressor cell-T-lymphocytes, according to the hypothesis advanced by Volpe /10/. Thus,clones originated through mutation cannot be eliminated by autoaggressive helper-T-lymphocytes ("forbidden clones"). They initiate both humoral and cellular immune processes. Clinically, two courses of Hashimoto-thyroiditis have been observed: I. hypertrophic thyroiditis with occasionally rapidly growing goitre, functionally often euthyroid, a number of the cases was marked by hypothyroidism, occasionally a hyperthyroid stage is initially found. II. atrophic thyroiditis with absence of goitre, the patients have no complaints for long periods of time as long as symptoms of hypothyroidism appear. An important diagnostic procedure for Hashimoto-thyroiditis is the determination of auto-antibodies against thyroid-binding globulin (TAK) and thyroid microsomes (MAK) /7/. The simultaneous incidence of both antibodies with high titres has an important diagnostic value for Hashimoto-thyroiditis. Low-titrated or even absent thyroid auto-antibodies do not exclude autoimmunothyroiditis. The following case report demonstrates a phase-like progress of auto-antibody titres over an observation period of 11 years with an almost unchanged cytomorphological finding of florid Hashimoto-thyroiditis of the clinically hyperplastic form with an euthyroid course.

The present case report is considered to be a contribution to the discussion on pathogenesis and diagnostic strategies for Hashimoto-thyroiditis.

Methods of investigation

The thyroid fine needle puncture was performed using the puncture-smear- and staining technique described earlier /11/. MAK-antibodies were determined using a commercial test (Fa. Wellcome, passive haemagglutination) semiquantitatively. TAK-antibodies were quantitatively measured using a radio-immunological method /2/, calibrated according to standard A 65/93 of the Medical Research Council, which contains per definitionem 1 megaunit per 1 litre (MU/l). Progressive examinations of autoantibodies were carried out of the same laboratory under identical conditions.

Patient data and results of the study

The female patient St. H., born on January 15, 1919 was 59 years old, when she underwent her initial examination at our clinic in 1978. Thyroid diseases were unknown in the medical history of her family. The patient retired with a pension due to mitral stenosis of degree III with a slight aortic insufficiency. For 3 months the patient had observed thyroid enlargement involving a globus feeling, which gave rise to her visit to the thyroid outpatient-department. The patient was clinically euthyroid at the initial examination. Both thyroid lobes were palpatorily enlarged, above the jugulum and in the area of the right thyroid lobe there were tough nodules palpable. The thyroid scintigram of March 21, 1978 (figure 1) revealed nodular goitre with inhomogeneous nuclide distribution in both lobes and a representation of cold nodules in the isthmus region and of the right thyroid lobe centrally. The fine needle puncture of the isthmus nodule and the nodule located in the right lobe, carried out on March 31, 1978, yielded (puncture-No. 134/78 A/B) the following cytologic findings: The cytologic smears obtained from scintigraphically

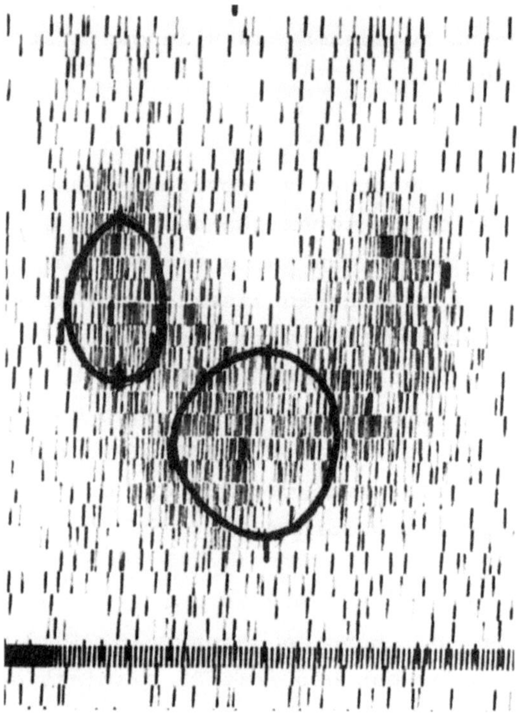

Figure 1

Thyroid scintigram with 37 MBq Tc-99m enlarged, bilobular thyroid with inhomogeneous storage pattern, cold nodules in isthmus region and centrally located in the right thyroid lobe

cold nodules of the right thyroid lobe and the isthmus, reveal similar pictures. However, the punctuated sample of the isthmus nodule contains considerably more cells. The smears are characterized by colorful, inflammable appearing cell pictures with oncocytes, degeneratively altered thyrocytes, pyknotic thyrocytes, cytolyses and a considerable number of group-cell and single cell necroses, apart from this, also normal thyrocytes. There are large numbers of lymphocytes and lymphoblastomas as well as some plasma-cells - cytologically the typical picture consists of florid Hashimoto-thyroiditis - group II (figure 2).

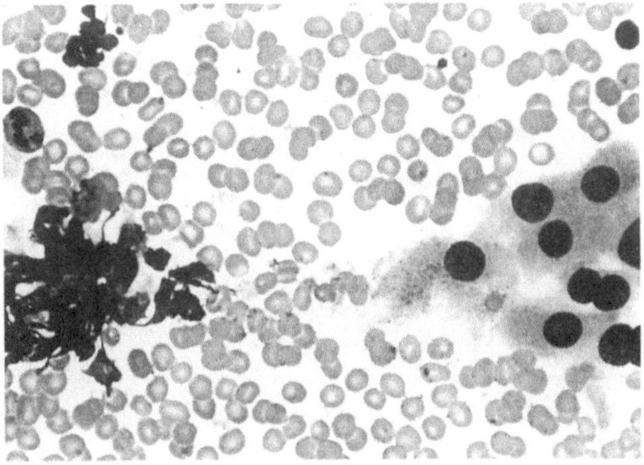

Figure 2

Cytological findings of fine needle punctuated sample of Hashimoto-thyroiditis

2a: Complex of oncocytes and cell necrotic focus

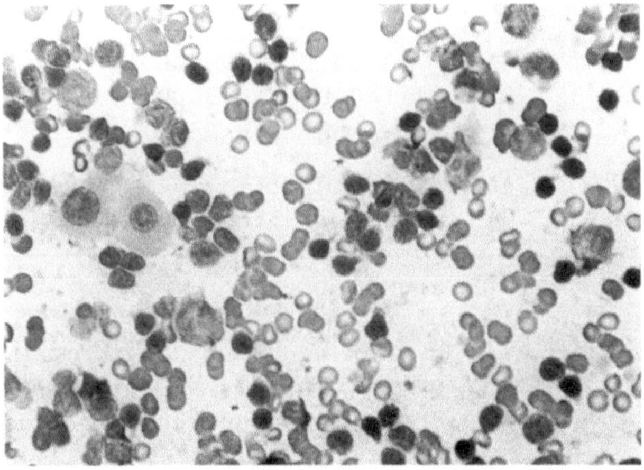

2b: Lymphocytes and lytic thyrocytes

The fine needle puncture was repeated twice during the observation period (table): 1983 the isthmus nodule was punctuated (puncture-No. 737/83) and in 1989 the isthmus nodule as well as a sonographically established echo-poor region in the left thyroid lobe was punctuated (puncture-No. 434/89 A/B). The cytological findings of the different localizations revealed the picture of florid Hashimoto-thyroiditis; compared to the initial examination of 1978 there was no change of the cytological picture.

Table: In vitro and cytological results in the follow up of 11 years (patient St. H.)

Date	T_3 nmol/l	TSH mU/l	Tg-AK IE	Ms-AK Titer	Cytology
11.07.78			neg.	neg.	Hashimoto-th.
13.05.80			neg.	neg.	
14.04.81		1.1	neg.	neg.	
13.10.81		1.0	neg.	neg.	
15.11.82		1.7	neg.	1:25000	
13.10.83		2.6			Hashimoto-th.
29.04.85		3.0	3000	1:409600	
30.03.87	2.4	1.7	14000	1:409600	
01.02.88		2.6	20000	1:25600	
13.06.89	2.9	1.6	neg.	1:6.5Mill.	Hashimoto-th.
03.10.89	4.4		neg.	1:6.5Mill.	

The cytological findings gave rise to the determination of TAK-antibodies and MAK-antibodies (table). Both results were negative and also the medical check-ups produced negative results in the following years until 1981. Only 4 years after cytological diagnosis of Hashimoto-thyroiditis MAK-antibodies occurred in the lower titre region, which remained constant in further annual medical check-ups, but were detectable

with variable titre levels. Lower TAK-values were present for the first time in the 7th year after initial diagnosis; they rose somewhat in the 9th and 10th year, whereas the TAK-value became negative again at the 11 th year.
During the observation period two thyroid sonograms of the patient were performed: on May 13, 1980 - both thyroid lobes revealed a homogeneous reflex pattern, in the isthmus a solid echo-rich nodule was found; on April 4, 1989 - echo-poor region in the right thyroid lobe, inhomogeneous, almost echo-normal nodule in the isthmus, normal echo structure in the left thyroid lobe (figure 3). The patient received thyroid hormones during the whole observation period. For this reason, a scintigraphical progressive control was not possible.

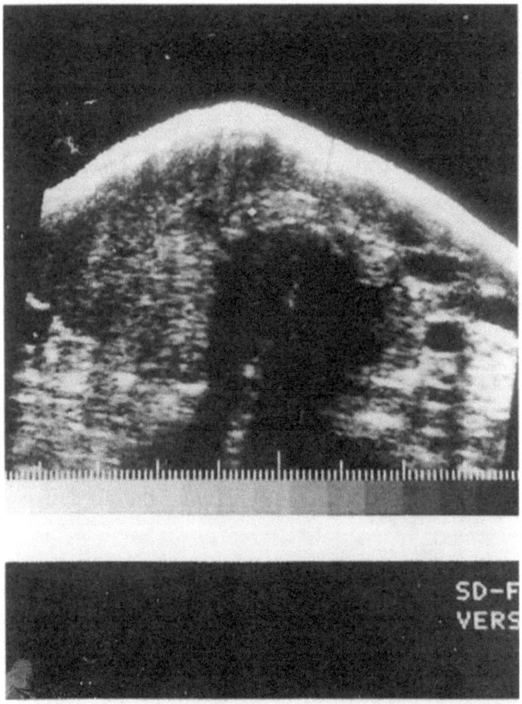

Figure 3
3a: echo-normal nodules in the isthmus
(transversal section)

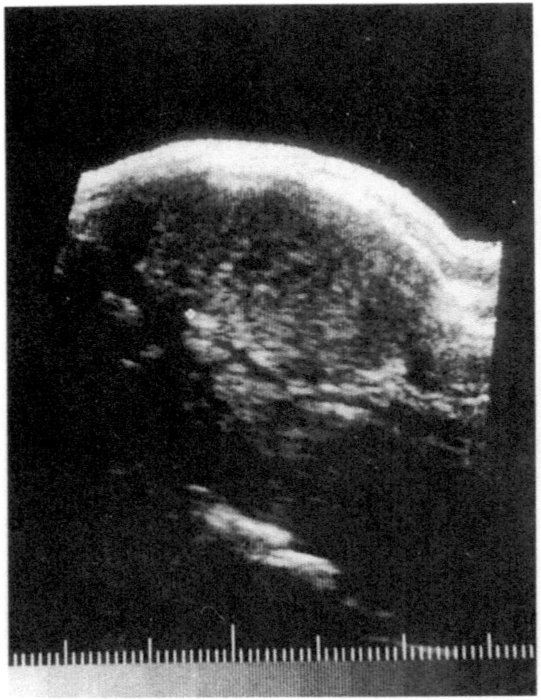

Figure 3b:

Echo-poor region in the right thyroid lobe (longitudinal section)

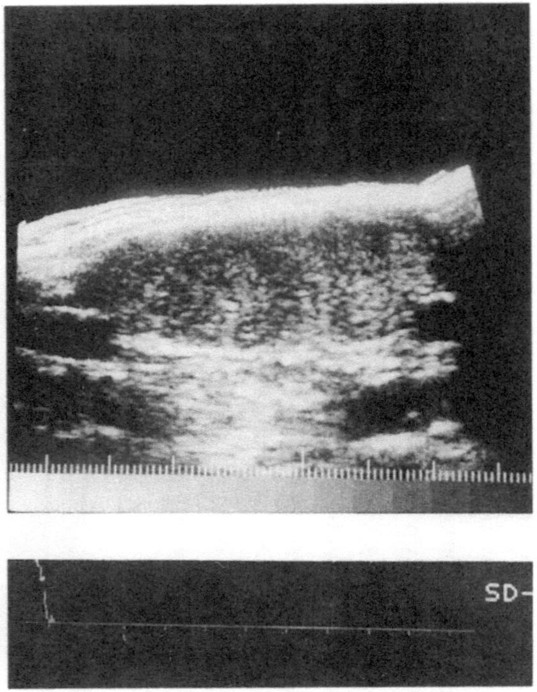

Figure 3c:

Normal echo-structure of the left thyroid lobe (longitudinal section)

Discussion

The remarkably delayed prevalence of thyroid auto-antibodies (MAK 4 years, TAK 7 years), observed in this case report, after reliable cytological diagnosis of Hashimoto-thyroiditis has so far not been described in the literature available to us. An explanation of this phenomenon can be the phase-like course of autoimmune thyroiditis, which is generally known; however, the cytological picture reveales constant signs of floridity in the whole process. It has to be taken into account that the cytological findings represent only the morphological condition of the punctuated region circumscribed and not the entire thyroid. As a reason for "false"-negative antibody findings of Hashimoto-thyroiditis also the detection sensitivity of determination procedures is to be discussed. In this reported case the progressive antibody examinations were carried out in the same laboratory under identical conditions. further explanations for the negative antibody findings are:

- immune complexes can form in circulationg antigens; therefore the antibodies cannot be determined,
- antibodies appear only in the blood, if they are not used up at the site of lymphocytic infiltration and immunoreactive activity /9/.

This casuistics is also interesting with regard to the discussions on the frequency of cytologically and/or histologically determined cases of Hashimoto-thyroiditis with negative auto-antibody determination. In the international literature /1,4-6/ this constellation of findings, although in most cases studied only on small populations, is described with a wide range of 0 % up to 37 %. Most studies present a value of some 15 %. Of the patient population studied by us (85 cases of cytologically established Hashimoto-thyroiditis) were with 16.5 % MAK and TAK negative /12/.
None of the cited publications contains data on logitudinal

controls so that in progressive examinations the percentage of patients with negative auto-antibody findings of Hashimoto-thyroiditis would decrease.
Although the determination of high auto-antibody levels is of marked importance for the diagnostics of Hashimoto-thyroiditis, the missing detection of auto-antibodies is not to be used as exclusion diagnostics. Here fine needle puncture cytology closes is an important diagnostic gap.

References

1. Becker, W., Chr. Reines, W. Börner: Therapiewoche **35** (1985), 1167. - 2. Blottner, A., S. Spitz, D. Fabian: In: Proceedings of the Second Multilateral Symposion on Thyroid, Reinhardsbrunn 1984, Schriftenr. wiss. Tagungen in der DDR, Isocommerz 1985, 4. - 3. Crockford, P.M., G.O. Bain: Canad. med. Assoc. J. **110** (1974), 1029. - 4. Droese, M., M. Bähre, D. Emrich u.a.: Dt. med. Wochenschr. **104** (1979), 875. - 5. Emrich, D., M. Droese, D. Hofmann u.a.: Med. Klinik **74** (1979), 516. - 6. Friedman, M., K. Shimaoka, U. Rao et al.: Acta cytol. **25** (1981), 513. - 7. Schatz, K., K. Federlin: Med. Welt **30** (1979), 614; 654. - 8. Schatz, H.:Die Thyreoiditiden. Diagnose und Therapie. Verh. dt. Gesellsch. inn. Med. 87. Tg., München: Bergmann, 1981, 398. - 9. Seif, F.J.: Akt. Endokr. Stoffw. **5** (1984), 112. - 10. Volpe, R.: In: Autoimmunity in the endocrine system/ed. by R. Volpe, Berlin (West) u.a.: Springer, 1981, 19. - 11. Weiss, M.L., E. Kleinau, E. Hamann u.a.: Dt. Gesund.-Wesen **31** (1976), 2186. - 12. Weiss, M.L., R. Pilz, A. Blottner u.a.: Radiobiol. Radiother. **25** (1984), 759.

Combination of Hashimoto- and de Quervain thyroiditis

K.P. Schmidt, Eva Deckart, R. Pilz, E. Strehlau
Klinikum Berlin-Buch, Clinic for Nuclear Medicine and Endocrinology

Two patients of our outpatient department are presented with an acute thyroiditis de Quervain in typical clinical and paraclinical symptomatology. Both patients had a severe course with a remission after intensive treatment (salicylate, corticosteroids) after about six months. In both patients the preexistent ultrasound diffuse echopoor pattern was not changed within this period (figure 2, 7). Increasing basal TSH represented hypothyroidism leading to thyroid hormone substitution.

The simultaneous occurrence of both forms of thyroiditis - immunogenic Hashimoto form just as thyroiditis de Quervain - was verified by persistent increase of thyroglobulin antibodies (TAK > 40 ng/ml) and negative TRAK, the persistence of diffuse echopoor behaviour of the total thyroid gland and cytologic characterization: in the acute phase granulomateous thyroiditis, later thyroiditis Hashimoto. This disease seemed to be preexistent, as hypothyroidism was observed in the beginning of acute phase just as echopoor immunogenic ultrasound pattern.

Recherching literature with Medline over a period of the past ten years only two references were found /1, 2/.

Case I: Female patient, 25 years of age, suffered from an acute and painful inflammation of goiter. Highly increased blood sedimentation rate, but no changes in differential blood cell smear; normal immune electropherogram. Increased basal TSH level, and highly increased antithyroglobulin- and microsomal antibodies (table 1).

Table 1

Date	BSR mm	TT_3-RIA nmol/l	TT_4 nmol/l	TSH mU/l	MAK	TAK mg/l	TRAK U/l	Therapy
23.03.90	60/120	2.2	46	16	1:6.5 mill.	> 40		Corticoid +
05.04.90	55/103		44	18				L-Thyroxin 10
24.04.90	47/87	2.0	219	15	1:6.5 mill.	> 40	10	" 10
07.05.90	20/37	2.5	141	18				" 12
05.06.90		2.2	109	3.7				" 17
27.09.90		3.1	99	5	1:6.5 mill.	> 40		
19.04.91		3.3	134	4.7	1:409600	> 40		III/90-IX/90 Corticoid

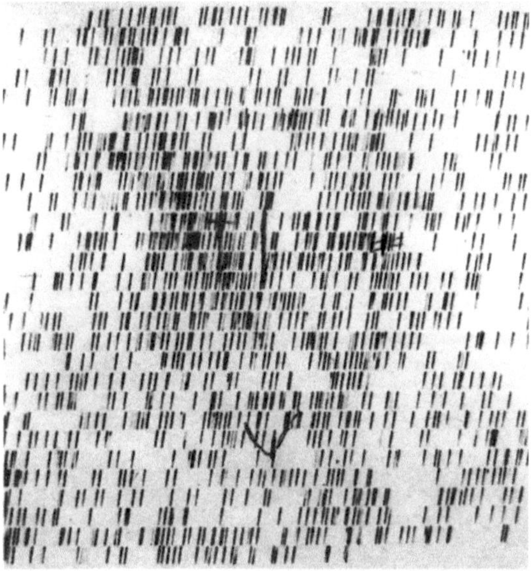

Figure 1

Extremely reduced pertechnetate uptake in thyroid scintigram

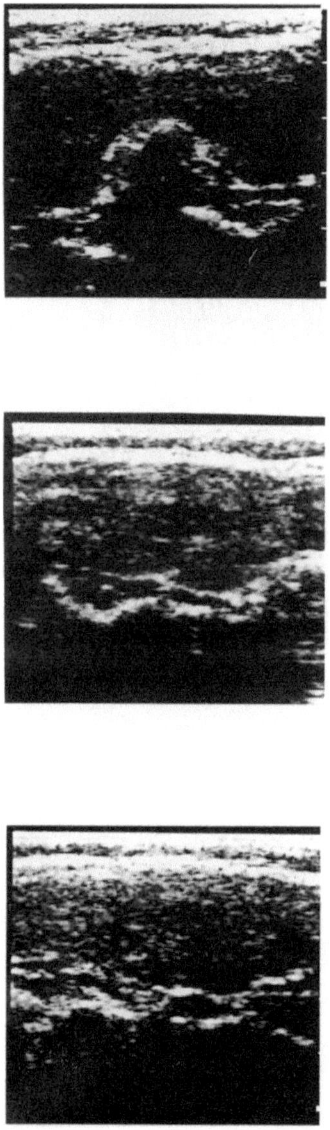

Figure 2

Hypothyroidism was replaced by thyroid hormone substitution. After remission of clinical symptoms corticoid release after six months of treatment. Persistence of high thyroid antibody values and diffuse echopoor pattern

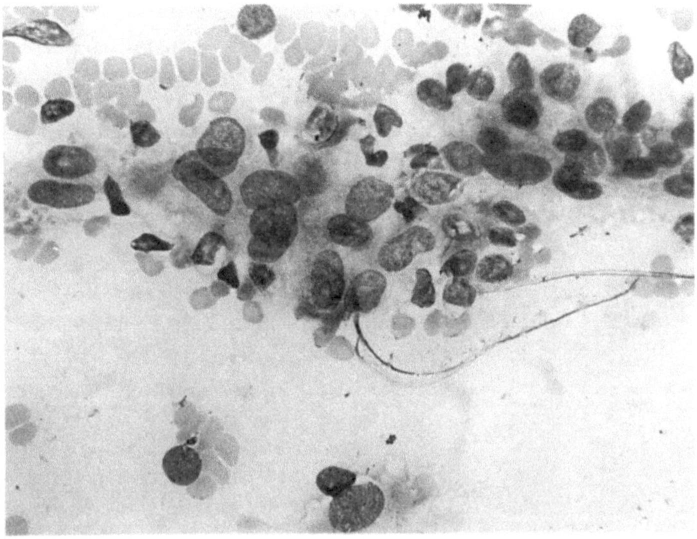

Figure 3

Cytological results
Case I:
1. Complex of epitheloid cells, inflammation cells, recent necrotic material as typic representation of thyroidis de Quervain.

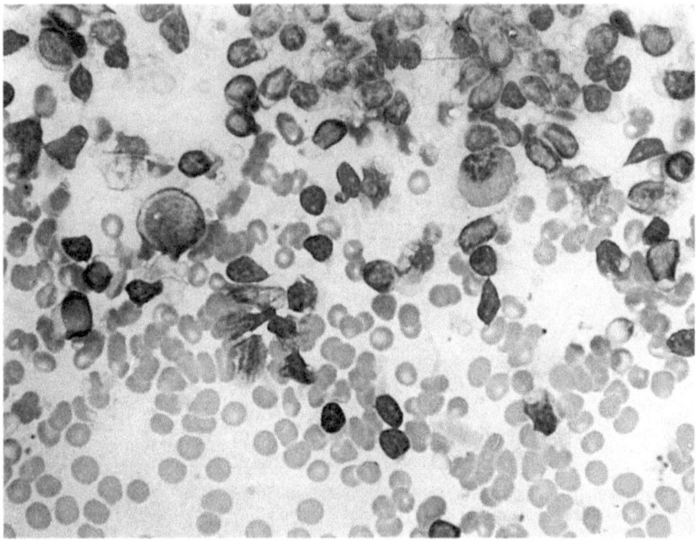

2. Lymphocytes, lymphoblasts and plasma cells together with cell-lysis represent the thyroiditis Hashimoto

Control puncture after 1 year was twince negative because of fibrotic changes and scar development

Long lasting weakness and general apathy: Insufficiency of adrenal cortex function could be excluded (normal cortisol day-night profile), normal stimulation test, performed 6 weeks after corticosteroid withdrawal).

Case II: Female, 39 years aged, has caught a cold in August 1990. Six weeks later acute pain in the neck with swelling of thyroid gland. Increase of sedimentation rate.

Table 2 shows a to case one similar behaviour of hormone and immune parameters in the course and during treatment with corticoids just als thyroid hormone substitution.

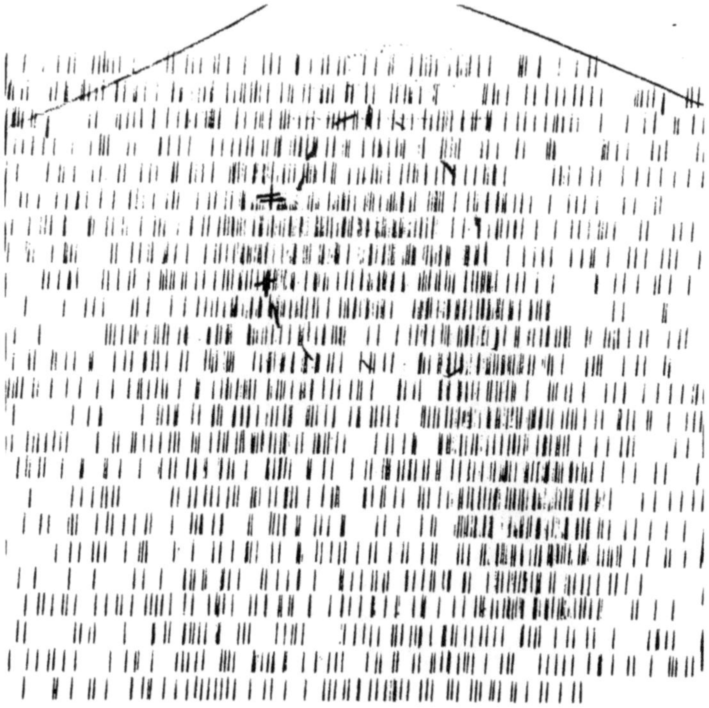

Figure 4
Scan extreme low pertechnetate uptake

Table 2

Date	BSR mm	TT_3-RIA nmol/l	TT_4 nmol/l	TSH mU/l	MAK	TAK mg/l	**TRAL** U/l	Therapy
05.10.90	85/102	1.6	76	34				
06.10.90	25/36			79	1:6.5 mill.	> 40	5	Corticoid
01.11.90	10/25	2.7	162	11				L-Thyroxin 100
03.04.91	10/22	2.9	56	6.3	1:102400	> 40	8.7	" 150 X/90 - I/91 Corticoid

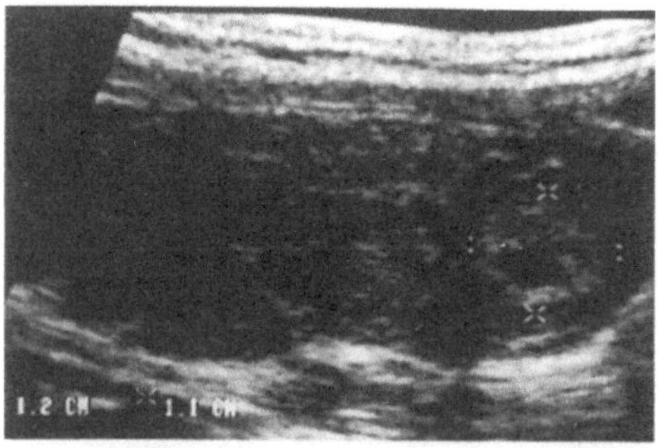

Figure 7a

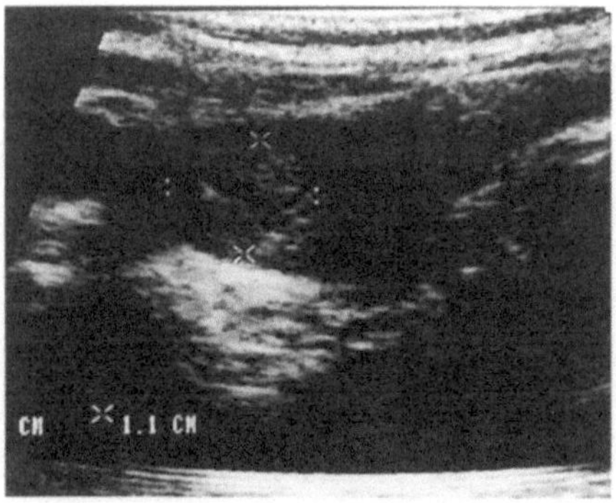

Figure 7b

Figure 7

Ultrasound shows diffuse echopoor pattern with small nodule at the beginning of the disease (7a), unchanged after 6 months (7b)

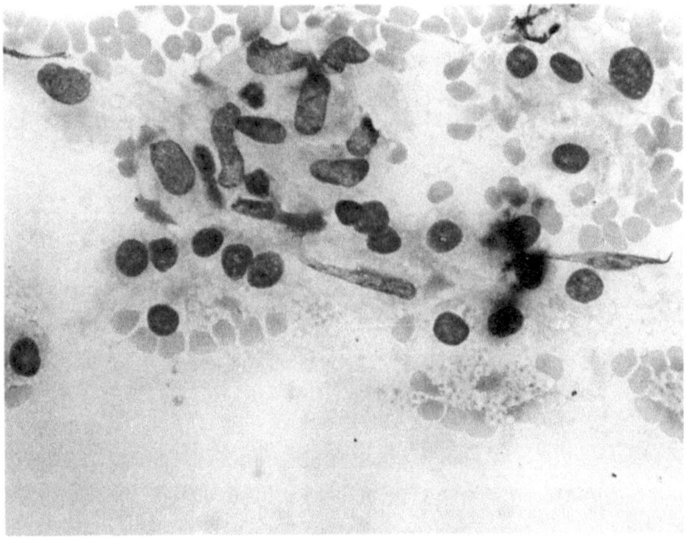

Case II:

1. Granulomateous thyroiditis with epitheloid cells

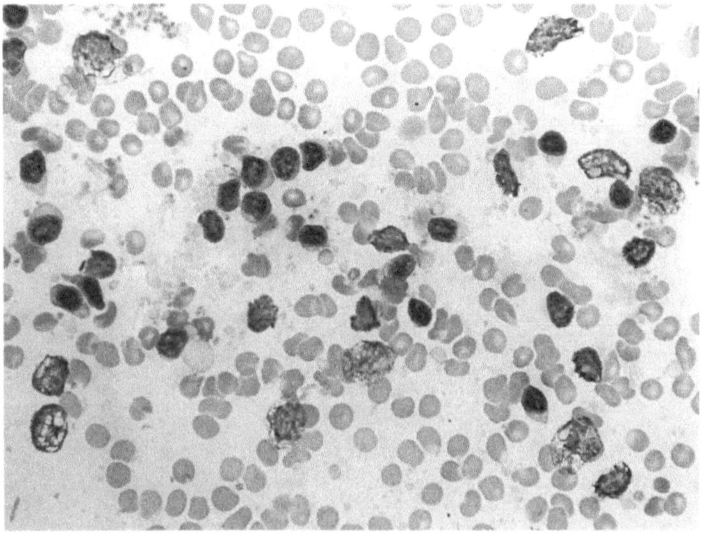

2. Concentration of lymphoid cells and cell-lysis represent chronic-lymphocytic thyroiditis Hashimoto

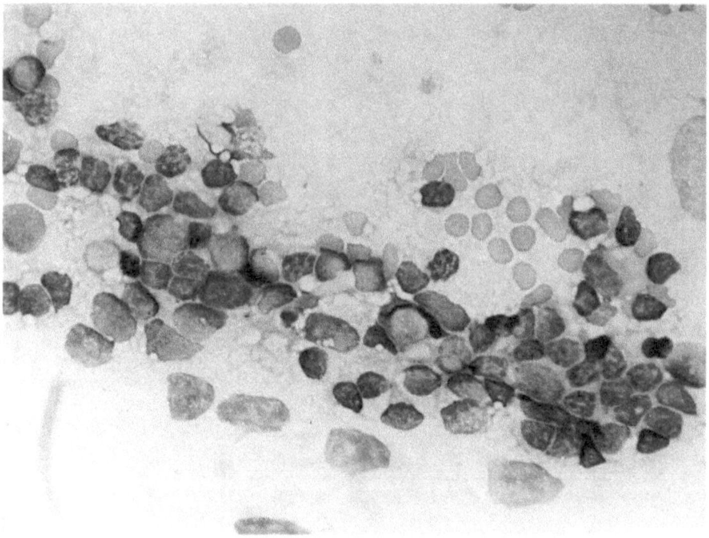

3. Control puncture one year after. Detritic cells and lymphoid cells representing thyroiditis Hashimoto. Cytologic parameter of thyroiditis de Quervain are not more visible

Conclusion

Presentation of rare cases of combined form of Hashimoto's and de Quervain's thyroiditis, cytological verified, leading to hypothyroidism.

Reference

1. Lenng, A.K., K. Hegde: J. Adolese Health Care **9** (1988), 434.

Occurrence of goitre and diffuse lymphoid thyroiditis (DLT) in secondary school adolescents in Bratislava

J. Podoba, P. Hnilica, M. Srbecký
Postgraduate Medical Institute, Bratislava, CSFR

Prophylaxis of endemic goitre by iodinated salt has been implemented in Czechoslovakia since 1947, resp. 1951. The original dose of KI was increased two times. Since 1965 common salt contains 25 mg KI/kg. This prophylactic measure has yielded remarkably good results /1-3/, nevertheless some authors in our country have recently argued for a more intensive prophylactic programme /4,5/. Similarly as in several other countries with iodine prophylaxis of endemic goitre /6-8/, the incidence of DLT keeps increasing also in the CSFR.

In light of these conditions we decided to establish the following parameters in adolescents aged 14.5. - 18 year in Bratislava: 1. occurrence rate of goitre by palpation and inspection; 2. mean thyroid volume ultrasonographically; 3. involvement rate of DLT in the occurrence of goitre.

Subjects and methods

Series 1:

Subjects: 358 boys (B), 360 girls (G) from five secondary schools in Bratislava.

Age: range 14.5 - 18 years, mean 16.1 y (B), 16.1 y (G), median 16.0 y (B), 16.0 y (G).

Body weight: mean 65.4 kg (B), 56.0 kg (G), median 65.0 kg (B), 56.0 kg (G).

Examination methods: inspection, palpation, ultrasonography.

USG equipment used: real time grey scale scanners using 7, 7.5 and 10 MHz transducers.

Series 2:

Subjects: 13 boys and 44 girls - outpatients with Gr. I goitre.

Age: same as in series 1.

Examination methods: inspection, palpation, fine needle biopsy.

Definition and classification of goitre (Perez et al., WHO 1960, modified according to Delange /9/).

Gr. 0 - goitre absent
- 0a - thyroid not palpable
- 0b - thyroid palpable, but lobes not exceeding the size of the terminal phalanx of the thumb in the subject examined

Gr. I - goitre palpable, not visible at normal position of the neck
- Ia - not visible at hyperextended neck
- Ib - visible at hyperextended neck

Gr. II - goitre visible at normal position of the neck
- III - very large goitre, visible from the distance of 10 m

Volume of the thyroid was calculated according to Brunn et al. /10/. DLT diagnosis was established by means of aspiration cytodiagnostics (criteria according to Persson). Fine needle biopsy was performed only in patients with Gr. I goitre.

Results

Tables 1a, 1b give the results of prevalence of goitre and thyroid volume parameters in adolescents, In boys goitre was found in 2.0 %, palpable thyroid not meeting the criteria to be classified as goitre in 21.5 % (Gr. 0b). The mean thyroid volume was 11.2 ml, the mean relative thyroid volume 0.17 ml/kg. In girls goitre was identified in 11.2 % of the series 1, palpable thyroid not classified as goitre in 26.5 % (Gr. 0b). The mean thyroid volume was 8.4 ml, the mean relative thyroid volume 0.15 ml/kg. The mean relative thyroid volume was statistically significant higher in boys compared to girls ($p < 0.001$). In both sexes a positive correlation was established between thyroid volume and body weight.

Table 1a: Prevalence of goitre and thyroid volume parameters in male adolescents

Boys n = 358

Diffuse goitre gr (palp.)	Occurrence rate (%)	thyroid volume (ml) median	mean	s	mean relative thyroid volume (ml/kg)
0a	76.5	10.7	11.0	0.2	0.17
0b	21.5	11.1	11.6	0.5	0.17
Ia	1.4) 2.0	13.3	13.1	1.7	0.19
Ib	0.6)	17.1	17.1	0.1	0.26

mean thyroid volume 11.2 ± 0.2 ml
mean relative thyroid volume 0.17 ± 0.02 ml/kg
No case of diffuse goitre gr II or III nor of nodular goitre was detected.

Table 1b: Prevalence of goitre and thyroid volume parameters in female adolescents

Girls n = 360

Diffuse goitre gr (palp)	Occurrence rate (%)	thyroid volume (ml) median	mean	s	mean relative thyroid volume (ml/kg)
0a	62.2	7.7	8.0	0.2	0.14
0b	26.6	8.2	8.6	0.3	0.16
Ia	6.4) 11.1	8.8	9.2	0.7	0.17
Ib	4.7)	9.6	11.4	1.0	0.21

mean thyroid volume 8.4 ± 0.1 ml
mean relative thyroid volume 0.15 ± 0.02 ml/kg
A single case of diffuse goitre gr II was recordered, no case of gr III or nodular goitre was detected.

Fine needle biopsy and cytologic examination was performed in 57 outpatients (aged 14.5 - 18 y) with gr. I diffuse goitre (table 2). Of the 13 boys examined DLT was established in 5 (38 %) and of the 44 girls in 25 (56.8 %). From the prevalence of gr. I goitre in series 1 and from the DLT ratio in series 2 the minimal occurrence rate of DLT in the population of adolescents aged 14.5. - 18 years was calculated to be 0.8 % in boys and 6.3 % in girls.

Discussion and conclusion

In the period of last 20 years of iodine prophylaxis only sporadic locally orientated epidemiologic studies were carried out assessing the prevalence of goitre in adolescents in CSFR /4,5/. The authors reported a 24 - 40.7 % prevalence of gr. I goitre in children and adolescents in original endemic areas and argued for a more intensive prophylactic programme. On using the classification according to Perez et al. (WHO 1960), our results proved to be more optimistic. While in adolescent girls the prevalence of goitre was still to be classified as endemic, boys exhibited only minimal occurrence rate. The finding of a statistically significant higher mean relative thyroid volume in boys compared to girls was however surprising. On considering the higher food intake (and perhaps relatively increased iodine supply) in boys this finding might be accounted for by the presence of some new as yet unknown nutritional goitrogens. In adolescent girls DLT proved to have a high occurrence: minimally 6.3 % of the given subpopulation is affected. The involvement of both genetic and potential environmental factors in the ethiopathogenesis of DLT should be investigated.

Table 2: Results of fine needle biopsy and cytologic examination in series 2 of 57 outpatients with diffuse goitre gr. I

Boys		Girls	
Total	13	Total	44
DLT	5 (38 %)	DLT	25 (56.8 %)

References

1. Podoba, J., R. Śtukovský: Acta endocr. panamer. **3** (1972), 1935. - 2. Podoba, J., R. Reisenauer: In: Schilddrüse 1981 (Eds. Scriba, P.C., K.H. Rudorff, B. Weinheimer), Stuttgart, Thieme Verlag, 1982, 239. - 3. Gutekunst, R., P.C. Scriba: J. Endocrinol. Invest. **12** (1989), 209. - 4. Felt, V., J. Křemenova, J. Bednár: Exp. Clin. Endocrinol. **86** (1985),207. - 5. Tajtáková, M. et al.: Klin. Wochenschr. **66** (1988), 749. - 6. Jensch, E. et al.: Dt. med. Wochenschr. **104** (1979), 838. - 7. Stubbe, P. et al.: Münch. Med. Wochenschr. **126** (1985), 857. - 8. Mäenpää, J. et al.: J. Pediatr. **107** (1985), 869. - 9. Thilly, C.H. et al.: In: Endemic Goiter and Endemic Cretinism (Eds. Stanbury, J.B., B.S. Hetzel), NY, J. Wiley, 1980, 155. - 10. Brunn, J. et al.: Dt. med. Wochenschr. **106** (1981), 1338.

Spontaneous course of Graves' Basedow's disease into hypothyroidism (case report)

Eva Deckart
Klinikum Berlin-Buch, Clinic for Nuclear Medicine and Endocrinology

A 50 years old woman suffered from an acute virus-infection in July 1989. After reconvalescence symptoms as tachycardia, tremor, arthralgia persisted.

Clinical examination: At her first visit in our outpatient department she demonstrated typical symptoms of severe thyrotoxicosis with general weakness, loss of concentration ability. No signs of endocrine-immunogenic orbito- or dermatopathy.

The diagnosis of an immunogenic hyperthyroidism was verified by high pertechnetate uptake in normally sized thyroid gland, a diffuse echopoor pattern in thyroid ultrasound, an increase of TRAK and pathologic hormone parameters (table, figure 1).

The patient was treated with low doses of Methimazole (15 mg/d at onset, rapidly decreased to 2.5 mg/d).

10 weeks later recurrence of hyperthyroidism occured, treated symptomatically with ß-blocking agent. Signs of beginning cardial decompensation initiated again Methimazole treatment beginning with 5 mg/d reduced to 2.5 mg/d. Further self-treatment without physician's consultation up to November, 1990. Again she visited the outpatient department in a state of severe hypothyroidism: At that time scintigraphy control showed no pertechnetate thyroid uptake at all. In ultrasound the diffuse echopoor pattern at onset had changed into homogeneous echonormal tissue characterization without loss of thyroid size (figure 2).

Table: Course of hormone and immune parameter

Date	TT_3 nmol/l	TT_4 nmol/l	TSH mU/l	MAK	TAK mg/l	TRAK U/l	Therapy
VII/89	6.5	240	< 0.4	1: 6400	neg.	54	
11.09.89	4.5	259	0.5				15 mg Methimazol
28.09.89	1.1	13	17	1: 400	neg.		5 mg " "
17.10.89	2.2	69	22				2.5 mg " "
17.01.90	5.1	108	< 0.4				Ø Therapy
14.03.90	5.1	192	< 0.4	1: 1600	neg.		"
27.04.90	5.6	160	< 0.4	1: 25600	neg.		5 mg Methimazol
29.11.90	0.9	23	39				" "
10.01.91	0.4	< 14	80	1:102400	neg.	< 405	since 18.12.90
24.01.91	2.9	39	45			< 405	no Therapy
18.02.91	2.6	170	0.5				125 L-Thyroxin

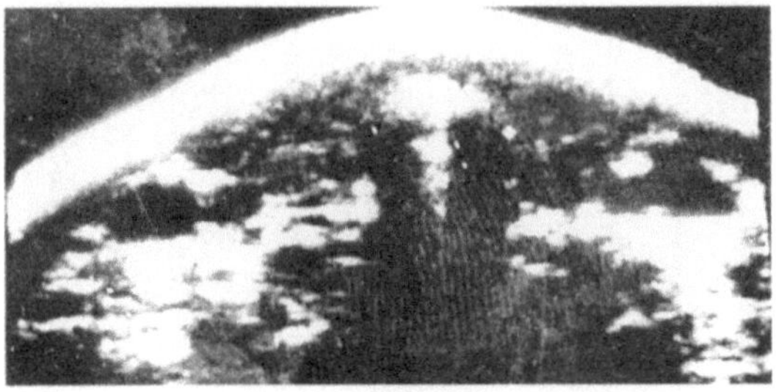

Figure 1a

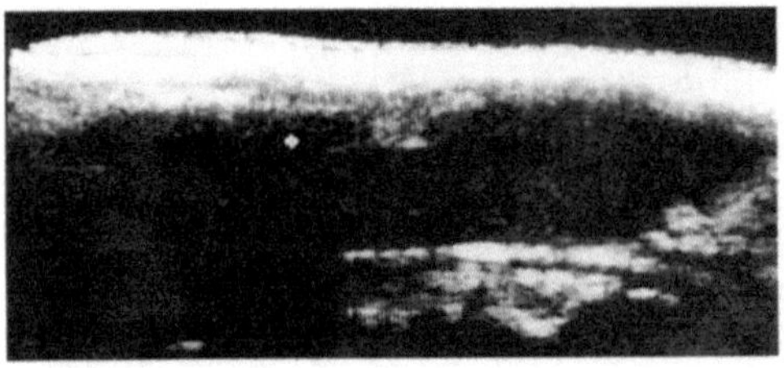

Figure 1b

Figure 1: Diffuse echopoor pattern, July 1989. Hyperthyroidism

a) transverse section

b) longitudinal section of left lobe

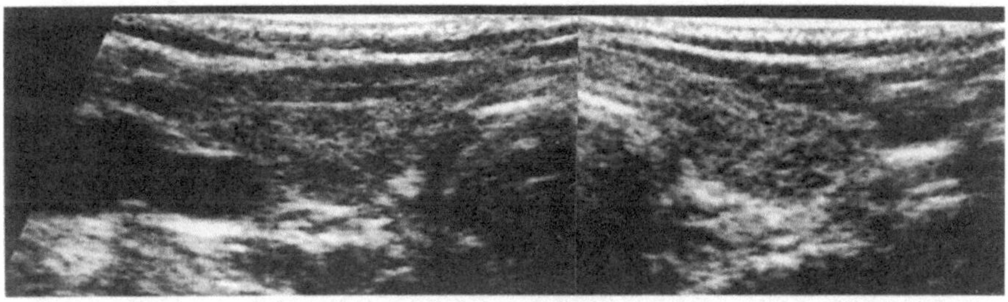

Figure 2a

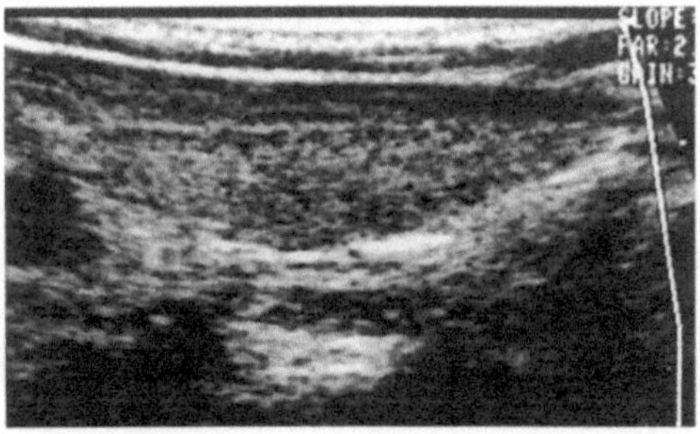

Figure 2b

Figure 2: Homogeneous echonormal structure, November 1990; hypothyroidism

a) transversal

b) longitudinal section

Discussion

The rapid change of immunogenic hyperthyroidism into hypothyroidism after only short time effect of thyrostatic drug is an example of self perpetuing character of Graves'-Basedow's disease. The enormous increase of thyroid stimulating/blocking antibodies (TRAK assay: 54 U/l (July 90) to above 405 U/l (January 91) within 5 months) may give the explanation: An increase of thyroid blocking antibodies (methodically not to be differentiated from stimulating immunoglobulins by TRAK assay) has caused hypothyroidism.

A similar case was newly reported by Tamai et al. /1/: According to their experience those cases have to be carefully followed-up, because as thyroid hormone substitution has to be adapted as thyroid-blocking activity can decrease by time and even recurrence of hyperthyroidism may be possible.
Another explanation might be the overwhelming of tissue destructive immunogenic process into hypothyroidism: in this situation a definite persisting hypothyroidism would be induced.
This example may be supported by another report /2/, in which in 4 of 5 similar cases cytologically chronic lymphocytic thyroiditis Hashimoto and in one case rheumatoid arthritis showed the coexistence of two autoimmune processes with tissue destructive character.
In contrast to these observations the opposite development can occur: initial hypothyroidism can change into transient or even persisting immunogenic hyperthyroidism - as Takasu et al. /3/ have reported. The development of thyroid stimulating antibodies accompanied hyperthyroidism in 7 cases (blocking antibodies negative), while in another patient the presence of thyroid stimulating - blocking antibodies prevented change from hypo- to hyperthyroid state.

References

1. Tamai, H., K. Kasagi, T. Hara et al.: Endocrinol. **33** (1990), 699. - 2. Serafinov, N., Nina Simova, I. Tadzer: Endocrin. Iugoslav. **11** (1988), 89. - 3. Takasu, N., T. Yamada, A. Sato et al.: Clin. Endocrinol. **33** (1990), 687.

Epidemiology, clinical syndrome, follow up, and prognostic factors in medullary carcinoma

Friedhelm Raue and the MTC Study Group*
Medizinische Universitätsklinik Heidelberg,
Heidelberg, Germany

Medullary thyroid carcinoma (MTC) is a malignancy of the thyroid parafollicular or calcitonin producing cells (C-cells) /1/. It exists in two forms: sporadic and hereditary (table 1). The hereditary form is one component of the multiple endocrine neoplasia type 2 syndrome (MEN 2) which is divided into the variant MEN 2a consisting of MTC, pheochromocytoma and parathyroid tumor and the variant MEN 2b consisting of MTC, pheochromocytoma, mucosal neuromata, and a marfanoid body habitus /2,3/. A third hereditary variety of MTC is the non-MEN familial MTC, a hereditary MTC without any other endocrinopathies . 32 years after the first description of MTC by Hazard, 1959 /4/ pathological and chemical techniques allow a save discrimination of MTC from other thyroid cancers. This neoplasm has distinct characteristics that separate it from malignancies of the follicular epithelium and make it necessary to discuss this tumor as a separate entity. MTC is highlighted by the fact that it:

---

*Members of the German MTC Study Group are: Prof. Bay, Hamburg, Prof. Becker, Erlangen, Prof. Benker and Prof. Reinwein, Essen, Prof. Buhr, Heidelberg, Dr. Dorn, München, Dr. Frilling and Prof. Röher, Düsseldorf, Prof. Heinze, Karlsruhe, Dr. Heissen, Mühlheim, Prof. Herrmann, Bielefeld, Prof. Höfer, Wien, Dr. Hornig, Münster, Prof. Klempa, Bremen, Dr. Kotzerke and Prof. Dralle, Hannover, Dr. Langer, Homburg/Saar, PD Dr. Neumann, Freiburg, Dr. Passath, Graz, Prof. Pfannenstiel, Wiesbaden, PD Dr. Raue and Prof. Ziegler, Heidelberg, Dr. Ritter, München, Prof. Schober,Münster, Prof. Schröder, Hamburg, Prof. Seif, Tübingen, PD Dr. Stracke, Gießen, Dr. Vogt, Augsburg, Prof. Wahl, Frankfurt, Dr. Winter and Prof. Trede, Mannheim, Prof.Zabaransky,Homburg/S.

- secrets calcitonin (important tumor marker),
- does not trap iodine (therapeutic implication),
- has a hereditary variety (screening program),
- is associated with other endocrine tumors (diagnostic and therapeutic implication).

Table 1: Varieties of medullary thyroid carcinoma

	% of all MTC cases	
sporadic (non-hereditary) MTC	75	
familial (hereditary) MTC	25	
- MEN IIa	-	15
- MEN IIb	-	3
- only MTC	-	6

*Data from the Registry German MTC Study Group /14,15/, n = 600

Epidemiology

The estimated proportion of MTC among all malignant tumors of the thyroid varied between 3 and 9 % /-12/. There have been only few investigations of the incidence rate in a defined population /8,12/. A population-based study of MTC in Sweden based in annual obligatory reports given by physicians and pathologists to the National Cancer Registry revealed that MTC constituted 5.2 % of all reported thyroid carcinomas with an overall age-standardized incidence rate per 105 inhabitants of 0.21 and of 0.1 in Norway. The lower incidence in Norway reported 1977 /8/ might have been caused by missing cases and therefore underestimating the real incidence. Family screening with the tumor marker calcitonin and genetic linkage studies had led to an increase in diagnosis of early cases /11,12/. These familial cases will represent an increasing fraction of patients with MTC, about 25 % in recently done studies /10,13,14/. Based on the better diagnostic criteria within the last three decade the overall incidence of MTC have increased as well as the distribution of the different varieties of MTC have changed to the more hereditary cases with better prognosis. Among the hereditary MTC MEN 2a is the most frequent syndrom (15 %) followed by the only MTC. A rare minority of patients suffered from MEN 2b syndrome (table 1, data from the German MTC registry /14, 15/). The female to male ratio varied between 1.4 to 1 /6/ to 1.06 to 1 /10/. The age of all patients at diagnosis of MTC varied from 9 months to 83 years with an average in the fifth decade, familial MTC is diagnosed earlier with a highest incidence in the third decade for MEN 2a and only MTC while MEN 2b is diagnosed in the second decade.

Clinical syndrome

There are three major types of clinical presentation for MTC. More than 50 % of MTC will be diagnosed as a result of evaluation for a thyroid nodule found incidentally during routine examination or metastatic carcinoma with an unknown primary source /1,10/. In the majority of patients with MTC the presenting symptomes and clinical findings are non specific and do not differ from those of other thyroid tumors. The only clinical feature that may lead clinicians to suspect MTC are the presence of hormone mediated diarrhoea especially in patients with wide spread tumor. A small percentage will be identified as a result of family screening for MEN 2a. The least common but most distinctive presentation is the clinical syndrome of MTC mucosal neuromata and marfanoid body habitus classified as MEN 2b /16,17/.

The current recommendation for screening family members at risk for hereditary MTC include the performance of a pentagastrin test (0.5 /ug intravenous pentagastrin per kilogram body weight with measurement of CT before and 2 and 5 minutes

after injection). This should be done systematically in all family members of a apparently sporadic MTC, as a negative family history in a patient presenting with MTC is not reliable in excluding familial disease /12/. This is because of the relatively low clinical penetrance of MEN 2a as only 40 % of gene carriers in known families will have presented clinically by the age of 50. There has been sustained progress towards the identification of the gene for MEN 2. Closely linked and flanking DNA markers have been identified, and it is now possible to assign gene carier states in informative families at risk with high percentage certainly by the use of molecular genetic technique /18-20/.
Before operating the MTC in MEN 2 patients an often bilateral pheochromocytoma has to be excluded or diagnosed by urinary and serum catecholamine screening. The sensitivity of the screening process can be improved by radioisotope scanning with MIBG.
Hyperparathyroidism is the last common manifestation of MEN 2. Periodic measurement of serum calcium concentration and if elevated intact PTH is probably adequate for screening process /1,2,21/.

Follow up

Perhaps the most difficult problem associated with the management of MTC is what to do with the patient who has a persistant elevation of serum CT concentration after an apparently adequate surgical procedure (figure 1). The first question to be considered is the adequacy of the primary surgical procedure (total thyroidectomy?, central neck dissection?, lateral lymph nodes examined for the presence of metastases?). Prior to reoperation a thorough evaluation should be done to define the extent of local and distant metastases disease /22,23/. Ultrasound of neck and liver, computerized tomography or MR imaging techniques of neck, chest and abdomen and selective venous catheterization with blood sampling for calcitonin determination are advocated. These procedure provide an anatomic region for the surgeon to focus upon and to exclude surgery as a treatment modality in patients in whom wide spread metastatic disease is found.

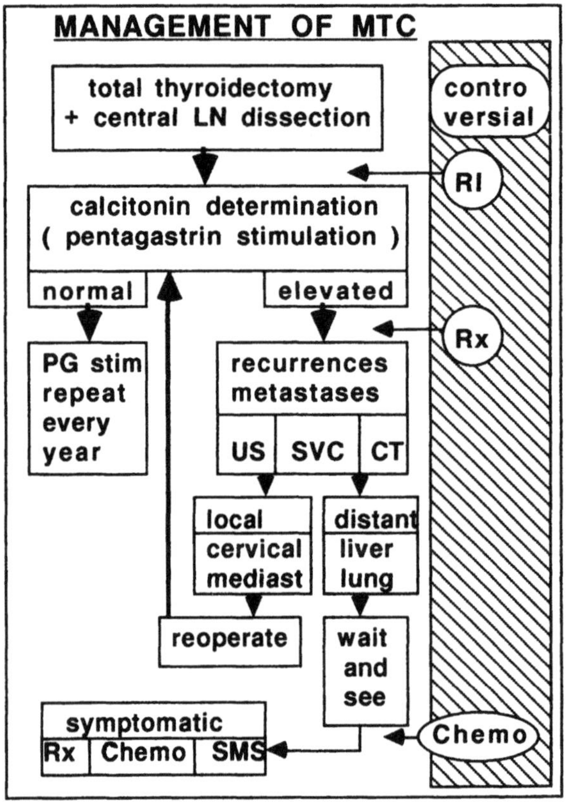

Figure 1

Management of medullary thyroid carcinoma. Abbreviations: LN = lymph node, PG = pentagastrin, US = ultrasound, SVC = selective venous catheterization, CT = computerized tomography, Rx = external radiotherapy, chemo = chemotherapy, RI = radioactive iodine therapy

The experience with other therapeutic modalities in the management of metastatic MTC has been disappointing as prophylactic external radiation /24/, radioactive iodine treatment /25/ or chemotherapy /26/.

Prognostic factors

The relative indolent clinical course of untreated MTC is likely to include progressive growth of the primary tumor, local (cervical, mediastinal) and distant (hepatic, pulmonary and bone) metastasis, and in a large percentage of cases (82 % in the German MTC Study Group /14,15/, deaths related to MTC. There is a general agreement that surgical management has favourably influenced the clinical course of the disease. The 5 and 10 years survival rates for all patients were 80 and 60 % (German MTC Study Group) and varied between 65-80 for 5 years and 25-67 for 10 years survival /4,7-10,14/. The most important factor that influenced the prognosis were the type and the stage of the disease. Patients with MEN 2a had a better survival rate than those with sporadic disease (5 years survival 77.5 % versus 87 %) while survival of patients with MEN 2b does not differ from patients with sporadic MTC.

The stage of the disease at presentation is another major prognostic factor, patients with stage I have a 100 % survival after 5 years in contrast to 75 % for patients with state IV (figure 2). The involvement of cervical lymph nodes is correlated with the probability of distant metastases and local recurrence. Patients younger than 40 years old at the time of diagnosis of MTC had a better survival than those who were older, also women have a better prognosis than men. This might be probably due to the better clinical stage depending on earlier diagnosis in women and younger patients, indicating that the stage of the disease at diagnosis was a more important prognostic factor than sex and age /13/. Diarrhoea as a bad prognostic sign is more commonly in patients with advanced disease and its presence may reflect the presence of a large tumor mass. The type of treatment was not a significant prognostic factor, especially external radiotherapy, radioactive iodine therapy and chemotherapy. The type of surgery did not influence the survival but patients had total thyroidectomy and modified neck dissection have lower incidences of recurrences.

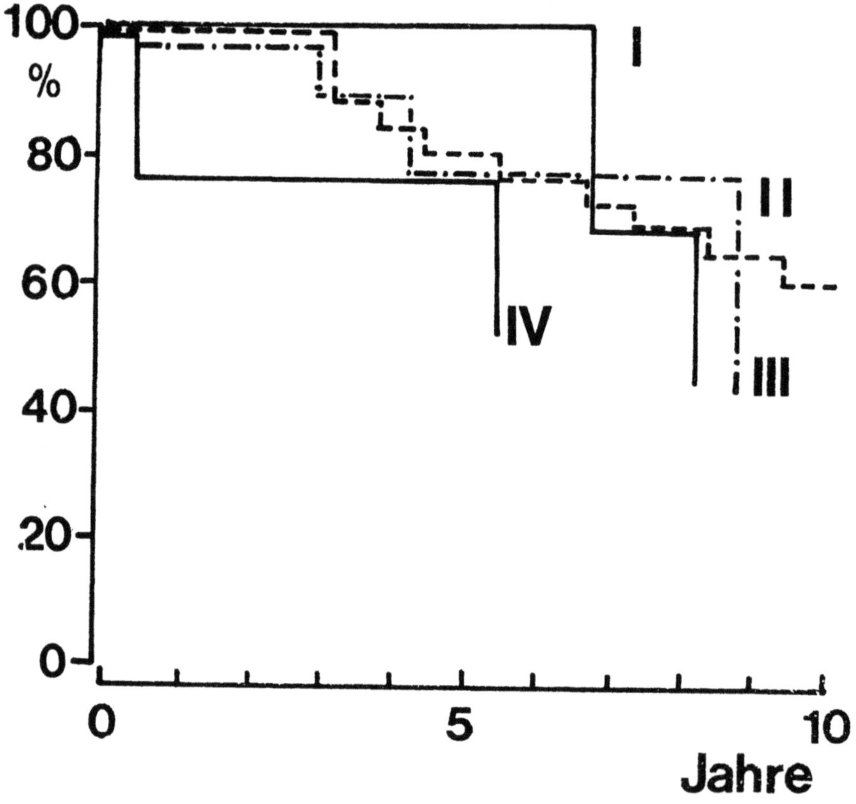

Figure 2

Survival curves for patients presenting with different stages of MTC (stage I = tumor localized to the thyroid gland, stage II = tumor localized to the thyroid gland and movable regional lymph nodes, stage III = direct local invasion or fixed cervical lymph nodes, stage IV = distant metastases)

References

1. Grauer, A., F. Raue, R.F. Gagel: Endocr. Metab. North Am. **19** (1990), 613. - 2. Raue, R., R.F. Gagel: Endokrinologie, Innere Medizin der Gegenwart. Band 5, Hrgb. R.D. Hesch, Urban und Schwarzenberg Verlag, München (1989), S. 1109. - 3. Raue, F, R. Ziegler: Endokrinologie, Innere Medizin der Gegenwart. Band 5, Hrgb. R.D. Hesch, Urban und Schwarzenberg Verlag, München (1989), S. 1073. - 4. Hazard, J.B., W.A. Hawk, G. Crile: J. Clin. Endocrinol. **19** (1959), 152. - 5. Fletcher, J.R.: Archievs of Surgery **100**(1970), 257. - 6. Hill, C.S., M.L. Ibanez, N.A. Samaan, M.J. Ahearn, R.L. Clark: Medicine **52** (1973), 141. - 7. Chong, G.C., O.H. Beahr, L.H. Woolner: Cancer **35** (1975), 695. - 8. Norman, T.: Acta Pathol. Microbiol. Scand. (A) **85** (1977), 775. - 9. Rossi, R.L., B. Cady, W.A. Meissner, M.S. Wool, C.E. Sedgewick, J. Werber: Am. J. Surg. **139** (1980), 554. - 10. Saad, M.F., N.G. Ordonez, R.K. Rashid, J.J. Guido, C.S. Hill, R.C. Hickey, N.A. Samaan: Medicine **63** (1984), 319. - 11. Calmettes, C., A. Chaventre, N. Feingold, B. Franc, J.M. Guliana: Henry Ford Hosp. Med. J. **37** (1989), 120. - 12. Ponder, B.A.J., N. Finer, R. Coffey, C.L. Harmer, M. Maisey, M.G. Ormerod, M.E. Pembrey, M.A. Ponder, P. Rosswick, Shalet: Quart. J. Med. **67** (1988), 299. - 13. Bergholm, U., H.O. Adami, R. Bergström, H. Johansson, G. Lundell, M. Telenius-Berg, G. Akerström: Cancer **63** (1989), 1196. - 14. Raue F., M. Späth-Röger, J. Winter, G. Benker, P. Buhr, R. Dorn, H. Dralle, A. Frilling, J. Herrmann, I. Hornig, H. Meybier, I. Klempa, J. Kotzerke, P. Pfannenstiel, D. Reinwein, M. Ritter, H.D. Röher, O. Schober, S. Schröder, F. Seif, M. Trede, H. Vogt, R. Wahl, R. Ziegler: Med. Klinik **85** (1990), 113. - 15. Kohlwagen, R., F. Raue, J. Winter: Acta Endocr. **124** (1991), Suppl. 1, Abstr. 7. - 16. Frank, K., f. Raue, J. Gottswinter, U. Heinrich, H. Meybier, R. Ziegler: Europ. J. Pediatr. **143** (1984), 112. -17. Raue, F.: Dt. med. Wochenschr. **110** (1985), 1334. - 18. Gagel, R.F.: Trend Endocr. Metab. **2** (1991), 19. -19. Mathew, C.G.P., D.F. Easton,

Y. Nakamura, B.A.J. Ponder: Lancet **I** (1991), 7. - 20. Sobol, H., S.A. Narod, Y. Nakamura: N. Engl. J. Med. **321** (1989), 996. - 21. Raue, F.: Dt. med. Wochenschr. **110** (1985), 1337. - 22. Frank, K., F. Raue, D. Lorenz, Ch. Herfarth, R. Ziegler: Henry Ford Hosp. Med. J. **35** (1987), 122. - 23. Raue, F., J. Winter, K. Frank-Raue, D. Lorenz, Ch. Herfarth, R. Ziegler: Horm. Metab. Res. Suppl. **21** (1989), 31. - 24. Samaan, N.A., P.N. Schultz, L.R. Hickey: J. Clin. Endocrinol. Metab. **67** (1988), 801. - 25. Saad, M.F., J.J. Guido, N.A. Samaan: J. Clin. Endocrinol. Metab. **57** (1983), 124. -26. Scherübl, H., F. Raue, R. Ziegler: Onkologie **13** (1990), 198.

Discussion

Szybinski:

- How is the sensitivity and role of fine needle biopsy in early diagnosis of medullary thyroid cancer?
- How is the sensitivity of pentagastrin test in comparison to calcium infusion test in early diagnosis of MTC?
- How is the percentage of MTC in total thyroid malignancies in Germany?
- Did you observe uneven distribution of medullary thyroid cancer (MTC) in terms of rural and urban areas in Germany?

Raue: The incidence on popular base is a problem, in Germany we have no register for cancer. So it can be only calculated from the national registry we have in some countries, in the Saarland and in Hamburg. From these data we can calculate how it looks in whole Germany. There are about 2000 new cases of thyroid cancer may be calculated. You see that about 50 new cases of medullary thyroid carcinoma are reported by the centers. If you look for big studies, for instance the group of Reinwein and Benker in Essen, who had about 1000 patients with thyroid cancers and they have an incidence of about 6 or 7 % of MTC in that and I think thats an impressive percentage.

The clinical presentation does not differ from other different thyroid cancers, so as in other thyroid cancers you do a fine needle biopsy if you have a cold nodule with a low echogenetity in ultrasound and then perhaps if you have a good pathologist he will do the diagnosis medullary thyroid carcinoma before operation. But in the most of the cases the diagnosis in sporadic cases is done after the operation. In familiar cases the pentagastrin stimulation test is the best method because you don't see any at the time when the test is pathologic. That is the only thing and the surgeon has to beleve that you are right and he has to do a total thyroidectomy.

The distribution is a problem as we don't know all the cases of medullary thyroid carcinoma it depends on the center which reported to us. There is an increasing number of familiar cases starting with this project, telling people doing the screening and so on. It depend on the doctor who is interested in this. But if we add all together, we get about 25 % of familiar cases. And from our data we can not look for urban regions or the countryside if there is difference in these distribution.

We think that the pentagastrin test is the most sensitive test, we have done calcium stimulation test and the increase in calcitonin is smaller if we use it. The side effects in pentagastrin test are tolerable.

Neradilova: Two short comments:

1. Our own modification of CT stimulation test is quickly for studying out-patients in medical practice: A one minute i.v. injection of 3-5 /ug calcium and simultaneously pentagastrin (Peptavlon) in a dose of 5-7 /ug/kg subcutaneously. And in 5 minutes we have the highest level of calcitonin. This test has been shown to be a reliable and well tolerable screening procedure for MTC (blood sample collection after 5 min. The elevation of CT is in this condition maximal.

2. Screening in family members should be made not only in familial but also in sporadic variants of MTC - incomplete expression of genetic information is very important in epidemiology of MTC.

Groth: I can give an answer to the question of Dr. Szybinski about the incidence of MTC: We have found an incidence of 1 per 100 000 inhabitants in the north of East Germany.
Raue: It is a very high incidence, because the data from the Swedish and Norwegian group say 0.1 per 100 000 in a year. Your results are tenfold more!
Limanova: May I ask you a question, if there are some special clinical signs in patients with medullary carcinoma, as we are performing fine needle biopsy to all solitary nodules, and we can not use a calcitonin screening (also to use calcitonin antibodies to smears from FNB), it would help to concentrate to patients only with special clinical signs.
Raue: The clinical sign is diarrhoea and it is only seen in an advanced stage of the disease. If you do the fine needle biopsy at this point, the patient has distant metastases. It does not differ from the other different thyroid cancer and as it is very rare we do not do screening of calcitonin in all patients with cold nodules. It is to expensive, we do it only if there is in fine needle biopsy a sign of possible medullary carcinoma.
There is no early diagnostic clinical sign for these patients.
Bergant: Can you tell me something about side - effects in your stimulation test?
Raue: In pentagastrin test within 30 seconds the patients started to crampling, abdominal pain, they got something like a flush. This has a duration about 30 seconds and then it is over. There is a problem with cancer families to give information to the patients. But when the patient is intelligent he says, I have a 50 % chance to get a cancer and there is a very sensitive test.
Deckart: Do you compare the intravenously and subcutaneously injection of pentagastrin? We only use the subcutaneous method as Dr. Neradilova and we have no problems with side effects.

Raue: I think the problem of subcutaneous method is the time interval. You got the maximum of calcitonin stimulation within two minutes after intervenous. And most of the european groups use the intravenous test. But the greater problem is to define normal ranges. Every group has to test, what is a normal test after pentagastrin injection.

Heberling: How often do you found a pheochromocytoma and hyperparathyroidism in patients with MEN?

Raue: In our 25 patients with MEN-A there are 5 patients with pheochromocytoma and one patient with a primary hyperparathyroidism. Thats relatively rare. And in the five MEN-2B patients there is one hyperparathyroidism and two pheochromocytomas. It depends on the observation time, I think some of them develop pheochromocytoma and we screen for it.

Neue Entwicklungen in der chirurgischen Therapie des Sipple-Syndroms: die Kompartment-orientierte systematische Mikrodissektion der Lymphknoten beim medullären Schilddrüsenkarzinom

H. Dralle, I. Damm, G.F.W. Scheumann
Klinik für Abdominal- und Transplantationschirurgie, Medizinische Hochschule Hannover, Germany

Die chirurgische Behandlung der Multiplen Endokrinen Neoplasie Typ 2A (Sipple-Syndrom) integriert die unterschiedlichen Strategien für die Therapie der synchron oder metachron auftretenden Erkrankung der C-Zelle und des Sympatho-adrenalen Systems. Während für die meist benigne Nebennierenmarkserkrankung in den letzten Jahren von vielen Zentren bevorzugt konservative, das heißt Nebennierenrinden-funktionserhaltende Behandlungsformen gewählt wurden /1/, stellt die C-Zell-Erkrankung der Schilddrüse den prognostisch entscheidenden Schrittmacher des genetischen Syndroms dar; zurückhaltende Operationsverfahren werden hierbei als onkologisch nicht ausreichend eingestuft. Letzteres betrifft vor allem das Ausmaß des chirurgischen Eingriffs an den regionalen Lymphknoten, deren metastatischer Befall das wesentliche prognostische Kriterium der Erkrankung darstellt /2,3/. Aufgrund operativer Ergebnisse nach sehr ausgedehnter cervicaler Lymphadenektomie /4/ ist die Mikrometastasierung, die selektiven oder symptomatischen Formen der Lymphadenektomie meist entgeht, als Ausgangspunkt für Tumorrezidive bzw. persistierende Hypercalcitoninaemien anzusehen.

Mit einer für dieses Krankheitsbild entwickelten Systematik einer Kompartment-orientierten Mikrodissektion der cervicalen und mediastinalen Lymphknoten /5/ haben wir seit 1986 33 Patienten operativ behandelt. Über die Ergebnisse dieser neuen chirurgischen Behandlungsmethode des sporadischen und familiären medullären Schilddrüsencarcinoms (MTC) soll im Vergleich mit den operativen Ergebnissen von 40 Patienten, die in den Jahren von 1970 bis 1986 unter Einsatz konventioneller Formen der Lymphadenektomie behandelt wurden, berichtet werden. Ziel der Arbeit ist es, in das möglicherweise unterschiedliche biologische Verhalten sporadischer und hereditärer medullärer Schilddrüsencarcinome neue Einblicke zu bekommen, die vor allem aus chirurgisch-therapeutischer Sicht von wesentlicher Bedeutung sein dürften.

Patientengut, Methoden

73 Patienten mit medullärem Schilddrüsencarcinom (49 sporadisch, 24 hereditär) wurden von 1970 bis 1990 in unserer Klinik operativ behandelt. Bis 1986 wurde bei primärem Lymphknotenbefall zusätzlich zur totalen Thyreoidektomie eine selektive Entfernung der befallenen Lymphknotengruppe en bloc mit umgebendem Fettgewebe durchgeführt (selektive oder symptomatische Lymphadenektomie). Seit 1986 erfolgt beim medullären Schilddrüsencarcinom unabhängig von der Pathogenese und Tumorgröße mit der totalen Thyreoidektomie eine systematische Lymphadenektomie des zentralen Lymphknoten-Kompartments (K 1a + b) und bei Tumoren über 1 cm Größe bzw. Befall der zentralen Lymphknoten eine systematische Lymphadenektomie der primärtumorseitigen lateralen Lymphknoten-Kompartimente (K 2 bzw. K 3, siehe Abbildung 1). Die systematische Lymphadenektomie besteht in der mikrochirurgischen Ausräumung des gesamten Lymphknoten-Fettbindegewebskompartimentes. Für die Ausräumung einer Halsseite wird durchschnittlich eine Operationszeit von ca. 4-5 Stunden benötigt.

Die Operationspräparate wurden nach Kompartimenten getrennt histologisch und immunhistochemisch hinsichtlich Anzahl der entfernten und der tumorbefallenen Lymphknoten aufgearbeitet. Die Tumoren wurden entsprechend der WHO-Klassifikation (1988) und TNM-Einteilung der UICC (1987) dokumentiert. Von allen Patienten wurden Nachsorgedaten erhoben und statistisch ausgewertet (BMDP und SAS Computerprogramm). Die Überlebenswahrscheinlichkeiten wurden nach Kaplan und Meier bzw. Mantel-Cox und Wilcoxon berechnet.

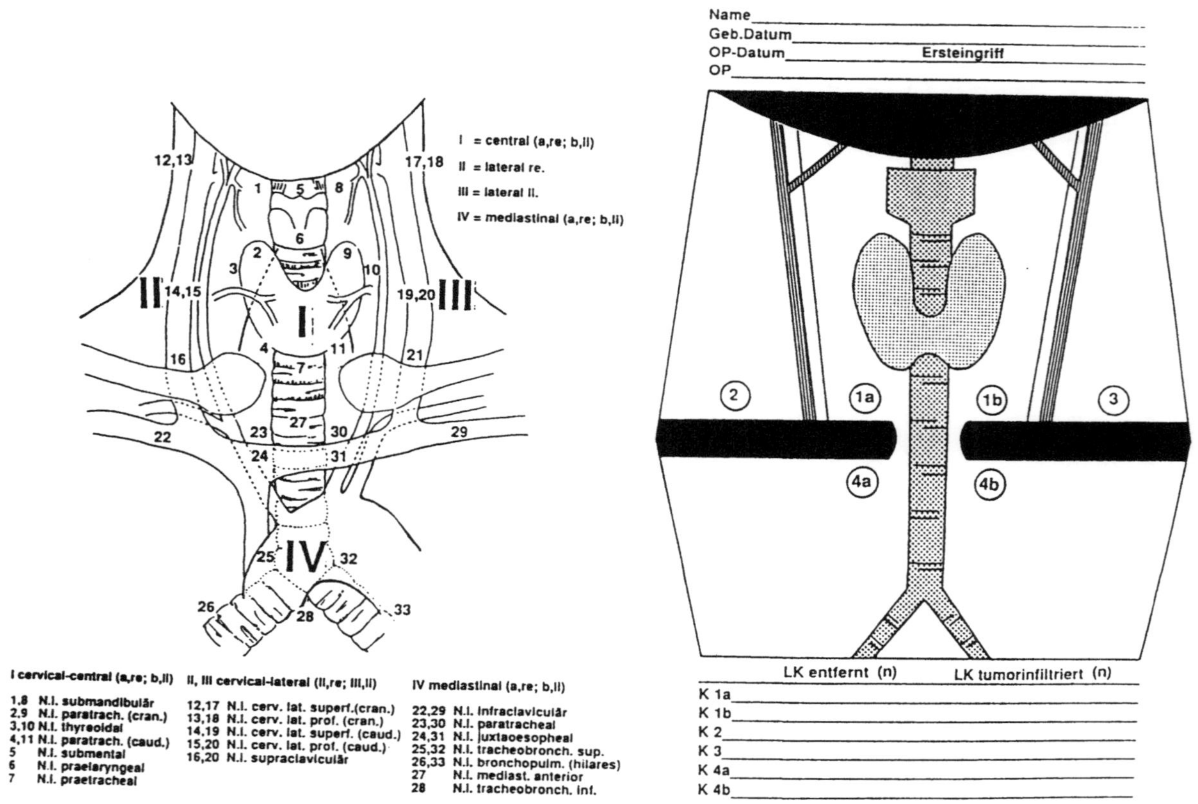

Abbildung 1

Schema der Kompartment-orientierten systematischen cercico-mediastinalen Lymphadenektomie beim medullären schilddrüsencarcinom. K 1-4, Kompartimente zentral (rechts, links paratracheal), lateral (rechtes bzw. linkes laterales Halsdreieck) und mediastinal

Sporadic MTC

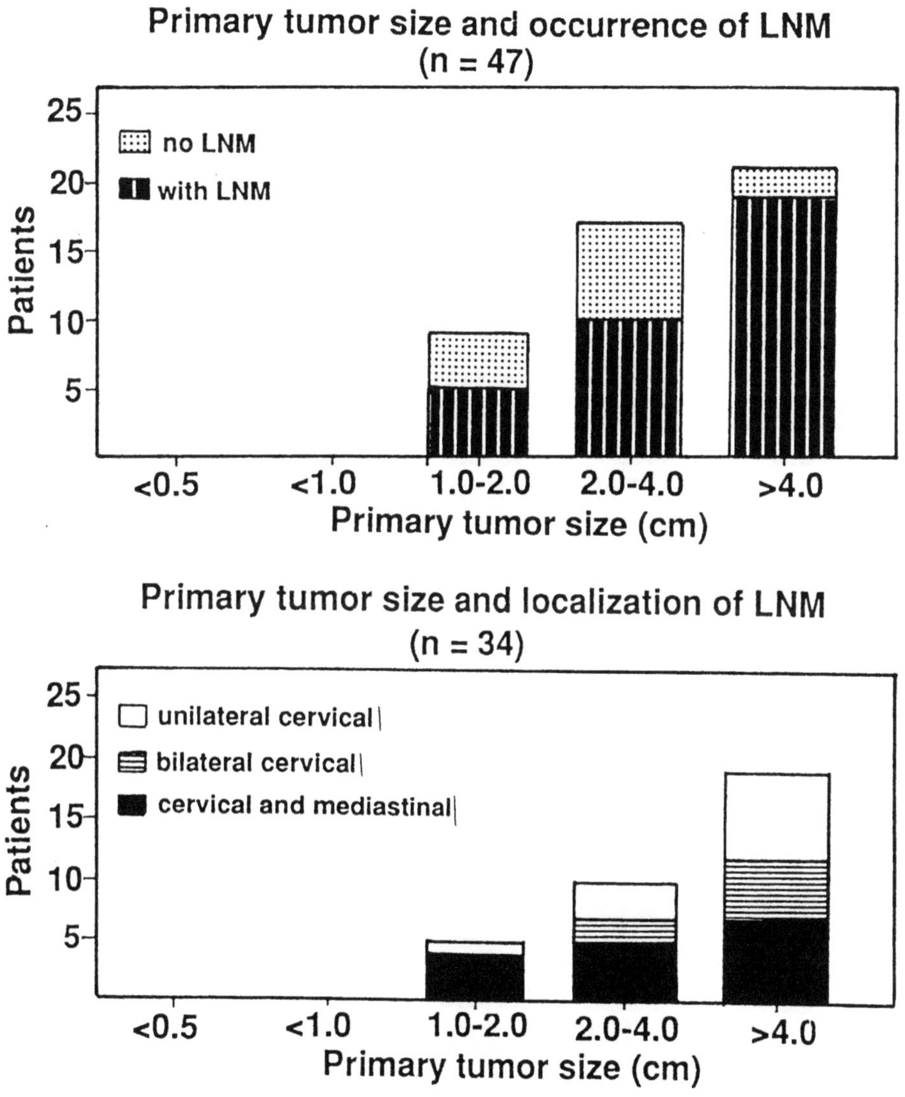

Abbildung 2
(a) Primärtumorgröße und Häufigkeit von Lymphknotenmetastasen beim sporadischen MTC
(b) Primärtumorgröße und Lokalisation regionaler Lymphknotenmetastasen beim sporadischen MTC

Familial MTC

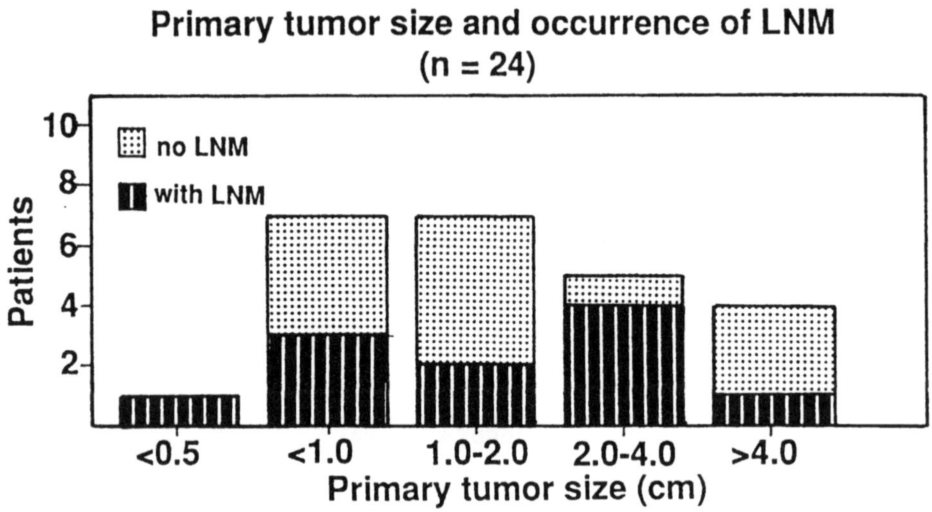

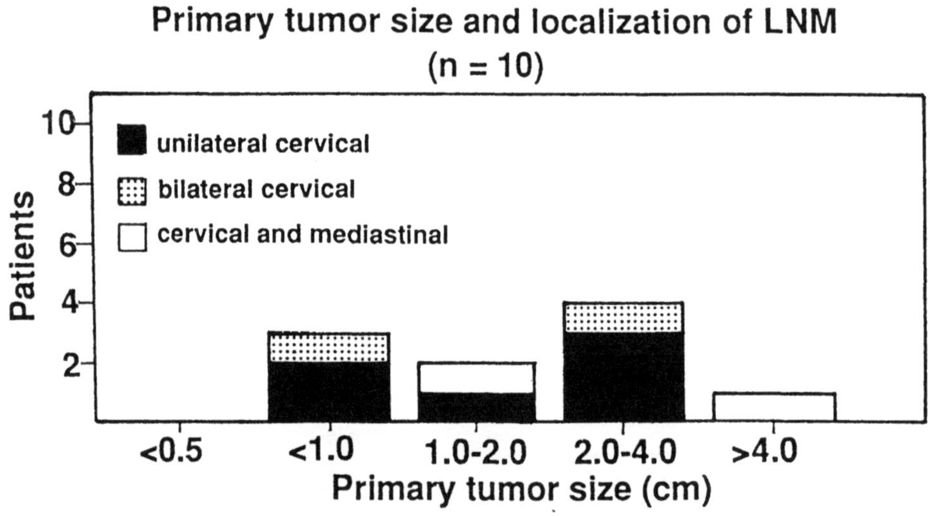

Abbildung 3
(a) Primärtumorgröße und Häufigkeit von Lymphknotenmetastasen beim familiären MTC
(b) Primärtumorgröße und Lokalisation regionaler Lymphknotenmetastasen beim familiären MTC

Systematic versus symptomatic lymphadenectomy in MTC
(MHH 1970 - 1990, n = 73)

Calcitonin

	syst. LA	sympt. LA
Primary patients [1]	22	16
LN removed	20.9 (1-63)	6.4 (1-22)
LNM	6.9 (0-37)	5.1 (0-17)
Calcitonin negativity [2]		
pT < 2.0 cm	9/10	0/ 3
pT 2.0-4.0 cm	5/ 7	1/ 3
pT > 4.0 cm	0/ 5	0/10

1) without reoperations 2) Pentagastrin-stimulated Calcitonin

Abbildung 4

(a) Anzahl der primär (beim Ersteingriff) entfernten und der tumorinfiltrierten Lymphknoten sowie postoperative Serum-Calcitonin-Konzentrationen nach Pentagastrin-Stimulation in Abhängigkeit von der Primärtumorgröße bei allen Patienten mit sporadischem und familiärem MTC. Vergleich der Ergebnisse nach systematischer versus symptomatischer Lymphadenektomie

Ergebnisse

Bei 22 Patienten wurde mit dem Ersteingriff, bei 11 Patienten mit dem Rezidiveingriff eine Kompartment-orientierte systematische Lymphadenektomie durchgeführt, bei den übrigen Patienten erfolgte die Lymphadenektomie als sogenannte selektive, symptomatische Lymphknotenentfernung. Die klinische und morphologische Auswertung der prae- und postoperativen Befunde führte zu folgenden Resultaten:

1. Es bestand keine Korrelation zwischen Primärtumorgröße und der Anzahl der primär aufgetretenen Lymphknotenmetastasen (R = 0,39). Insbesondere bei zwei Patienten mit einem MTC im Rahmen einer MEN 2b-Erkrankung fanden sich hohe Lymphknotenmetastasenzahlen bei kleiner Primärtumorgröße.

2. Das Vorkommen von regionalen Lymphknotenmetastasen korrelierte mit der Primärtumorgröße beim sporadischen, nicht jedoch beim hereditären MTC (Abbildungen 2a + 3a).

3. Bezüglich des Zusammenhangs von Primärtumorgröße und primärem Lymphknotenmetastasen-Status mit den peripheren Serum-Calcitonin-Konzentrationen konnte eine positive Korrelation der Serum-Calcitoninspiegel sowohl mit der Primärtumorgröße (R = 0,69) als auch mit der Anzahl der tumorbefallenen Lymphknoten (R = 0,67) nachgewiesen werden.

4. Die Analyse der Überlebenszeiten aller 73 MTC-Patienten ergab signifikante Unterschiede in der Überlebenswahrscheinlichkeit von Patienten ohne regionale Lymphknotenmetastasen gegenüber Patienten mit unilateralen oder bilateralen Halslymphknotenmetastasen oder Patienten mit mediastinalen Lymphknotenmetastasen (jeweils $p < 0,0001$ zwischen allen vier Gruppen).

5. Bei Patienten mit Primärtumoren von über 2 cm im Durchmesser fand sich eine ausgedehnte regionale Lymphknotenmetastasierung häufiger, wenn eine sporadische, als wenn eine hereditäre Tumorpathogenese vorlag (Abbildungen 2b + 3b).

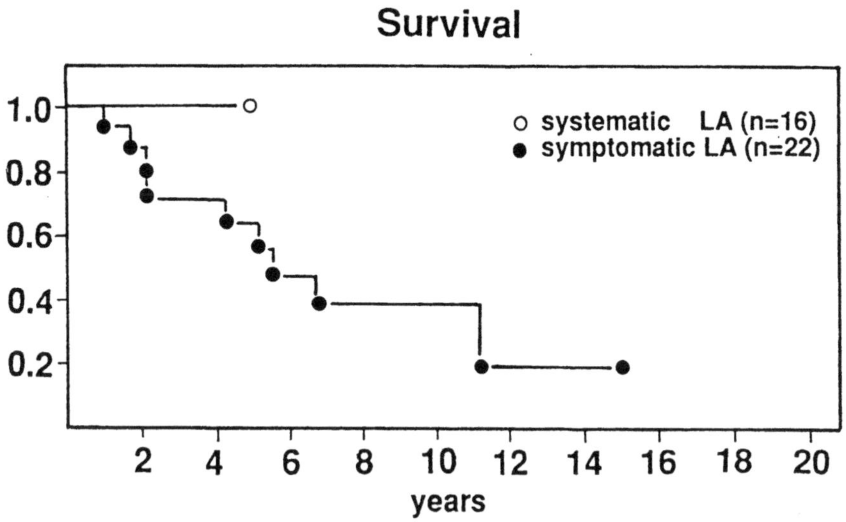

Abbildung 4

(b) Überlebenskurven von Patienten mit MTC nach systematischer versus symptomatischer Lymphadenektomie

6. Die Zahl der beim Ersteingriff chirurgisch entfernten Lymphknotenmetastasen war bei systematischer Lymphadenektomie deutlich höher als bei symptomatischer Lymphadenektommie. Die Anzahl der postoperativ Pentagastrin-stimuliert Calcitonin-negativen Patienten war nach systematischer Lymphadenektomie deutlich höher als nach symptomatischer Lymphadenektomie, wenn die Primärtumoren eine Größe unter 4 cm im Durchmesser aufwiesen. Kein Unterschied hinsichtlich der postoperativen Rate Calcitonin-negativer Resultate fand sich bei systematisch oder symptomatisch lymphadenektomierten Patienten mit Primärtumoren über 4 cm im Durchmesser (Abbildung 4a).

7. Die vorläufige Analyse der Überlebenswahrscheinlichkeiten von Patienten mit MTC ergibt einen deutlich positiveren Trend für systematisch lymphadenektomierte Patienten gegenüber solchen, bei denen lediglich eine symptomatische Lymphadenektomie durchgeführt wurde. Der Unterschied ist jedoch aufgrund der noch begrenzten Patientenzahl und Beobachtungszeit nicht signifikant (Abbildung 4b).

Diskussion und Schlußfolgerungen

Die systematische Kompartment-orientierte Mikrodissektion der regionalen Lymphabflußgebiete beim medullären Schilddrüsencarcinom stellt eine chirurgisch-onkologische Behandlungsform dar, die - wie bereits bei anderen Organtumoren gezeigt /6/ - zum einen bestmögliche Voraussetzungen zur tumortypspezifischen Analyse des Metastasierungsverhaltens und zur individuellen Bestimmung des Lymphknotenstatus (staging) schafft, zum anderen ohne wesentliche Erhöhung der chirurgisch bedingten Morbidität nicht nur eine höhere Erfolgsrate hinsichtlich der Tumorrezidiv- bzw. Tumorpersistenzrate erzielt, sondern wahrscheinlich auch eine deutliche Prognoseverbesserung zumindest bei Patienten mit primär begrenzt lymphogen metastasierten MTC erreichen kann. Ausgehend von den Ergebnissen zur postoperativen Calcitonin-Negativität, die Primärtumorgrößenabhängig keinen Effekt der systematischen Lymphadenektomie bei Tumoren über 4 cm im Durchmesser zeigte, ist zu vermuten, daß die systematische Lymphadenektomie als prognoseverbessernde chirurgische Maßnahme bei allen Patienten unter 4 cm im Durchmesser anzusehen ist, bei Primärtumoren über 4cm im Durchmesser diese chirurgisch-technisch und zeitlich aufwendige Technik jedoch keinen Vorteil gegenüber symptomatischen Formen der Lymphadenektomie erbringt. Die systematische Lymphadenektomie stellt damit beim medullären Schilddrüsencarcinom, und hier durchaus mit den Ergebnissen beim Magencarcinom vergleichbar /6/, einen Fortschritt in der Behandlung früher und mittlerer Tumorstadien dar; sie verbessert jedoch wahrscheinlich nicht die Prognose fortgeschrittener Tumorstadien.

Zusätzlich zu diesen primär therapeutischen Aspekten der systematischen Lymphadenektomie beginnt die morphologische Analyse der Lymphknoten-Gesamtkompartimente die Kenntnisse über das regionale Metastasierungsverhalten sporadischer und familiärer medullärer Schilddrüsencarcinome zu erweitern. So konnte gezeigt werden, daß familiäre MTC eine frühzeitigere cervicale, jedoch seltenere mediastinale Manifestation der Lymphknotenmetastasierung aufweisen. Hierbei ist auffällig, daß eine cervical-bilaterale Lymphknotenmetastasierung seltener ist, als von der thyreoidal-bilateralen Primärtumormanifestation beim familiären MTC hätte erwartet werden können. Welche Schlußfolgerungen hinsichtlich des generellen und individuellen chirurgischen Vorgehens insbesondere beim familiären MTC hieraus zu ziehen sind, ist derzeit noch nicht sicher zu formulieren; möglicherweise handelt es sich jedoch beim familiären MTC überwiegend um biologisch günstiger verlaufende Tumorformen des MTC, so daß bei diesen Patienten möglicherweise nicht in jedem Fall grundsätzlich eine bilateral-cervicale komplette Lymphknoten-Ausräumung aller drei Kompartimente erforderlich ist, sondern ein individuell von der Primärtumorgröße und dem primären Metastasierungsverhalten bestimmtes Ausmaß der systematischen Lymphadenektomie angezeigt ist.

Beim sporadischen medullären Schilddrüsencarcinom findet sich dagegen eine sehr deutliche Zunahme des Ausmaßes der regionalen Lymphknotenmetastasierung mit zunehmender Tumorgröße, so daß bei dieser Tumorform gerade auch bei makroskopischem Hinweis einer nur auf das zentrale Lymphknotenkompartment beschränkten Metastasierung grundsätzlich zusätzlich zur zentralen eine tumorseitige laterale systematische Lymphadenektomie vorgenommen werden sollte.

Der mediastinale Tumorbefall stellt bei beiden Formen des MTC ein prognostisch sehr ungünstiges Tumorstadium dar, das wahrscheinlich nicht durch mehr als symptomatische Tumorresektionen beeinflußbar ist.

Die vorliegenden Ergebnisse zeigen zusammenfassend, daß mit Hilfe der vorgestellten operativen Technik der systematischen Lymphadenektomie unter Erweiterung und Verfeinerung bisheriger Formen der selektiven bzw. symptomatischen Lymphadenektomie neue Einblicke in das Metastasierungsverhalten medullärer Schilddrüsencarcinome gewonnen werden konnten. Die Kompartment-orientierte systematische Lymphadenektomie wird als Standardverfahren zur Lymphknotendissektion empfohlen, da sie als wirksame Maßnahme zur Prophylaxe und Therapie einer möglicherweise Prognose-entscheidenden Mikrometastasierung dieser Erkrankung anzusehen ist. Weitere Untersuchungen sollen zeigen, ob ein Tumortyp- und Tumorstadien-gerechte Differenzierung des chirurgischen Behandlungskonzepts beim Primär- und Rezidiveingriff möglich und sinnvoll sein wird.

Literatur

1. Dralle, H., Th. Schürmeyer, J. Kotzerke, J. Kemnitz, H. Grosse, A. von zur Mühlen: Horm. Metab. Res. **21** (Suppl.), (1989), 34. - 2. Woolner, L.B., O.H. Beahrs, B.M. Black et al.: In: Young, S., O.R. Inman (eds.), Thyroid Neoplasia,

New York, Academic Press, 1968, p. 51. - 3. Schröder, S., W. Böcker, H. Baisch, C.G. Bürk, H. Arps, I. Meiners,H. Kastendieck, Ph.V. Heitz, G. Klöppel: Cancer **61** (1988), 806.- 4. Tisell, L.E., G. Hansson, S. Jansson, H. Salander: Surgery **99** (1986), 60. - 5. Dralle, H., S. Becker, G.F.W. Scheumann: In: Schilddrüse 1989, Thieme (im Druck). - 6. Meyer, H.J., J. Jähne, H. Wilke, R. Pichlmayer: Langenbecks Arch. Chir. Suppl. **2** (1990) (im Druck).

Discussion

Hehrmann: What are the operation times for compartment-ectomy (1 - 2 - 3): Dr. Tysell from Stockholm reports on dissection times of more than 8 hours?

Dralle: For one side the operation time is about four hours, and both sides eight hours, with the mediastinum about 14 to 16 hours.

Deckart: I thank you very much for these presentation, I think it's very important to perform this in that way. We see it from the bad results in those patients where this microdissection is not been performed. Please tell me, how is the outcome of the movebility of patients after surgery? We have some who have not the possibility to move enough the neck and they have pains and a very disagreeable situation. It took up to now some month.

Dralle: It's an important question, I think its very important to discuss this problem of mobility and I think we reach this results only with these sophisticated technical methods as I said: with magnifiing glasses and these form of coagulation. And with these techniques we have no morbidity than in former times without these extensive lymphnode dissection. And so I think you can reach these results with the same morbidity as in earlier times, regarding the mobility of the neck, there is no problem. We divide both sternocleidoid muscles in two side compartment ectomies and the patients have no problems. You have more problems after external radiation than after surgery.

Raue: May I ask you, what are you doing with patients you operated adequately and who have still elevated calcitonin levels, wait and see or reoperate - what do you prefer?

Dralle: This is a problem in treatment of MTC patients, if I have by myself performed the first operation or the preceding operation, I know completely what I've done and there is also a development in the surgical technique. I think, in first patients I did not remove the lymph node tissue posterior to the cervical branches of the nerves and this is a very important thing in the lymph node resection. And now also these posterior parts behind these cervical branches of the cervical plexus are removed. But the decision: reoperate or "wait and see" still remains very difficult. There is a report on 22 patients with the method of "wait and see" and they have also very good results. Patients without imaging results but slidely elevated calcitonin levels have still a good prognosis.

Nemec: I agree, that the lymphnode involvement in MTC is extremely important for the faith of patients. On your last slide you have shown that you perform these dissections even in patients; with distant metastatic lesions - it is correct?

Dralle: Yes, we perform also in these patients with distant metastasis the lymph node dissection but not in the mediastinal space. But in the cervical space we always perform a lymphnode dissection. Although we do not know, if we can improve the prognosis of the patient out if you have no increased morbidity, you give the patient the chance to remove all tumor tissue.

Medullary cancer in histopathological view

H.G. Peschel, T. Decker
I. Institute of Pathology, Klinikum Berlin-Buch,
Berlin, Germany

Medullary cancer of the thyroid gland arises from the parafollicular so-called C cells because these cells are able to produce calcitonin. They belong to the APUD cell system of Pearse /9/ and are of neuroendocrine origin. They enter the thyroid via ultimobranchial body. Synonyms are: The term medullary carcinoma was coined by Hazard et al. in 1959 /4/. Its rate of incidence from 3 to 10 percent of all thyroid malignancies. In institutions where in relatives with familial forms of the neoplasia are traced and treated, the percentage will be higher than the average of 5 percent. The tumour is slightly more common in women with the majority in the fourth and fifth decade. It occurs in a sporadic and in a familial form with the ratio of 2 to 1.
In the last 15 years we have investigated 434 cases of thyroid cancer in biopsies obtained by surgical treatment. In 24 patients medullary carcinoma was diagnosed, that is in 5.5 percent, which is in keeping with the figures given in the literature (table 1). Grossly, the tumour is solid, firm, grey-white to yellow, usually quite well circumscribed but seldom encapsulated. Granular calcification may be seen. Most cases are located in the upper half of the gland corresponding to the areas of highest C cell concentration. Microscopically, the number of cytoarchitectural variations is very large. Polygonal, round or spindle shaped cells with abundant acidophil cytoplasm are clustered into solid irregular groups and cords. The nuclei are relatively uniform in size and shape. Mitoses are sparse. In the same tumour you may have different pattern: carcinoidlike, palisading, serpentine, rosette, trabecular, glandular and even pseudopapillary. The stroma is hyaline and variable in amount. It characteristically contains amyloid which is demonstrable by the usual stains.

Table 1: Medullary thyroid carcinoma in biopsies
Period 1. 1. 1977 - 31. 3. 1991
I. Institute of Pathology, Klinikum Berlin-Buch
Thyroid cancer total: 434
Medullary cancer: 24 (5.5 %)

Age	n	sex
11 - 20	3	3 x f
21 - 30	1	m
31 - 40	9	5 x f, 4 x m
41 - 50	6	2 x f, 4 x m
51 - 60	3	3 x f
> 60	2	f, m

f : m = 1.4 : 1
7 x Sipple's syndrome (adrenal pheochromocytoma)

This APUD amyloid is apparently a product of the tumour cells and may be found in metastases, too. Occasionally, there is a foreign body giant cell reaction to the amyloid. True psammoma bodies with calcification are often present.
Most of the cells contain cytoplasmic secretory neuroendocrine granules which are usually argyrophilic with Grimelius' stain or other methods.
Immunohistochemically, the tumour cells are reactive for epithelial markers such as cytokeratin, for pan-endocrine markers such as chromogranin, synaptophysin and the so-called neuronspecific enolase, and for the specific product of C cells, calcitonin. They also are positive for CEA, but negative for thyroglobulin. The differential diagnosis of tumours with follicular or C-cell differentiation is most often possible by visualizing thyroglobulin in tumours with follicular differentiation. Calcitonin, chromagranin A and especially carcinoembryonic antigen (CEA) are typical markers of

medullary carcinomas /1,2,6/. Synthesis of various peptide hormones, e. g. somatostatin, ACTH and HCG can take place. These products may be absent as can amyloid.

In the last ten years some authors /3,7/ reported a mixed medullary-follicular carcinoma with the morphological features of both medullary and follicular carcinoma together with immunoreactivity for calcitonin and thyroglobulin. This mixed type probable exists, but it remains a controversial entity, as medullary carcinoma may entrap thyroid follicles with incorporation of thyroglobulin /8,10/.
Small cell carcinoma of the thyroid, identical to the equally named lung tumour, is regarded as small cell variant of medullary carcinoma. Those which are calcitonin-negative seem to represent the most undifferentiated type; their behaviour is quite aggressive. In medullary carcinoma vascular invasion is quite common. The tumour metastasizes both by lymphatics and by blood stream into lymphnodes and distant organs.
The familial forms of medullary carcinoma are often multiple and bilateral (5 of our cases). Their proportion is increasing compared to the sporadic forms when relatives are screened and carefully investigated.
The association of medullary carcinoma with adrenal pheochromocytoma and other endocrine tumors was first described by Sipple in 1961 /11/. This condition is known as Multiple Endocrine Neoplasia type II b /5/. In Sipple families medullary carcinoma may be remarkably positive in course. We investigated biopsies of 7 patients that is from 3 families, with MEN type II a.
C cell hyperplasia, occasionally with elevated serum calcitonin, is the preneoplastic disorder of medullary carcinoma. These cells exhibit greater calcitonin immunoreactivity than the cells of medullary carcinom itself. We diagnosed two additional cases with such lesions. Finally, the diagnosis of medullary carcinoma can be established with conventional histological and histochemical methods to detect the neuro-

endocrine origin of the cells and their production of amyloid. Nevertheless, morphological variability with occasional possession of microfollicular architecture represents some risk of a "missed" diagnosis, especially when amyloid is not found with usual stains. The knowledge about elevated serum calcitonin and possible familial forms of the disease allow the pathologist to confirm the diagnosis even in frozen sections without any doubt as a helpful information for the surgeon. Immunhistochemical methods are left for amyloid-free, solid and for undifferentiated tumour types when conventional histology is not convincing enough.

References

1. De Lellis, R.A. et al.: Am. J. Clin. Pathol. **70** (1978), 587. - 2. De Lellis, R.A., M. Wolfe: In: De Lellis, R.A. (ed.): Diagnostic immunohistochemistry, New York, 1981, Masson Publishing USA Inc., 61. - 3. Hales, M. et al.: Cancer **50** (1982), 352. - 4. Hazard, J.B., W.A. Hawk, G. Crile: J. Clin. Endocrinol. Metab. **19** (1959), 152. - 5. Keiser, H.R. et al.: Sipple's syndrome: Ann. Intern. Med. **78** (1973), 561.- 6. Krisch, K. et al.: Histopathology **9** (1985), 1077. - 7. Ljungberg, O. et al.: Cancer **52** (1983)m 1053. - 8. Lloyd, R.V., J.C. Sisson, P.J. Marangos: Cancer **51** (1983), 2234. - 9. Pearse, A.G.E.: Pathol. Ann. **9** (1974), 27. - 10. Schröder, S., G. Klöppel: Am. J. Surg. Pathol. **11** (1987), 100. - 11. Sipple, J.H.: Amer. J. Med. **31** (1961), 163.

Discussion

Finck: You told about tumors with calcitonin - free cells in histology. Does this mean that we should not expect elevated levels of calcitonin in blood serum in these patients? And if it is correct, is this type of tumor a rare one?
Peschel: I think so, this remarks were given in the literature. It is a rare tumor, it is the most undifferentiated form of the tumor as have been shown as small cell carcinoma

of the thyroid and it may be of neuroendocrine origin.

Cytological view of medullary cancer

Marie-Luise Weiss
Klinik für Nuklearmedizin und Endokrinologie,
Klinikum Berlin-Buch, Germany

The importance of cytology to the diagnostics of medullary thyroid cancer is to be assessed differently depending on the clinical question formulated. The medullary thyroid carcinoma is detected cytologically most frequently in connection with routine punctures when assessing the potential malignancy of thyroid nodules. The diagnosis of medullary carcinomas is in such cases more a surprise finding, because often clinical symptoms, which would indicate a medullary thyroid carcinoma, are absent. In the case of suspected medullary thyroid carcinomas as heriditary disease, detected during family examinations, fine needle puncture of the thyroid can also be applied. In the presence of positive paraclinical findings puncture, however, is only useful, if palpatorily, sonographically or scintigraphically a nodule in the thyroid has been localized. In the follow up treatment of patients, who were already operated on a medullary thyroid carcinoma, fine needle puncture can be occasionally useful in detecting a relapse or metastases. The presurgical, cytological diagnosis of a medullary carcinoma is clinically of great importance, as the radical degree of surgical intervention can be planned accordingly. Moreover, in the case of a cytologically suspected medullary carcinoma further endocrine tumors have to be searched for presurgically, e.g. phaeochromocytomas, in order to avoid surgical complications. The cytological diagnosis requires of course confirmation by quick section histology.

Histologically, in the medullary carcinomas several growth patterns and a considerable variability of cell forms are observed so that the cytological picture can be shaped very differently. Characteristic are monomorphic or pleomorphic cell populations, isolated situated cells or tissue fragments.

The cells are round, oval, plasmacytoid, triangular, polygonal or spindle-shaped. The nuclei are located frequently excentrically; single-, bi- and multi-nuclei have been observed. They are round or ovally shaped, occasionally they are bizarre. The chromatin is dense to granular; both micronucleoly and macronucleoly are observed. Occasionally intranuclear cytoplasmic inclusions are visible. The cytoplasma varies from light to fine-granular. Typical and diagnostically decisive are eosinophil granules in the cytoplasma, as they are especially clearly visibles in air-dried and Giemsa-stained smears. These granules can be immunocytologically identified as calcitonin. The background can occasionally reveal homogeneous material, which reminds of colloid but with the Congo-red staining it is characterized as amyloid. The determination of amyloid is an important criterion for histology; it is in the field of cytodiagnostics of minor importance. However, decisive is the determination of azurophilic granulation in smears. This feature, however, occurs optionally also in other tumors of the APUD-cell system. That's why the differential diagnosis can yield no findings considering a lymph node metastasis of a medullary carcinoma and a paraganglioma of the glomus caroticum. According to Droese /2/, approximately 60 % of medullary carcinomas can be reliably diagnosed in applying conventional Giemsa-staining. If there is no determination of granules available the diagnosis can be made immunocytologically by determining calcitonin and/or CEA or by determining the intermediary filaments cytoceratin, vimentin and neurofilamentes. The coexpression of these three intermediary filaments has so far been found only in medullary thyroid carcinomas. Also the rare and with conventional methodology applied differential diagnosis between a lymph node metastasis of an occult medullary carcinoma and a paraganglioma of the glomus caroticum should yield a finding by means of intermediary filaments. To determine neurosecretory granules the immunocytochemical representation of chromogranin is available which contrary to neuron-specific enolase and silver staining according to Grimelius can be observed in all C-cell carcinomas. Under this procedure also medullary carcinomas can be detected, which produce no calcitonin but other polypeptides. Although in most C-cell carcinomas a stronger cell- and nuclear polymorphism is absent, occasionally anaplastic variants are observed. Whether, however, in the group of anaplastic carcinomas C-cell tumors are to be found with the frequency as reported by Nieuwenhuejzen-Krusemann and coworkers /5/ remains controversial. This group of authors reports that in a follow up examination 9 out of 14 anaplastic carcinomas were identified as medullary carcinomas. Three further publications of groups of authors /1,4,6/ have detected very rarely or no calcitonin production in anaplastic carcinomas. If anaplastic tumor cells are diagnosed in cytological smears of patients of middle and younger age, cytochemical methods should be applied to search for a medullary carcinoma. Small cell thyroid carcinomas can, even though rarely, conceal medullary carcinomas. However, more frequently metastases of bronchial cancer or lymphomas are found. The papillary variant and glandular, tubular and follicular variants of medullary thyroid carcinomas will be interpreted as follicular or papillary carcinomas by conventional cytological diagnostics. Here even in a histological examination the relevant classification can be achieved only by the determination or absence of calcitonin or thyroglobulin. Genuine mixed forms of medullary and follicular thyroid carcinomas occur rarely, whose tissues reveal both calcitonin and thyroglobuline. Difficulties occur occasionally through misinterpretation of this constellation of findings by invasion of the medullary carcinoma into the normal thyroid tissue. The clear diagnosis of a follicular/medullary mixed form of tumor can actually only be made with metastases using the definite histochemical determination of both tissue components.

Since 1974 we have performed the fine needle puncture of the thyroid and we have evaluated some 18000 punctures cytologically. Among these there were 10 patients, whose histological examination yielded a medullary thyroid carcinoma (table 1). The findings obtaines by Kini and coworkers /3/, who have reported on the largest group of medullary thyroid carcinomas in the cytological literature, are demonstrated on table 2. Half the medullary carcinomas were recognized by us rightly as such. Two further smears were recognized as malignant tumor or as suspected malignant cells and thus as surgical indication. In a smear with anaplastic tumor cells a relapse nodule had been punctured in the cervical region at the state after surgery of a medullary carcinoma. Three smears have to be classified as false negative. In these three patients the diagnosis of a medullary thyroid carcinoma was definite based on clinical and paraclinical criteria: In one case a medullary carcinoma was diagnosed during the puncture of hepatic metastases. Thyroid puncture was carried out for localization of the primary tumor. A large, scintigraphically cold nodule was punctured in the right thyroid lobe, which revealed cytological retrogressive changes. A small echo-poor nodule in the cranial sections of the left thyroid lobe was not punctured. Here after surgery a primary tumor was found histologically. Two patients with Sipple-syndrom showed a cytological finding false negative or no cell material was taken. This two patients, who were operated on, because the presence of a medullary carcinoma had been paraclinically definitely confirmed, histology yielded multifocal, medullary thyroid carcinomas. Both in the patient group presented by Kini and in our patient population one false positive interpreted smear has been found. We detected the typical azurophil granules, which could not be clearly differentiated from the granules of active thyrocytes. An additional cytochemical calcitonin representation could have avoided this false diagnosis.
The patient group examined by Kini reveals two medullary carcinomas which have been falsely interpreted as follicular

adenomas.

Table 1: Cyto-histologic correlation of MTC
(KNME Klinikum Berlin-Buch

MTC Histology N 10

N 5 typical cytologic feature

N 1 anaplastic cells

N 1 atypical thyroid cells

N 1 normal thyroid cells (miplaced puncture)

N 1 retrogressive changes (Sipple syndrome)

N 1 acellular (Sipple syndrome)

one case false positive - Histology: follicular adenoma

Table 2: Cyto-histologic correlation of MTC
(Kini, S.R. et al.: Arch. Pathol. Lqb. Med.
108 (1984), 156)

MTC Histology N 17

N 10 typical cytologic feature

N 1 papillary cancer

N 3 anaplastic cells

N 2 follicular adenoma

N 1 acellular

one case false positive - Histology: nodular goiter

To summarize the importance of puncture cytology for the diagnostics of medullary thyroid carcinomas:

1. With fine needle punctures as secondary screening methods for scintigraphically cold and sonographically echo-weak thyroid nodules the cytological diagnosis of medullary thyroid carcinomas has an important diagnostic value, even though occasionally false positive findings are reported.

2. For localization of the primary tumor in the hereditary forms of MTC cytology can be applied only partly. Provided a definite localization of the nodules these can be punctured. However, all foci, which can sonographically be represented, have to be punctured regardless of their size. The diffuse or nodular C-cell hyperplasia as precancerosis can cytologically be not determined.

3. For cytologically detected anaplastic carcinomas in patients of younger age we recommend the cytochemical determination of calcitonin in order not to overlook a medullary carcinoma.

References

1. Carcangiu, M.L., T. Steeper, G. Zampi, J. Rosai: Amer. J. Clin. Pathol. **83** (1984), 135. - 2. Droese, M., H. Schicha: Internist **28** (1987), 542. - 3. Kini, S.R., M. Miller, J.I. Hamburger, M. Smith: Arch. Pathol. and Lab. Med. **108** (1984), 156. - 4. Myskow, M.W., A.S. Krajewski, A.E. Deware, E.P. Milar, K. McLaren, J.W. Fabre: Clin. Endocrinol. **24** (1986), 335. - 5. Nieuwenhuijzen-Kruseman, A.C., F.T. Bosman, J.C. van Bergen Henegouw, G. Cramer-Knijnenburg, G.B. de la Rivere: Amer. J. Clin. Pathol. **77** (1982), 541. - 6. Schäffer, R., S. Finkler, E. Goss: Verh. Dt. ges. Pathol. **70** (1986), 286.

Discussion

Raue: May I ask you, are there in this calcitonin free medullary carcinoma reports about measurements of calcitonin values in the serum of these patients? Are these cells which produce calcitonin and don't have granuals of calcitonin?
Weiss: I know a paper from the cytological literature where is a comparison of cytochemical calcitonin punctures and the blood calcitonin.
Deckart: You told us about the histochemical staining of cytologic smears?

Weiss: Yes, it's a fine method and I have contacted our collegues and I hope we can do it. We start with thyroglobulin in smears where the primary tumor is not known and we will continue. The method is not different to histologic staining.

Imaging techniques in detection and follow up of MTC

H.F. Deckart, Katharina Djakowa, H. Marciniak, E. Strehlau, Marie-Luise Weiss
Klinikum Berlin-Buch, Clinic for Nuclear Medicine and Endocrinology

Imaging methods play an important role in the preoperative staging and follow up of MTC. The detection of the disease is primarily done with tumor markers: increase of calcitonin and/or CEA serum level resp. the positive stimulation of calcitonin with pentegastrin, alcohol or calcium infusion are more sensitive than all imaging methods together.
These are necessary tools in the localization of tumor and metastases if postsurgical tumor marker levels persist high or increase once during the lifelong follow up.
Tc-99m-pertechnetate thyroid scan can detect MTC preoperatively as cold nodule which will be characterized by ultrasound in the next step. In the follow up this method is unimportant.
Ultrasound will detect size and extension of nodules within the thyroid much more precise than thyroid scan.
With high resolution realtime technique (10 MHz transducer) lesions with some mm diameter can be seen. Ultrasound guided fine needle aspiration biopsy can increase the accuracy to find contents of tissue or fluid specimen. Ultrasound itself is absolute unspecific; though differentiated thyroid carcinoma and MTC show mostly echopoor pattern, or mixed resp. solid nodules with echopoor margin, the so called "halo-sign" (figure 1). The histologically detected calcification in papillary cancer and the calculus deposits within amyloid-stroma in MTC (figure 2) can be observed with ultrasound within the thyroid just as in distant metastases of the liver (figure 3). In this context we may point out that an indication for surgery under the suspicion of malignancy will never be set up from the result of ultrasound investigation alone but from cytological diagnosis of fine needle biopsy.

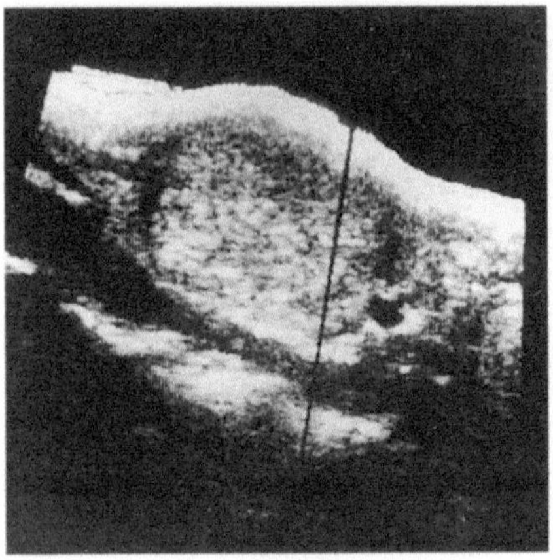

Figure 1

Ultrasound: solid nodule with echopoor rim ("halo-sign"), histologically proven MTC

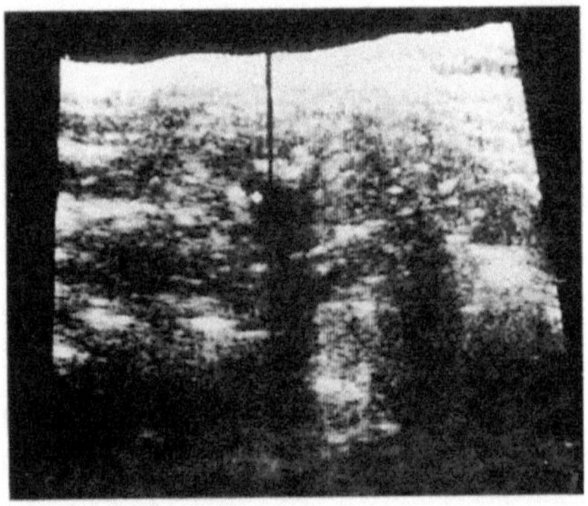

Figure 2

Ultrasound: calculus deposits within thyroid tissue with echoless shadow behind (MTC)

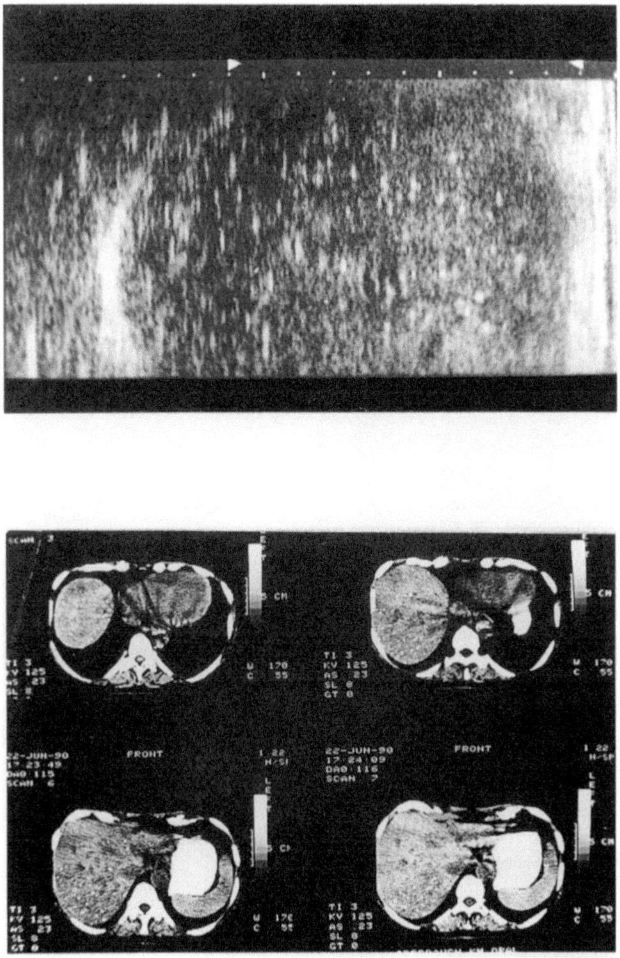

Figure 3

Ultrasound (3a) and computed tomography (3b): calcified metastases of MTC in the liver

In an analysis from 376 cases out of literature echopoor pattern was seen in 85.2 % of thyroid tumor /1/. Ultrasound can give additional information on the relation of tumor nodule and surrounding tissue: sharp delineation (figure 4a) or infiltration with blurred pattern (figure 4b). In our series of 85 cases we have seen echopoor pattern in 32/85, halo sign in 13/85, cysts within solid lesion (figure 5) in 7/85. Calcification was detected sonographically in 6 out of 9 MTC and in 3 out of 52 papillary carcinomas.

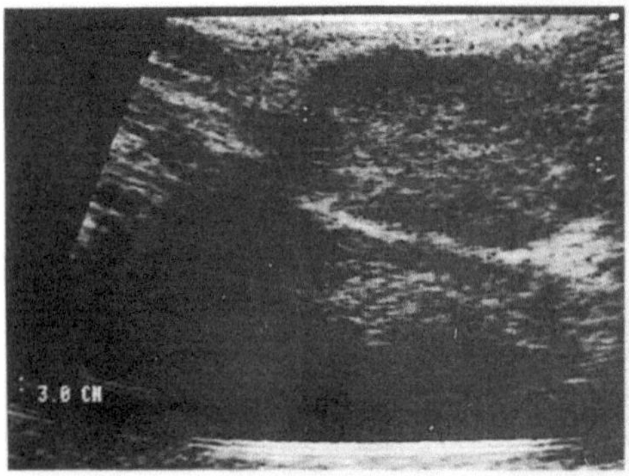

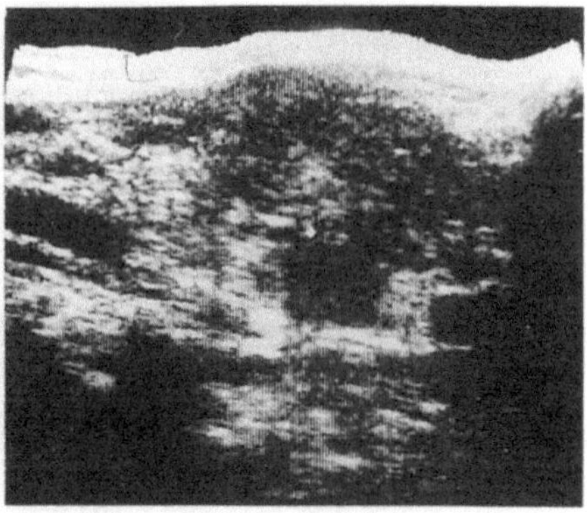

Figure 4

Ultrasound: tumor nodule, echopoor, with sharp delineation (figure 4a), with infiltration of surrounding tissue (figure 4b); both MTC histologically verified

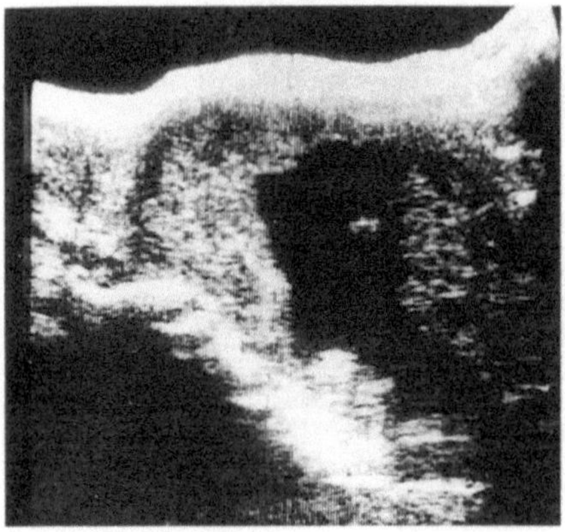

Figure 5

Ultrasound: cystic lesions in solid tumor nodule (histologically proven MTC)

In three cases of familiar MTC we observed members with increased calcitonin level bilateral small echopoor lesions with 3 to 5 mm diameter, postsurgically - histologically proven as MTC - non palpable, and undetectable by scintigraphy.
Ultrasound is most helpful in the postsurgical follow up in the verification of complete or uncomplete resection of thyroid mass, in the volumetry of thyroid remnants, and in the early detection and localization of lymph node metastases in the neck, detected as small echopoor or hyperechogenic lesions (figure 6).

We have analyzed 106 patients with differentiated thyroid carcinoma before surgery to compare ultrasound pattern with 85 patients preoperatively with postsurgical histologically proven thyroid adenoma(s) and the corresponding pertechnetate scans. The occurrence of either echopoor, complex, solid (echonormal) characterization between malignant and benign tumor was equal (no significant difference, table 1). In this retrospective study the diagnostic accuracy could be increased in the combined interpretation of scan and sonography (table 2).

Scintigraphy

The detection of liver metastases with conventional liver-rhs-scintigram and bone metastases with osteotropic radiopharmaceuticals is generally known. As the MTC cells secrete physiologically calcitonin and CEA and have shown to produce a variety of peptides, biogenic amines somatostatine derivatives one has tried to use various radiopharmaceuticals for the detection of occult metastases. Pacini et al. /2/ have found an expression of the following five antigens in primary MTC resp. its metastases (in percent): calcitonin 100/100, CEA 100/93, neuron specific enolase (NSE) 90/71, somatostatin 63/39 and thyroglobulin 59/13.

Table 1: Comparison of ultrasound echopattern in histologically proven thyroid adenoma (85 patients) and differentiated thyroid carcinoma (106 patients) after surgery

	Adenoma	%	Carcinoma	%
echopoor	39	(45.9)	50	(47.2)
complex	32	(37.6)	31	(29.5)
solid or echonormal or total	14	(16.5)	25	(23.6)
	85		106	

chi^2-test: unsignificant

	Sensitivity	Specificity
echopoor	0.47	0.46
complex	0.29	0.38
solid/normal	0.24	0.16

Table 2: Comparison of results with combination of scintigraphy and ultrasound in patients with thyroid adenoma versus differentiated thyroid carcinoma

Adenoma (N 85) vs. Carcinoma (N 106)

1. Echopattern — no significant differentiation

2. Echopattern and Scan

echopoor	no significant differentiation
complex	in carcinoma significant more cold lesions
solid	in adenoma significant more warm lesions

US	Scan	Ca.	Aden.	Sens.	Spec.
echopoor	cold	32	27	0.80	0.31
	warm	8	12		
complex	cold	33	9	0.92	0.72
	warm	3	23		
solid)	cold	8	3	0.62	0.79
normal)	warm	5	11		

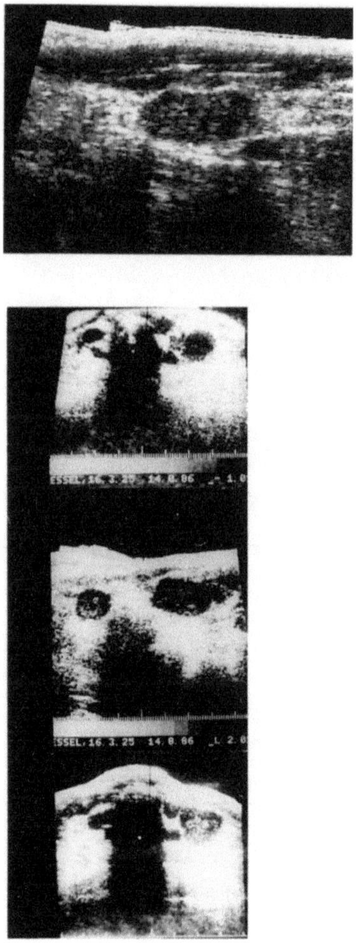

Figure 6

Ultrasound: MTC-lymph node metastases.
Status after total thyroidectomy. Bilaterally
multiple metastases in lymph nodes from MTC

According to the thyroglobulin expression the scintigraphic detection with Iodine-123 or 131 might be possible - though generally not used - Hoefnagel et al. /3/ have reported a sensitivity of 0.3 in 123 cases.
One has used the guanethidine analogue I-123 (I-131)-meta-iodobenzylguanidine (MIBG) since 1984 /4/, which is concentrating in the neurosecretory granules of chromaffine cells in tissue of neurocrest origin, as it is used for the imaging of adrenal medullary hyperplasia and pheochromocytoma, which is connected with MTC in Sipple's syndrome. The pentavalent dimercaptosuccinic acid (Tc-99m(V)DMSA) was proposed in 1984 /5/, Tl-201-chloride (figure 7) was used just as Ga-67-citrate /6/. Newest results are reported with positive accumulation in MTC-metastases with I-131- or Tc-99m-anti CEA immunescintigraphy (figure 8) or with In-111 labelled somatostatin or its derivatives /7/.
We observed 13 patients in our series who have developed an increase in basal calcitonin and/or CEA serum level in the follow up after total thyroidectomy and lymph node dissection after a period of tumor marker negativity. These patients we observe over years, most of them are well feeling and symptomless. From our experience we had positive staining with every of these 5 radiopharmaceuticals - but none was in favour:
In 13 patients with postoperatively increased CT levels metastases were detected in case I: Tl-201 positive, MIBG negative; case 2: Tl-201 positive, Ga-67-citrate positive, MIBG positive; case 3: Tc-99m(V)DMSA positive, anti-CEA positive, MIBG negative; case 4: anti-CEA positive, Tl-201, MIBG and DMSA negative; case 5: MIBG negative, DMSA negative, but verified metastases by ultrasound and computed tomography.
8 patients with negative results of imaging techniques (3 radiopharmaceuticals, CT, ultrasound). The low sensitivity of MIBG-scan in detecting MTC metastases was reported by Clarke et al. /4/ and Hoefnagel et al. /5/. The high sensitivity of

Tc(V)DMSA reported by some authors /6/ we didn't observe in our series.

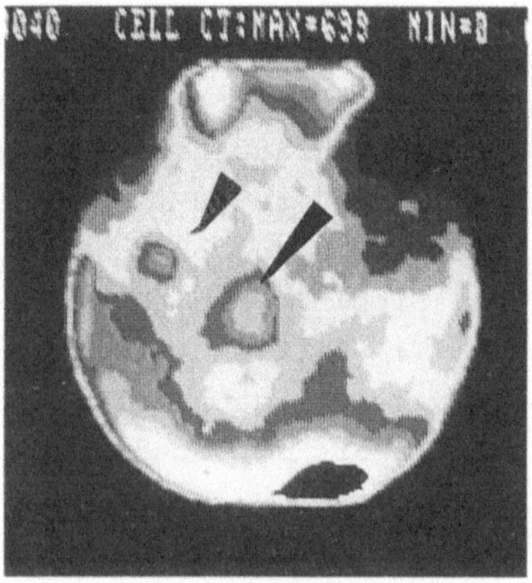

Figure 7

Tl-201-chloride scintigraphy of the mediastinum with two MTC-metastases

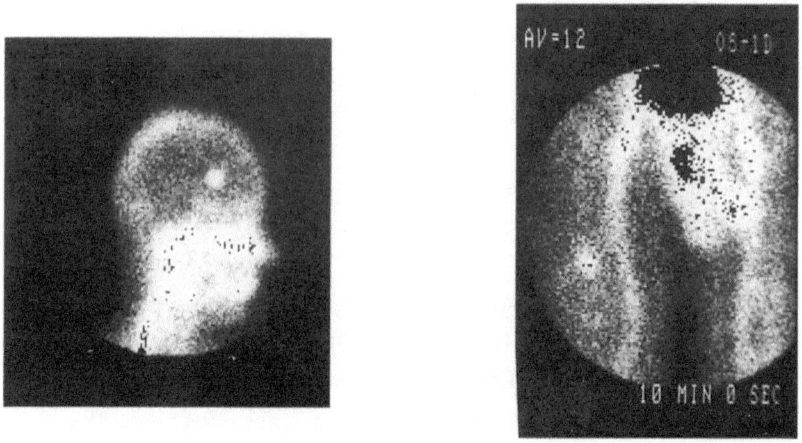

Figure 8

Whole body scintigraphy with I-131-anti CEA. MTC-metastases in brain and right thigh

Computed Tomography is the most precise technique for accurate morphological investigation of tumor masses in the neck in the relation to neighbouring organs and tissue especially in mediastinal extension which neither can be detected by scintigraphy or ultrasound (see ref. 1 and figure 9).
The combined interpretation of results of three methods is our general practice.

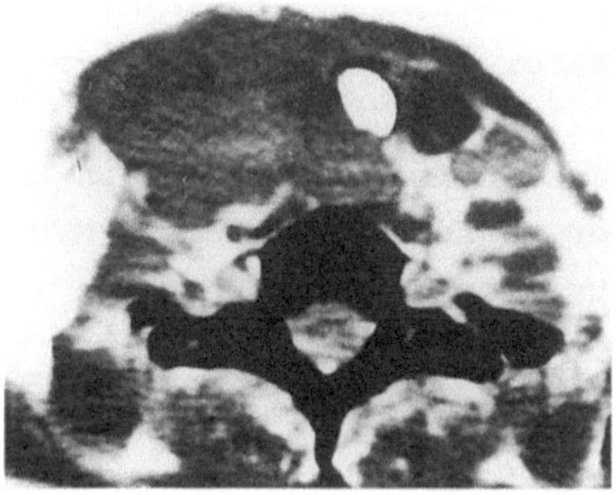

Figure 9
Computed tomography of the neck region: large thyroid tumor mass infiltrating surrounding tissue (MTC)

Summary

Early diagnosis of MTC as primary tumor or its metastases after radical thyroid surgery inclusive neck lymph node dissection is performed with tumor marker detection (calcitonin, CEA-assays). Tumor visualization can be performed in the neck by ultrasound high echopoor or mixed lesions with echopoor margin (halo-sign) may represent MTC, verified only by US-guided fine needle biopsy. Some tumors are marked by calcification especially in the genetic familiar form: tiny echopoor lesions (5 mm diameter and less) have represented MTC

proven by histology with step slice technique. Sensitivity in differentiation between malignant and benign thyroid nodules (inclusive MTC) in connection with scintigraphy retrospectively reviewed we calculated with 0.8 in comparing 106 malignant and 83 benign thyroid nodule bearing patients. Lymph node metastases can be localized by carefully performed ultrasound by an experienced examinator.
The detection of MTC-metastases distant the neck region can be tried by whole body scanning (planar in combination with SPECT) using different radiopharmaceuticals (Tl-201-chloride, Ga-67-citrate, Tc-99m(V)DMSA, I-123 (I-131)MIBG, In-111- or Tc-99m labelled anti-CEA or somatostatin derivatives) with variable success.
Computed tomography plays an important role in the anatomical differentiation of tumor masses derived from MTC before surgery and/or radiation treatment.

References

1. Deckart, H., E. Strehlau, H. Marciniak et al.: Schriftenreihe ISSN 0233-1268, Band 17, S. 31. - 2. Pacini, F., F. Basolo, L. Fugazzola et al. in "Medullary Thyroid Carcinoma". Eds. C. Calmettes, J.M. Guliana. Colloque INSERM Eurotext Limited **211** (1991), 81. - 3. Hoefnagel, C.A., C.C. Delprat, D. Zanin et al.: Clin. Nucl. Med. **13** (1988), 159. -
4. Endo, K., K. Shiomi, K. Kasagi et al.: Lancet II (1984), 233. - 5. Ohta, H., K. Yamamoto, K. Endo et al.: J. Nucl. Med. **35** (1984), 323. - 6. Kujat, Ch, K. Neidl, Ch. Müller-Leiss et al.: Fortschr. Röntgenstr. **153** (1990), 495. -
7. Krenning, E.P., S.W.J. Lamberts, J.C. Reubi et al.: 65th Meeting American Thyroid Association 1991, Abstract 126, p. 64.

Positive scintigraphy in medullary thyroid cancer

V. Holub, N. Neradilová, J. Němec*
M. Beňová, T. Blažek, P. Vlček**
Postgraduate Medical Institute, Prague, Institute of Endocrinology, Prague*
Department of Nuclear Medicine, Faculty Hospital, Prague-Motol, Czechoslovakia**

Medullary cancer of thyroid (further only abbreviation MCT) secretes many polypeptide products, usable as its markers. Evaluation of enhanced plasma levels of immunoreactive calcitonin (further iCT) remains the best criterion of tumour progression, but it fails to localize the site of tumorous spread for the surgical intervention. While the use of tagged iCT-antibody might be the best way to localize the tumorous tissue we were concentrated on comparing the results of two alternative ways to imagine it.

Material and methods

Between 1982 and 1991 we examined 51 patients. They were scanned by alcalized complex of dimercaptosuccinic acid, tagged by pentavalent Tc-99m (further only Tc (V) DMSA) 73-times, by Tl-201 chloride (further Tl-201) 43-times. In 18 cases was familial form of MCT diagnosed, out of them in 7 instances involved in MEA II and in one in MEA III, other cases were believed to suffer from sporadic disease. All were at least 4 months after surgical treatment or also irradiation of the neck region. The examination comprised estimation of iCT - basal and after pentagastrin and calcium stimulation, clinical and instrumental (sonography and or CT of the neck region) examination, followed by scintigraphy by Tc (V) DMSA or/and Tl-201. Static scintiscans were made using scintillation camera Gamma Müvek 9 101 A (Hungary) at 30. and 90 to 120 minutes following I. V. administration of 400 MBq Tc (V) DMSA or 74 MBq Tl-201. The DMSA complex (Rotop, Germany) was alkalized immediately before use by a decimolar solution of NaOH to pH 8.5 and tagged with Tc-99m.

Results

In the table are all cases (scanned by Tl-201 in parentheses) distributed into three groups:

- I - Clinically and by sonography (CT) positive cases - 22 (17) - (later confirmed bioptically 14 (11))
- II - Other iCT positive cases, without clinical and-or instrumental confirmation of recurrent MCT - 34 (18 cases)
- III - cases following succesfull treatment, with no sign of tumor recurrence with low iCT 17 (8).

As follows, sensitivity of scanning by Tc (V) DMSA was 0.59/ 0.95 for group I and only 0.35 for group II/- while sensitivity of scanning by TL-201 was 0.49 - only 0.7 for cases of group I and 0.28 for those of group II. No false uptake was found in 17 clinically negative cases with low iCT, scanned either by Tc (V) DMSA (17) or by Tl-201 (8).

Discussion

Plasma calcitonin level measurements are most important for the detection of tumour recurrence of MCT following therapy. Many methods were used for the localization of the source of high plasma iCT levels. The comparison of diagnostic efficacy for the detection of recurrent MCT for Tc-99m (V) DMSA and Tl-201 was reported for instance by Ohta et al. in 1984 /1/. Both Troncone et al. /2/ and Clarke et al. /3/ in 1989 found high sensitivity, but lower specifity of Tc (V) DMSA comparing with I-131-MIBG scanning.

Our results with Tc-99m (V) DMSA scanning confirm high sensitivity of this evaluation and are comparable to the data reported by Querra et al. in 1988 /4/. MCT scanning by Tc-99m (V) DMSA was found to be more sensitive and less expensive than that by Tl-201, and should be widely used in

Table 1: Uptake of Tc (V) DMSA (Tl-201) in cases, treated for MCT - N = 73 (43)

		DMSA + (Tl+)	DMSA-(Tl-)	sensitivity	
I	US (CT) + iCT positive	21 (12)	1 (5)	0.95 (0.70)	0.59 (0.49)
II	only iCT positive	12 (5)	22 (13)	0.35 (0.28)	
III	iCT negative	0 (0)	17 (8)		

this field. Most difficult for the interpretation are the results of patients with high plasma iCT levels without sonographical suspicion. Positive scan localized recurrent MCT in minority of cases only with repeatedly high iCT levels showing no clinical signs of recurrence for many years. While earlier we were inclined to indicate chemotherapy, we are now much more conservative as many patients live without clinical recurrence for many years in spite of high iCT levels.

Conclusion

56 clinically positive cases, following initial treatment for MCT, were scanned with Tc (V) DMSA for recurrent tumor with positive scans in 59 %, while Tl-201 uptake was found in 49 % of 35 scanned cases. Tc (V) DMSA was successful to prove sonographically positive cases of recurrent MCT in 95 % of 22 cases, while Tl-201 scans in only 70 % of 18 cases. No false positive uptake of both radiopharmaceuticals was found in 17 (8) clinically negative controls.

References

1. Ohta, J. et al.: J. Nucl. Med. **15** (1984), 43. - 2. Troncone, L. et al.: Henry Ford Hosp. Med. J. **37** (1989), 178. - 3. Guerra, U. et al.: J. Nucl. Med. All Sci. **32** (1988), 242.- 4. Clarke, S. et al.: Henry Ford Hosp. Med. J. **37** (1989), 167.

Discussion

Groth: Thank you for the very interesting results. We have found a very high sensitivity in pentavalent Tc-DMSA too.
In March this year at meeting of Cancer Research Campaign in London Mrs. Clark from Hammersmith Hospital has reported that Tc (V) DMSA has the highest sensitivity (86 %) in comparison to other investigations (e.g. Tl, MIBG etc.).

Holub: The London results are a little better in the sensitivity but a little smaller in the specificity in comparison with iodine and MIBG.
Bergant: DMSA is accumulating in soft tissue sarcomas, inflammatory processes and so on, so that interpretation of results must be careful discussed and to take this in respect.
Holub: We have made always whole body scanning and did not found any other accumulation in the body. There was the strict principle of scanning at least fore month after last surgery.
Simova: I could not hear your personal experience with the techniques with DMSA, with Tl and with technetium labelled. What is the dosage?
Holub: Thallium is not available for us for economic reasons. And the sensitivity is not quite well. So we used it only in other indications.
Weiss: I am interested in you experience with MIBG diagnostics. How is the percentage of positive cases because in our group it is not so good. We always saw in Sipple's syndrome the pheochromocytoma, the adrenals or extraadenals, but we never saw the primary or metastases of the medullary cancer.
Holub: We have performed in the last years only nine scannings with MIBG always in the field of MEN - 3 or MEN - 2 and we have not very good results to detect MCT tissue only pheochromocytoma. Only in one case of MEN - 2 we detected an accumulation in the region of thyroid.

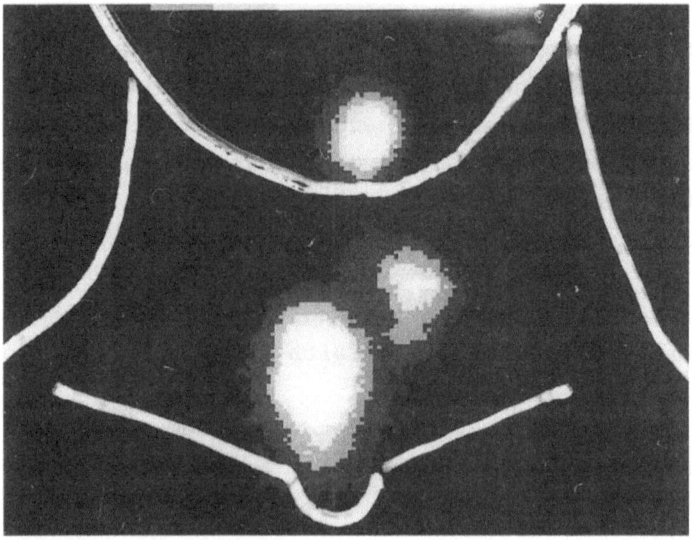

Figure 1

Positive Tc (V) DMSA scan of recurrent MCT (US posit., high iCT). Male 51

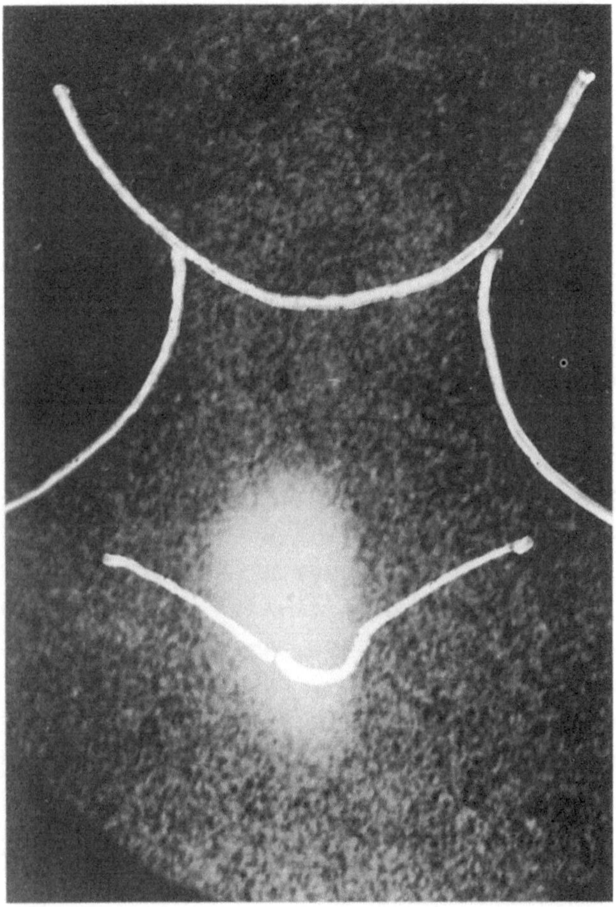

Figure 2

The same patient, 5 months following neck re-exploration (bioptically MCT in two metastatic lymphnodes; primary tumor in jugular region inoperable)

I-131-uptake in medullary thyroid carcinoma

G. Riccabona, A. Stöger, D. Ladurner, K. Schmid
Departments of Nuclear Medicine, Surgery and Pathology,
University of Innsbruck, Austria

Medullary thyroid carcinoma (MTC) is thought to develop from the parafollicular or C-cells within the thyroid gland and therefore should not take up radioactive iodine. Recently, however, I-131-uptake has been reported in metastases of "medullary carcinoma" and consequently some authors have suggested that these tumors can be treated with radioactive iodine. On the basis of observations in 5 patients out of 20 with MTC we would like to comment regarding this situation. From 1961 to 1990 there were 2153 patients with thyroid cancer treated in our hospital and about 1 % of these patients (n = 20) had MTC. From 1974 to 1989 we chose 5 well-documented cases as examples to discuss the question proposed in the title of this article. Two of these patients with MTC appeared to take up radioactive iodine (I-131) in their tumors. Preoperative thyroid isotope scans, neck and chest radiographs, aspiration biopsy cytology specimens and thyroid function tests were available in all patients. Serum calcitonin levels were measured in all patients by radioimmunoassay.

Thyroglobulin levels were measured by RIA in 4 patients. The thyroid glands and tumors were examined histologically in all patients. Four patients also had immunochemical analysis of the thyroid tumors for calcitonin, thyroglobulin, CEA and somatostatin. Two tumors were also examined by electron microscopy.

The relevant cases will be described after a tentative classification in 3 groups.

Group 1

Case No.1.1 G.S., a female, born 1951: a small, diffuse, euthyroid goiter was found in 1974. There was no family history

of goiter, MTC, or related disease.
She did not suffer from diarrhoea. In 1981 she was found to have a cold nodule in the left thyroid lobe on a Tc-99m-scan. Fine-needle biopsy showed a benign cell pattern. As the nodule grew further (in spite of thyroid hormone therapy) in the following years, a near-total thyroidectomy was performed in 1983. Chest radiographs were normal. Histologic examination revealed clusters of calcitonin-positive cells in the periphery of an undifferentiated thyroid tumor that usually suggests "medullary thyroid carcinoma". Postoperatively the patient was treated with telecurietherapy (60 Gy) and 2.7 GBq of I-131 of which 5 % were taken up in small thyroid remnants in the neck.
The patient has subsequently done well and has normal serum concentrations of thyroglobulin and calcitonin. There is also no clinical or radiological evidence of metastases or recurrence: no stimulation tests for calcitonin were performed. This tumor seems to be a nonspecified thyroid cancer in a gland with some C-cell hyperplasia. Many C-cells in the periphery of the tumor may therefore persist probably due to tissue compression and a higher resistance of C-cell against tumor invasion. It seems doubtful whether such tumors can be considered as medullary thyroid carcinoma per se.

Group 2

Two cases are described that can be classified as classic MTC patients, one belonging to MEN IIb, the other to the sporadic type.

Case No. 2.1 P.H., male, born in 1963, beginning growth of goiter in 1982, first examination at thyroid clinic in 1985. A multinodular goiter with a cold nodule on the left side was found, diarrhoea and marfanoid status as well as changes in oral mucosa typical for MTC in the context of MEN-syndrome. Two weeks later thyroidectomy, histology: MTC. Postoperatively telecurietherapy (60 Gy) and I-131-therapy (3.4 GBq)

because of minimal uptake in thyroid remnants. Only one person of the family could be checked for calcitonin in blood (negative). In 1987 hypertensive crisis, malignant pheochromocytoma of right adrenal gland and adrenalectomy. Serum calcitonin level rises to 13470 pg/ml, recurrence of neck tumor and multiple metastases, radiation therapy and chemotherapy without success, death in 1988.
In summary typical MTC in context of MEN-syndrome, no response to I-131-therapy.

Case No. 2.2 H.J., male, born in 1911, growth of a mass on the left side of the neck at 68 years of age. Otherwise he was asymptomatic and there was no family history of goiter, MTC or MEN. On physical examination a tender thyroid nodule was noted as well as multiple palpable lymph-nodes in his neck. A near-total thyroidectomy with radical neck dissection was performed in 1982 (age 71 years). Histological examination revealed medullary thyroid carcinoma. Telecurietherapy (60 Gy) and I-131-therapy (3.5 GBq) with a minimal uptake in thyroid remnants was given. His serum calcitonin level was 649 pg/ml. Eighteen months later he developed another nodule on the left neck side. At reexploration in 1984 metastatic MTC was removed. Chest radiographs and liver ultrasound were normal: however, his calcitonin level increased to 3.130 pg/ml. One year later he developed a swelling of the left parotid gland, had a reintervention, and the histological examination of the removed mass revealed an anaplastic tumor with a positive calcitonin stain. He also had a partially cystic parotid tumor. Chemotherapy was started with aclacinomycin. In summary he had classic sporadic MTC, and did not respond to I-131-therapy. Death with liver metastases in 1987.

Group 3

Another 2 patients are presented with obvious MTC but with definite radioiodine uptake in metastatic lesions.

Case No. 3.1 P.J., a male, born 1937, noticed the growth of a goiter at 35 years of age: there were no other complaints. Family history remained without evidence of goiter, MTC or MEN. At an examination in a thyroid clinic a nontoxic multinodular goiter (nodules partially cold by isotope scan) with normal cytologic findings was found. Conservative therapy with thyroid hormone was started, but the goiter continued to grow. Therefore a neartotal thyroidectomy was performed in 1974. The histological diagnosis was "medullary thyroid carcinoma". In a postoperative scan with I-131 multiple foci with tracer uptake were found in both lungs: the chest radiographs were normal. I-131-therapy and telecurietherapy were given. The following years he developed multiple metastases and two therapeutic I-131 doses were given as well as polychemotherapy. In spite of this the patient developed paraplegia and died. In summary the patient had histological rather than typical medullary thyroid carcinoma, which behaved clinically like a poorly-differentiated follicular thyroid carcinoma (with I-131-uptake in multiple metastases).

Case 3.2 R.M., a female, born 1921: no family history with MTC or MEN. In previous years the patient had been treated with antithyroid drugs for "hyperthyroidism". At 63 years of age she noticed a swelling on the left side of the neck. In a local hospital an excision of a lymph node was performed and revealed histologically a metastasis of MTC. A neartotal thyroidectomy was done a few weeks later: the histological diagnosis of MTC was confirmed. On I-131-scan there was radionuclide uptake in small thyroid remnants and in a lesion below the upper thoracic aperture on the left. Chest films and liver sonography were normal. Telecurietherapy (60 Gy) and I-131-therapy (4.1 GBq) were applied. Calcitonin and thyroglobulin levels have remained normal since then and there is no evidence of metastases or recurrence by clinical, radiological, laboratory or scintigraphic examinations. In summary this seems to be a case in which all histological and immunohistological parameters justify a diagnosis of MTC. There was, however, obvious I-131-uptake in a metastasis in the chest and the patient responded well to I-131-therapy.

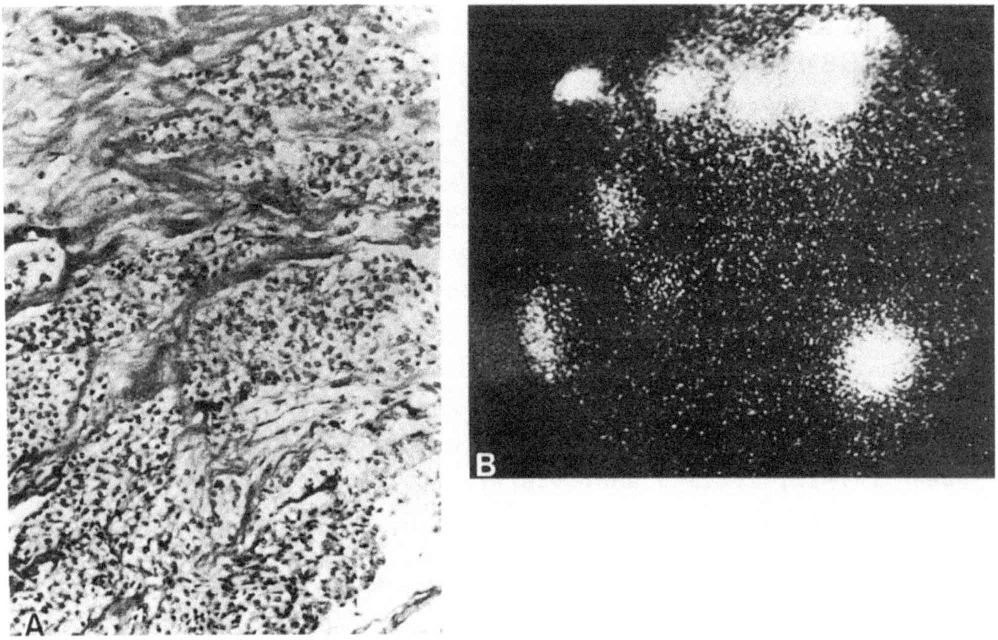

Figure 1

A. Typical histological pattern of medullary thyroid carcinoma with amyloid stroma, no evidence of papillae or follicles.
B. Multiple metastases in pelvis and femurs with I-131-uptake

Histologically (including immunohistochemistry) typical MTC with definite I-131-uptake in metastases, no calcitonin and thyroglobulin in serum and a positive response to radioiodine therapy can occur also (group 3). This most puzzling group - in which all possibilities of artifacts on scans could be ruled out - behaves clinically rather like poorly differentiated follicular carcinoma. The histogenesis of the tumor tissue remains unknown. This discrepancy between pathohistology, calcitonin content of tumor cells and I-131-uptake (just as in differentiated thyroid adenocarcinomas) cannot be explained at present but may represent a tumor of both follicular and parafollicular cell origin.

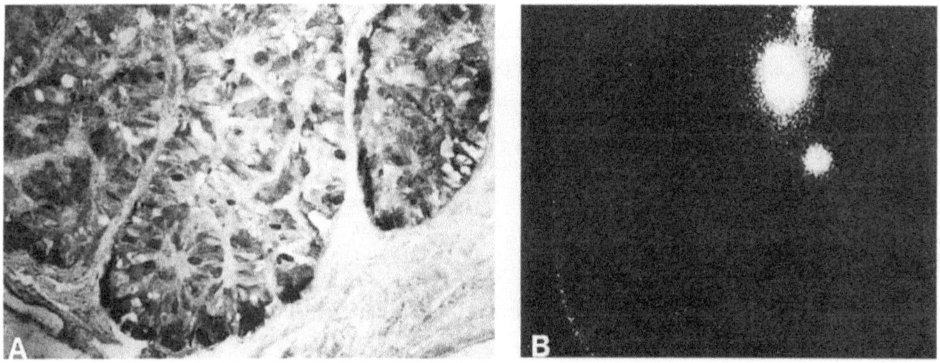

Figure 2

A. Diffusely positive staining for calcitonin in medullary thyroid carcinoma, thyroglobulin negative.
B. I-131-neck and chest scan with 7 MBq showing uptake in thyroid remnants after surgery and in chest focus. Chest lesion gone after large-dose I-131-therapy

Conclusion

The patient presented in this study reveal that medullary thyroid carcinomas can take up radioactive iodine and that MTC can be a heterogeneous tumor. Even with sophisticated techniques for diagnosis and follow-up (immunohistochemistry "specific" radioimmunoassays for tumor antigens) the histogenesis of MTC cannot be clarified in all cases.
It is possible that these tumors represent poorly differentiated thyroid carcinomas with C-cell metaplasia or mixed tumors originating from both follicular and parafollicular

cells. Other neoplasms classified as "medullary cancer " seem to be unspecified thyroid cancers with C-cell hyperplasia in the periphery of the tumor.
For the management of patients with medullary thyroid carcinoma we would suggest that histopathological and immunopathological criteria may not adequately reflect whether the tumor will take up radioactive iodine. One should therefore do whole-body I-131-scans using a large tracer dose in these patients: if abnormal tracer uptake is found one should treat the patients with I-131. Serum calcitonin, CEA and thyroglobulin will play an important role in the follow up examination of these patients as well as clinical and radiological examinations.

References

Williams, E.D.: J. Clin. Pathol. **19** (1966), 114. - 2. Oberdisse, K., E. Klein, D. Reinwein: Die Krankheiten der Schilddrüse. Stuttgart, New York, Thieme 1980. - 3. Hedinger, C., L.H. Sobin: Histological Typing of Thyroid Tumors. In: International Classification of Tumors, no. 11, Geneva, WHO,1974.-4. Bussolati, G., A.G.E. Pearse: J. Endocrinol. **37** (1967), 205.- 5. Deftos, L.J., M.F. Stein: J. Clin. Endocrinol. Metab. **50** (1980), 967. - 6. Wolfe, H.J., R.A. DeLellis: Clin. Endocrinol. Metab. **10** (1981), 351. - 7. Pearse, A.G.E., A.F. Carvalheira: Nature **214** (1967), 929. - 8. Benker, G., S. Dabag, D. Reinwein. In: Advances Field Educational Italia, Rome, 1981, p. 263. - 9. Stepanas, A.V., N.A. Samaan, C.S. Hill, R.C. Hickey: Cancer **43** (1979), 825. - 10. Sokal, M.M., C.L. Harmer: Clin. Oncol. **4** (1978), 3. - 11. O'Bryan, R.M., L.H. Baker, J.E. Gottlieb, S.E. Rivkin, S.P. Balcerzak, G.M. Grumet, S.E. Salmon, T.E. Moon, B. Hoogstraten: Cancer **39** (1977), 1940.

Discussion

Raue: I am not convinced on the I-131-uptake by MTC in your third group of patients, as it is not confirmed by histological examinations; these cases are anecdotal, a systematic I-131-scanning in all MTC patients in the follow-up could not be concluded from these observation.

Gembicki: Could you tell me please, how high was the I-131-uptake by metastases expressed in percent of activity, given or calculated on any other way?

Stöger: I can't give you an information about this, because it was from 1974 up to now before my time.

Our experiences with medullary carcinoma and MEN-syndrome

H.F. Deckart, S. Birke, E. Deckart, Ch. Koloc, W. Lobers,
R. Pilz, E. Strehlau, C. Wardius, M.L. Weiss
Clinic for Nuclear Medicine and Endocrinology,
Klinikum Berlin-Buch, Germany

The Clinic of Nuclear Medicine and Endocrinology is looking after patients with thyroid malignancy since 15 years. Diagnostic procedures (scintigraphy, ultrasound, fine needle aspiration biopsy, hormone and immune parameter analysis) and the clinical follow up examinations are performed in this clinic, while surgery was achieved in the 1st Surgical Clinic (J. Brandt, D. Geipel), percutaneous radiation in the Clinic of Radiation Treatment (R. Gremske) and the pathohistological investigation in the 1st Institute of Pathology (T. Decker, H.J. Peschel).

Incidence

Table 1 shows the analysis of 609 patients (pts) with thyroid tumor: 512 pts suffered from differentiated thyroid cancer (84 %), 48 pts from medullary thyroid carcinoma (MTC), these are 7.8 % - within the range varying in literature between 5 and 10 %.
These 48 MTC patients are subdivided in 28 (58.3 %) with the sporadic form and 20 (41.7 %) of the familial variety, which has an autosomal dominant hereditance.

Age- and Sex-Distribution

The peak age of incidence in MTC is the fifth decade - the mean age at time of diagnosis was calculated to 47.7 years of total MTC, 43.8 years in male and 47.8 years in female. The mean age of the familial form was lower: 4 pts with only familial MTC mean age 26.8 years, 14 pts with MEA IIa mean age 38.3 years, and 2 pts with MEA IIb mean age 18.5 years. The differentiated thyroid cancer and MTC showed differences in sex distribution (table 1): in MTC this is nearly equal,

Table 1a: Frequency of tumor types(differentiated)

in the series 1991

Histology	N	%	male : female
papillary c.	278	45.6	1 : 5.6
follicular c.	234	38.4	1 : 4.1
medullary c.	48	7.9	1 : 1.4
total	609		

Table 1b: Frequency of tumor type(undifferentiated, others)

Histology	N	%	male : female
squameous cell c.	3 (m)	1.9	
undifferent.c.	35	5.7	1 : 1.9
malignant lymphoma	4 (f)	0.7	
metastases	6	1.0	1 : 0.2
malignant struma ovarii	1	0.2	
total	609		

in differentiated thyroid carcinoma females were prefered.

Histological differentiation is in general possible with H-E staining alone, detection of argyrophilic cytoplasmatic granules with Grimelius stain and congored staining of amyloid, questionable cases verification can be accomplished with immunohistochemic methods of calcitonin, CEA-, chromogranin detection (see chapter Peschel/Decker).
In 5/48 cases two cancer types of medullary and follicular (2) or papillary (3) were observed, in 2 cases medullary in one and differentiated thyroid cancer in the opposite lobe.

The familiar form of MTC is frequently connected with uni- or bilateral pheochromocytoma and/or primary hyperparathyroidism (hyperplasia or adenoma of parathyroids). This so called Sipple-syndrome or multiple endocrine neoplasia (MEN II a) we observed in 11 patients (table 2): pheochromocytomas were seen in 5 patients, hyperparathyroidism in 3, and the combination of both in 3 patients. The autosomal dominant gen transfer can be demonstrated in four families, schematically seen in figure 2-5. The MEN type II b we observed in two cases characterized by multiple mucosal neurinomas of the tongue, thickening of the lips, a characteristic phenotype with marfanoid habitus (elongated face) together with bilateral pheochromocytoma.

Staging

The staging in our series at the time of surgery resulted in 23/48 patients $pT_{1-3}N_0M_0$. In 11 cases the tumor had penetrated the capsule (pT_4), 10 had metastases into ipsi- and contralateral lymphnodes (N_1, N_2) and 6 distant metastases ($M_{1,2}$). After treatment 11 patients developed metastases: 5 in local lymphnodes between 2 and 11 years of observation, 2 in the liver (after 3 resp. 8 years), 2 into the lung, 4 years after treatment, further 2 into lymphnodes and the skeleton after 3 resp. 4 years follow up.

Table 2: MTC series 1991: MEA 13 patients

MEA 1 a	11 patients
pheochromocytoma	5
prim. hyperparathyroidism	2
combined	4
MEA 2 b	2 patients
pheochromocytoma bilat.	
ganglioneuromatosis intestinalis	
Marfanoid habitus	

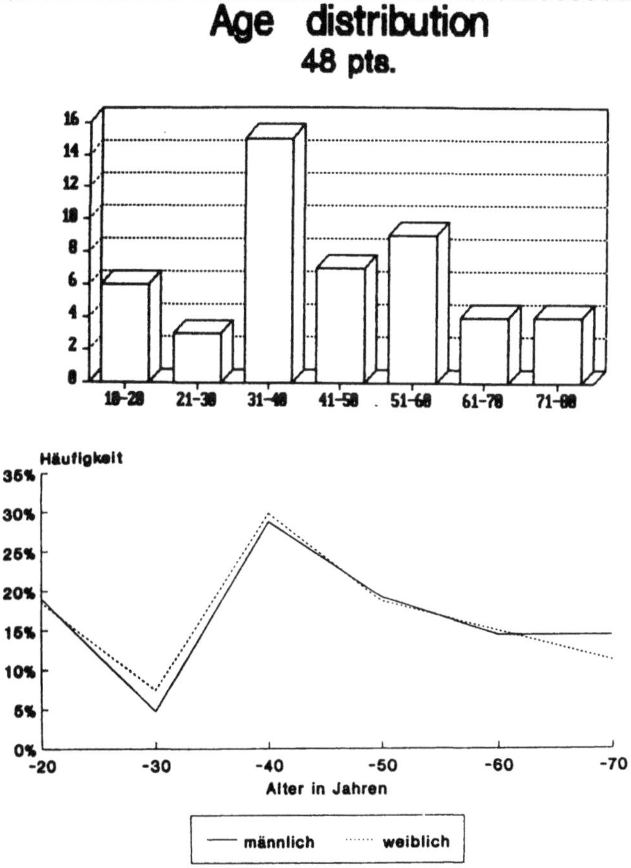

Figure 1

Age and sex distribution of our series of MTC-patients (male ----, female - - -)

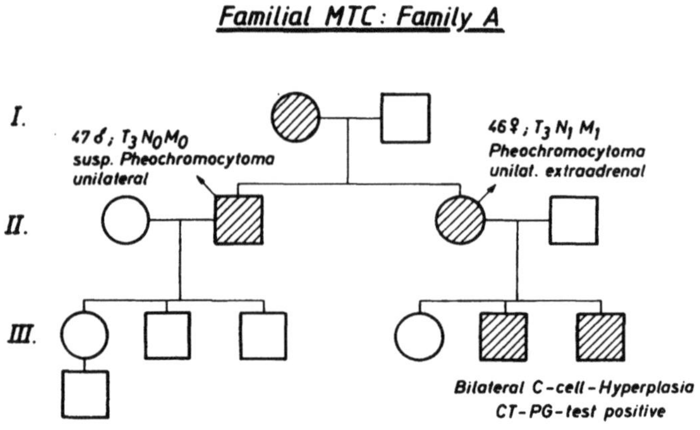

Figure 2

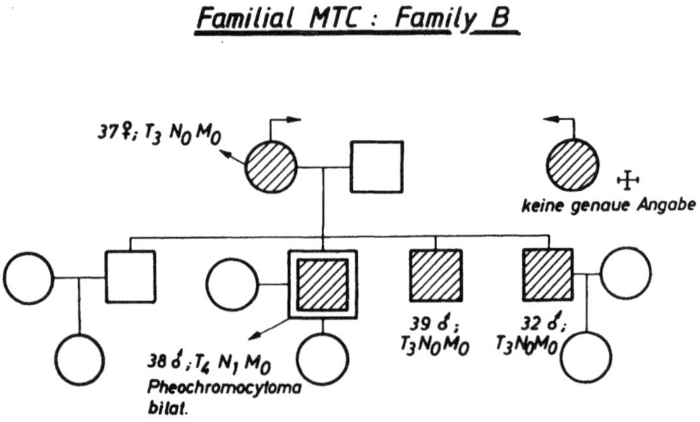

Figure 3

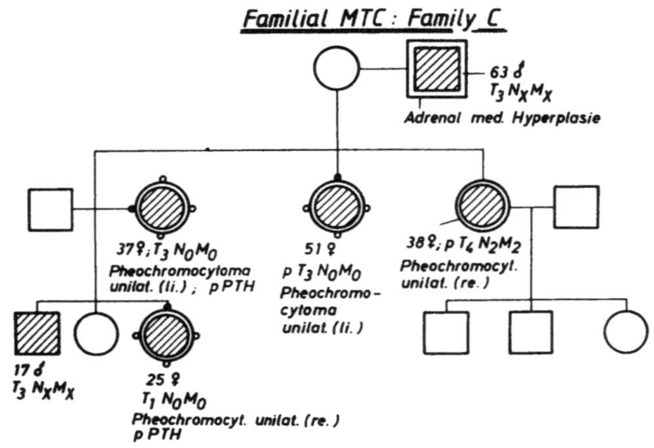

Figure 4

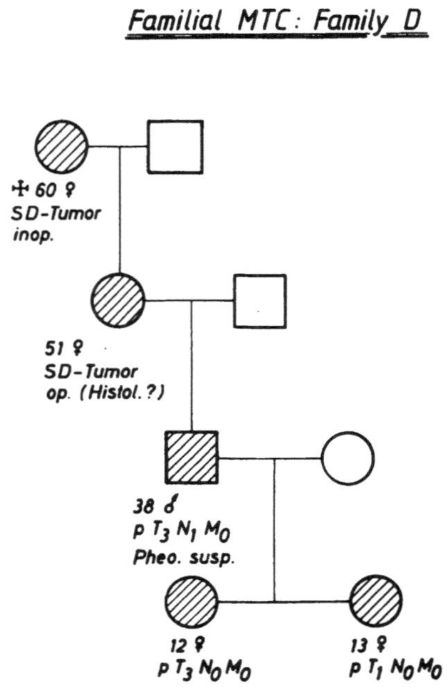

Figure 5

Figure 2-5

Genetic transfer of MTC, in 4 families A to D, additional occurence of C-cell hyperplasia (family A), hyperplasia of adrenal medulla (fam. C, and pheochromocytoma (fam. A to D)

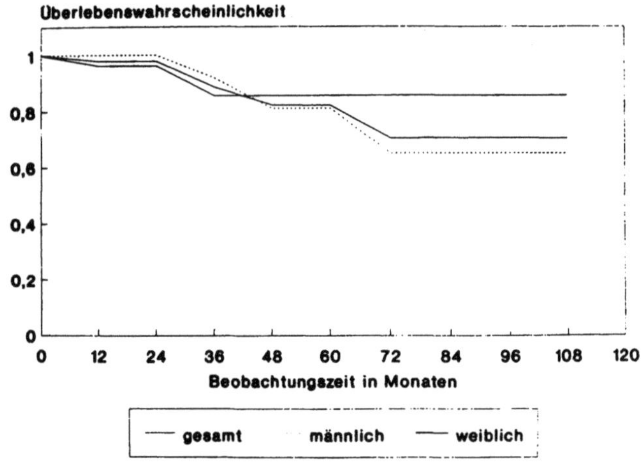

Figure 6

Life table analysis of 48 patients with MTC (according to Kaplan-Meyer): the 5-years survival rate was calculated to 0.82

The survival rate of our patients was 87.5 % (42/48 pts), these consisted out of 19 patients up to two years, 16 patients between 3 and 5 years and 6 patients with 7-12 years after surgery. 6 patients died (letality rate 12.5 %). The survival table analysis within five years was 0.82 (figure 6): two within 6 months of diagnosis and surgery, 4 between 2 and 5 years. All of them had ipsi(4)- or contralateral (2) lymphnode and distant metastases at the time of clinical cancer detection.

Surgery

As patients were transfered to our oncological centre after surgery from 14 different surgical clinics (25) only half of them (23) were operated according to special criteria in our 1st Surgical department. The generally accepted method of one-step thyroidectomy after cytological suspicion and diagnosis proven by intraoperative frozen-section histology was performed in 31/48 patients (64.6 %). 12/48 patients (25 %) received thyroidectomy in two steps, and in 5/48 patients (10.4 %) hemithyroidectomy, subtotal resection or palliative surgery was reported.
The now generally accepted bilateral neck dissection was performed in 13/48 patients (27.1 %), the unilateral form in 12/48 (25 %) with proven lymphnode metastasis. As the highly experienced staff in thyroid surgery could be effective in only half of our patients the rate of postsurgical complication was high: lesion of n. recurrence occured in 19/48 patients (39.6 %), unilateral left in 9, unilateral right in 10 cases. Persistent hypoparathyroidism has to be treated in 12 patients (25 %).

Radiation treatment

Radiation ablation of postsurgical remnants is not our general treatment concept as MTC is relatively radioresistant - it was performed in 16/48 patients (33.3 %) and the postsurgical percutaneous radiation therapy of lymph vessel drainage area in the neck with 40-60 Gy was given to 24/48 patients (50 %) in 7 different departments: in 20 patients with stage pT_{1-3}, $N_{1-2}M_o$ and in 4 patients with $pT_{1-3}N_oM_o$.

<u>MIBG-treatment</u> we performed in only one female case, 39 years of age, who received thyroidectomy with unilateral neck dissection 14 years ago, stage $pT_2N_1M_1$, accomplished with percutaneous Co-60-radiation treatment. 6 years ago a second lymph node dissection was performed. She was transfered to our clinic with disseminated liver metastases with calcification (see page 262), increased level of serum calcitonin (1312 ng/l and CEA (15 879/ug/l). Diagnostic MIBG biokinetic data resulted in high liver-uptake of 42 % (normal less 3 % of test dose) with long retention: the effective half time within the liver was calculated to $T_{eff(1)}$ 3 hours (42 % of injected activity), $T_{eff(2)}$ 19 hours (23 %), $T_{eff(3)}$ 49 hours (36 %). The patient received 200 mCi (7.6 MBq) I-131 MIBG intravenously resulting in a liver dose of 9 Gy and whole body dose of 0.8 Gy. As radiation effect 4 months later a decrease of liver volume and lack of liver pain (liver capsule compression syndrome) was observed, the long lasting diarrhea was stopped and CEA- as calcitonin level decreased. In conclusion MIBG-treatment led into a positive palliative amelioriation in patient's behaviour.

<u>Cytostatic drug treatment</u>

Six patients with metastases with progression of the disease despite of surgical and radiation therapy were treated with combination of Adriblastin + Vincristin. Three died, three are alive: one female (17 years, $pT_4N_2M_2$) with highly aggressive MTC died within 6 months after diagnosis, but 2 patients (male, 45 years, $pT_2N_oM_2$ and female, 34 years , $pT_2N_1M_2$) survived 2 years during drug treatment in quite valuable way of live. Three patients received Adriblastin and Cytostasan since 2-3 years (female, 58 years, $pT_4N_1M_1$; female, 38 years, $pT_4N_2M_2$; male, 18 years, $pT_1N_1M_2$) and are in a stable well feeling situation. Adriamycin was given with a total dose of 800 mg/m^2 body surface. Cytostasan in 100 mg single doses every 3 weeks over long time; its bone marrow depression is low and rare, the total dose not limited.

Follow up

Our patients are asked to visit our outpatient department twice a year to perform clinical investigation, ultrasound and to take blood samples for calcitonin-pentegastrin test: 13 out of 46 patients had or developed postsurgical increased calcitonin-levels and 10/46 patients increased CEA-levels. In these patients metastases could not be verified using different imaging techniques: ultrasound, CT, and whole body scintigraphy with Tc-99m(V)DMSA, MIBG, anti-CEA. This tumor-marker increase occured in 1 to 3 years, in 3, 4 to 5 years, in 3 patients 11 to 12 years after thyroidectomy.

Conclusion

1. The rare occurrence of MTC and the complicated genetic and biochemical behaviour of this disease makes concentration of patients in tumor centres with experienced staff necessary.
2. Prognosis is depending from tumor stage at first diagnosis: In 48 patients of our series 41.7 % had regional lymph node metastases at MTC-detection. 6/48 patients died (letality rate 22.5 %), they all had local and distant metastases at time of surgery.
3. Total thyroidectomy with bilateral neck dissection and careful histological examination can be proposed according to our experiences treatment of choice. The low radiation sensitivity of MTC doesn't propose radiation treatment as general therapy concept. But cytostatic drug therapy in cases with incurable metastases was encouraging to prolong life with well feeling over years. 4/6 patients with Adriblastin (and Cytostasan) therapy were treated with

positive results in our series.

4. The rate of familial variety in our series was higher then reportes in literature (about 25 %). Careful family screening and anually repeated biochemical tests may have caused this difference.

5. In the follow up we observe in 10/42 patients (23.8 %) continously elevated calcitonin-, and/or CEA-serum level up to 10 years. Metastases could not be detected using different imaging techniques. As similar observations with symptomless clinical behaviour are reported in literature, patients should not be informed about tumor marker values to avoid unnecessary disencouragement and negative influence on their will of life.

Possibilities and limitations of tumor-scintigraphy for follow up of medullary thyroid cancer

Chr. Reiners
Clinic for Nuclear Medicine, University of Essen, Germany

In many patients after surgery for medullary thyroid cancer (MTC), residual or recurrent tumor has to be suspected according to elevated serum levels of calcitonin or CEA. Frequently, conventional imaging procedures like sonography, X-ray or computed tomography are not able to localize the tumor lesions. It is not surprising therefore, that several radiopharmaceuticals were tested for tumor scintigraphy in MTC patients during the last decade. First attempts were made in 1980 with Tl-201 chloride /24/, which has been proven to be very useful in follicular, papillary and especially oncocytic thyroid cancer /21/. As early as in 1982, radiolabelled anti-CEA antibodies were used for immunoscintigraphy in MTC patients /4/. In 1984, accumulation of I-131 MIBG in MTC tumor tissue has been reported first /13/. In this very year, the japanese group of OHTA published first results with Tc-99m(V) DMSA scanning in MTC patients /22/.

Preparation of Pentavalent Technetium Dimercaptosuccinic Acid (Tc-99m(V) DMSA)

It has been recognized by Ikeda et al. /18/ that various Tc-99m DMSA complexes - in the trivalent, tetravalent and pentavalent state - behave biochemically quite different. The trivalent Tc-99m(III) DMSA complex with its high cortical accumulation is used routinely for renal scanning; it has to be prepared by reconstitution of Tc-99m Pertechnetate with DMSA at pH 5. The preparation at pH 8 yields the pentavalent Tc-99m(V) DMSA anion /10,18,27/, which has a structure comparable to the orthophosphate ion. It therefore has an affinity to bone structures, but to certain tumors like MTC as well /22,27,28,40/.

The preparation of pentavalent Tc-99m(V) DMSA by modification of commercial DMSA kits is quite simple /19,27,39/. The only manipulation consists in alkalization of the Tc-99m Pertechnetate solution before adding it to the preparation vial with "cold" DMSA (table 1). We check the radiochemical purity routinely by paper chromatography; the quality of the preparation was sufficient in more than 100 applications.

Table 1: Preparation of Tc-99m(V) DMSA

1. Bottle 925 MBq of Tc-$99mO_4$ (in 2.5 ml of 0.9 % NaCl) into an empty elution vial
2. Add 0.1 ml H_2O ad inj. + 0.2 ml $NaHCO_3$
3. Mix and check pH-value (set point pH 8)
4. Bottle this solution into a commercial lyophilized DMSA-Kit (1.2 mg DMSA, 0.31 mg Sn (ii)-Cl), mix gently for 15 min
5. Quality control: Paper chromatography with n-Butanol + Acetic Acid + H_2O

Patients and results

In 1987, we began an open prospective study in patients with recurrent or metastatic MTC, comparing Tc-99m(V) DMSA scintigraphy with clinical findings, tumor markers, sonography, computed tomography and with other scintigraphic procedures like Tl-201 scans or immunoscintigraphy using Anti-CEA antibodies /28/. Up to now, 62 MTC patients were investigated.

Including repeated scans, we performed more than 100 scans with Tc-99m(V) DMSA in MTC patients. 600 MBq of the pentavalent complex prepared with a commercial DMSA kit are injected (table 1). Routinely, we aquire multiple planar camera images of the whole body 6 hours after intravenous injection. In most cases, SPECT scans of neck and thorax are added.

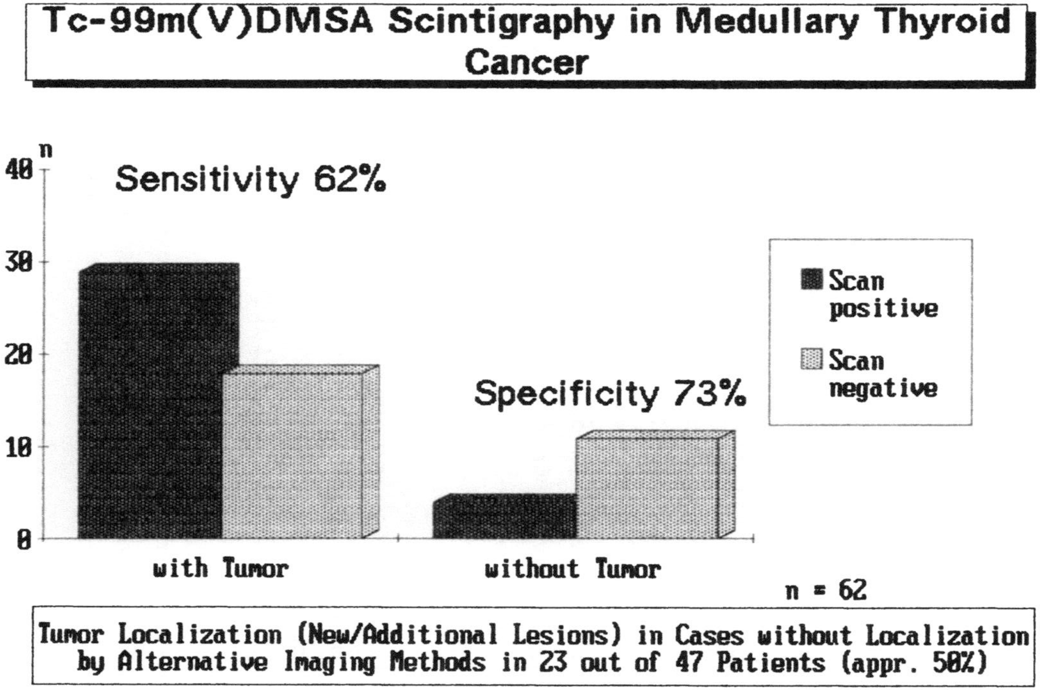
Tc-99m(V)DMSA Scintigraphy in Medullary Thyroid Cancer
n
40
30
20
10
0
Sensitivity 62%
Specificity 73%
Scan positive
Scan negative
with Tumor
without Tumor
n = 62
Tumor Localization (New/Additional Lesions) in Cases without Localization by Alternative Imaging Methods in 23 out of 47 Patients (appr. 50%)

Figure 1

Figure 1 summarizes the results of Tc-99m(V) DMSA scanning in follow-up of MTC: Tumor localization was possible in 29 out of 47 patients with elevated serum levels of calcitonin (sensitivity 62 %); 4 patients without elevation of the tumor marker showed unspecific uptake of pentavalent DMSA in sceletal lesions like fractures (specificity 73 %).

On the whole, a sensitivity of 62 % and a specifity of 73 % seem to be anything less than excellent. But it has to be stressed that in 23 out of the 47 patients with "active" tumor, DMSA scanning was the only imaging procedure which was able to detect and localize the tumor. Those patients were referred to the surgeon again; in only one case with a suspected metastases to the spine, the tumor lesion could not be confirmed by surgery. To conclude, DMSA scanning yields clinically very relevant informations in appr. 50 % of the patients with recurrent or metastatic MTC.

Discussion

The diagnostic efficacy of Tc-99m(V) DMSA scintigraphy for follow-up of MTC has to be compared to the performance of alternative scanning procedures using Tl-201 chloride, MIBG labelled with I-131 or I-123 or radiolabelled Anti-CEA antibodies.

Up to now, positive results of Tl-201 scans in 44 out of 70 patients with recurrent or metastatic MTC are reported in the literature (table 2). This yields an overall sensitivity of 63 %.

MIBG scans were performed in 150 patients with "active" MTC; the overall sensitivity of this imaging procedure is only 31 % (table 3).

Immunoscintigraphy with Anti-CEA antibodies offers the advantage of a relatively high specificity, as compared to the other radiopharmaceuticals used for follow-up of MTC. But its

Table 2: Sensitivity of Tl-201-Scintigraphy in follow-up of Medullary Thyroid Cancer

Talpos	1985 /35/	5/10
Arnstein	1986 / 1/	2/2
Holub	1987 /17/	20/34
Hoefnagel	1988 /16/	11/12
Rufini	1989 /31/	4/5
Sandrock	1989 /32/	2/7
		44/70 = 63 %

Table 3: Sensitivity of I-131-/I-123-MIBG-Scan in follow-up of Medullary Thyroid Cancer

Hilditch	1986 /15/	1/5
Coutris	1986 / 9/	2/2
Clarke	1987 / 8/	4/16
Baulieu	1987 / 2/	10/35
Hoefnagel	1988 /16/	3/11
Perdrisot	1988 /26/	2/6
Becker	1989 / 3/	0/5
Cabezas	1989 / 5/	2/8
Sandrock	1989 /32/	2/7
Guerra	1989 /14/	10/24
Troncone	1989 /36/	9/19
Verga	1989 /38/	1/12
		46/150 = 31 %

sensitivity of 60 %, established in 82 patients (table 4), is not higher than for Tl-201 or pentavalent DMSA.

The most extensive experiences with scintigraphy in follow-up of 253 MTC patients were gathered with Tc-99m(V) DMSA

Table 4: Sensitivity of CEA-Immunoscintigraphy in Follow up of Medullary Thyroid Cancer

Sullivan	1982 /34/	0/5
Parmentier	1984 /23/	4/10
Reiners	1986 /29/	3/6
Hoefnagel	1986 /16/	6/7
Edington	1988 /11/	1/1
Cabezas	1989 / 5/	7/10
Becker	1989 / 3/	0/5
Troncone	1989 /36/	2/3
Sandrock	1989 /32/	6/7
Scheidhauer	1990 /33/	7/12
Zanin	1990 /41/	1/1
		49/82 = 60 %

Table 5: Sensitivity of Tc-99m(V) DMSA-Scan in Follow up of Medullary Thyroid Cancer

Hilditch	1986 /16/	0/16
Endo	1987 /12/	14/19
Holub	1987 /17/	4/8
Hoefnagel	1988 /16/	2/3
Patel	1988 /25/	12/15
Becker	1989 / 3/	2/5
Clarke	1989 / 7/	28/32
Guerra	1989 /14/	16/19
Rodrigues	1989 /30/	14/10
Troncone	1989 /36/	11/14
Urcancioglu	1989 /37/	12/15
Verga	1989 /38/	3/12
Wulfrank	1989 /40/	1/5
Castellani	1991 / 6/	7/15
Mojiminiyi	1991 /20/	9/10
Reiners	1991	29/47
		174/257 = 68 %

(table 5). The overall sensitivity of 68 % corresponds quite well to the sensitivity of 62 % in our relatively large series.

Conclusions

1. Tc-99m(V) DMSA for scintigraphy in follow-up of MTC is easy to prepare, cheap and always available.
2. Tc-99m(V) DMSA is safe and may be applicated repeatedly (no adverse reactions, no problems with HAMA etc.).
3. Tc-99m(V) DMSA localizes lesions in appr. 50 % of the patients with residual tumor or metastases of MTC and negative results of alternative imaging procedures.
4. Tc-99m(V) DMSA therefore is the radiopharmaceutical of first choice for follow-up of MTC; radiolabelled Anti-CEA antibodies may be used additionally in special cases.

References

1. Arnstein, N.B., J.E. Juni, J.C. Sisson, R.V. Lloyd, N.W. Thompson: J. Nucl. Med. **27** (1986), 1564. - 2. Baulieu, J.L., D. Guilleteau, M.J. Delisle, R. Perdrisot, P. Gardet, N. Delepine, F. Baulieu, J.L. Dupont, J.N. Talbot, G. Coutris: Cancer **60** (1987), 2189. - 3. Becker, W., W. Börner, Chr. Reiners: Horm. Metabol. Res. Suppl. **21** (1989), 38. - 4. Berché, Ch., J.P. Mach, J.D. Lumbroso, C. Langlais, F. Aubrey, F. Buchegger, St. Carrel, Ph. Rougier, C. parmentier, M. Tubiana: Brit. med. J. **285** (1982), 1447. - 5. Cabezas, R.C., L. Berna, M. Estorch, I. Carrio, A. Garcia-Ameijeiras: Henry Ford Hosp. Med. J. **37** (1989), 169. - 6. Castellani, M.R., F. Crippa, L. Del Bo, M. Gasparini, M. Grassi, L. Mafioli, F. Cusumano, E. Baombardieri, G.L. Buraggi: In: Nuclear Medicine. The State of the Art in Europe, eds.: H.A.E. Schmidt, J.B. van der Schoot, Schattauer Stuttgart, New York (1991), 334. - 7. Clarke, S., C. Lacarus, M. Maisey: Henry Ford Hosp. Med. J. **37** (1989), 167. - 8. Clarke, S.E.M., C.R. Lazarus,

M.N. Maisey: Henry Ford Hosp. Med. J. **35** (1987), 124. - 9. Coutris, G., J.N. Talbot, G. Kabla, C. Calmettes, G. Milhaud: Eur. J. Nucl. Med. **12** (1986), 77. - 10. N.D. Dahir, S.R. Hesslewood, D.B. Jack: In: Nuclear Medicine. Trends and Possibilities in Nuclear Medicine, eds.: HA.E. Schmidt, G.L. Buraggi, Schattauer Stuttgart, New York (1989), 131. - 11. Edington, H.D., C.G. Watson, G. Levine, W.N. Tauxe, S.A. Yousem, M. Unger, C.D. Kowal: Surgery **104** (1988), 1004. - 12. Endo, K., H. Ohta, K. Torizuka, K. Horiucht, I. Yomoda, A. Yokoyama: J. Nucl. Med. **28** (1987), 252. - 13. Endo, K., H. Tanimura: Lancet (1984), 233. - 14. Guerra, U.P., C. Pizzocaro, A. Terzi, R. Giubbini, G. Maira, R.P. Pagliani, M. Bestagno: Nucl. Med. Comm. **10** (1989), 285. - 15. Hilditch, T.E., J.M.C. Conell, Th. Murray, N.S. Reed: J. Nucl. Med. (1986), 1150. - 16. Hoefnagel, C.A., C.C. Delprat, D. Zanin, J.B. van der Schoot: Clin. Nucl. Med. **13** (1988), 159. - 17. Jolub, V., J. Nemec, M. Neradilova, M. Benova, T. Blazek, M. Dusek: Radiobiol. Radiother. **28** (1987), 640. - 18. Ikeda, I., O. Inoue, K. Kurata: J. Nucl. Med. **18** (1977), 1222. - 19. Kujath, Ch., N. Panitz: Nuklearmediziner **12** (1989), 291.- 20. Mijominiyi, O.A., R. Udelsman, N.D.W. Soper, B.J. Shepstone, N.E. Dudley: In: Nuclear Medicine. The State of the Art in Europe, eds.: H.A.E. Schmidt, J.B. van der Schoot, Schattauer, Stuttgart, New York (1991), 344. -21. Müller, St. P., B. Guth-Tougelidis, B. Piotrowski, J. Farahati, Chr. Reiners: J. Nucl. Med. **31** (1990), 767. - 22. Ohta, H., K. Yamamoto,K. Endo, T. Mori, D. Hamanaka, A Shimazu, K. Ikekubo, K. Makimoto, Y. Iida, J. Konishi, R. Morita, N. Hata: J. Nucl. Med. **25** (1984), 323. - 23. Parmentier, C., J. Lumbroso, M. Schlumberger, P. Gardet, J.P. Mach, Ch. Berché, Ph. Rougier, B. Caillou, M. Tubiana: Ann. med. Interne **135** (1984), 345. - 24. Parthasarathy, K.L., K. Shimaoka, S.P. Bakshi, M.S. Razack: Clin. Nucl. Med. **5** (1980), 45. - 25. Patel, M.C., R.B. Petel, N. Ramymoorthy, B.A. Krishna, S.M. Sharma: Eur. J. Nucl. Med. **13** (1988), 507. -

26. Perdrisot, R., V. Rohmer, J.J. Lejeune, J.C. Bigorgne, P. Jallet: Eur. J. Nucl. Med. **14** (1988), 37. - 27. Ramamoorthy, N., S.V. Shetye, P.M. Pandey, R.S. Mani, M.C. Patel, R.B. Patel, P. Ramanathan, B.A. Krishna, S.M. Sharma: Eur. J. Nucl. Med. **12** (1987), 623. - 28.Reiners Chr.: Nuklearmediziner **11** (1988), 123. - 29. Reiners, Chr., Chr. Eilles, W. Spiegel, W. Becker, W. Börner: Nucl. Med. **25** (1986), 227.- 30. Rodrigue, M., M.R. Rieira, R. Santos, E. Limbert: Eur. J. Nucl. Med. **15** (1989), 522. - 31. Rufini, V., L. Troncone, A. Giordano, M.S. Daidone: Eur. J. Nucl. Med. **15** (1989), 473. - 32. Sandrock, D., H.Chr. Blossey, M. Steinroeder, D.L. Munz: Henry Ford Hosp. Med. J. **37** (1989), 173. - 33. Scheidhauer, K., C. Puskas, J. Sciuk, W. Brandau, P. Bartenstein, O. Schober: Nucl. Med. **29** (1990), A50. - 34. Sullivan, D.C., J.S. Silva, C.E. Cox, D.E. Haagensen, C.C. Harris, W.H. Birner, S.A. Wells: Invest. Radiol. **17** (1982), 350. - 35. Talpos, G.B., C.E. Jackson, J.W. Froelich, A.A. Kambouris, M.A. Block, A.H. Tashijan: Surgery **98** (1985), 1189. - 36. Troncone, L., V. Rufini, G. DeRosa, A. Testa: Henry Ford Hosp. Med. J. **37** (1989), 178. - 37. Urgancioglu, I., F. Üzüm, K. Özker: Eur. J. Nucl. Med. **15** (1989), 540. - 38. Verga, U., F. Muratori, G. DiSacco, F. Banfi, A. Libroia: Henry Ford Hosp. Med. J. **37** (1989), 175. - 39. Westera, G., A. Gadze, W. Horst: Int. J. Appl. Radiat. Isot. **36** (1985), 311. - 40. Wulfrank, D.A., K.H. Schelstrate, F. Small, C. J. Fallais: Clin. Nucl. Med. **14** (1989), 588. - 41. Zanin, D.E. A., A. Van Dongen, C.A. Hoefnagel, P.F. Bruning: J. Nucl. Med. **31** (1990), 1854.

Discussion

Raue: Is there a correlation between the size of metastases and the positive scanning? And in comparison to ultrasound, what method is better?
Reiners: If we have large lymphnodes, you can detect them better than small ones. I think it is not possible to loca-

lize lymphnodes smaller than 1 cm. But we perform both techniques (ultrasound and scanning) together. We have a center for follow up of cancer patients and they are quite experienced. The problem in ultrasound is the enlargement of lymphnodes by unspecific inflammations. In these cases we use especially the scanning. The other indication is detection of lymphnodes in mediastinal region.

Bergant: Do you have some experience with Re-DMSA complexes?

Reiners: I heard about it but we have no personal experience in this method. But I think, the unspecific uptake in the kidneys and in the bone marrow of this substance may be a problem. Then you have a high radiation exposure to organs which should not be irradiated.

Weiss: You demonstrated in your both slides of liver metastases with DTPA and with anti-CEA. The one slide was suspect. Did you see this CEA-positive metastasis also in the planar image or only in the SPECT?

Reiners: We did see it only in the SPECT-scan, therefore I demonstrated this. It was not be seen on the planar scan.

Scheidhauer: Do you see blood pool activity in the scans and does it interfere with the tumor uptake? Do you perform scans at several times after injection of (V)-DMSA?

Reiners: We use 600 MBq and we scan the patient routineously 6 hours after injection. In that time there is nearly no blood pool activity and we perform multiple images of the whole body in this patients and add SPECT scans of the neck and the thorax, because of the high probability for metastases in this regions. Sometimes if we are not sure we add scans 24 hours after injection.

Szybinski: Could it be possible to use Tc-99m(V) DMSA in early stage of thyroid cancer diagnostic procedure?

Reiners: It is not quite useful in early diagnosis which have not been operated. We found in patients with MEN 2a cold nodules as with pertechnetate as well. It has no special indication for early diagnosis, only for follow up.

Thyroid cancer - differentiated and medullary: the aftercare system

J. Němec, M. Neradilová, V. Zamrazil
Institute of Endocrinology and Department Nuclear Medicine
Faculty Hospital Praha 5-Motel, CSFR

Although both basic types of thyroid cancer arise from different cell system, follicular and parafollicular, they have some dissimilarities as well as similarities in the clinical behaviour: the most important thing may be the relatively long survival with higher incidence than mortality, leading thus to considerable cumulation of surviving patients. As both cancers are known not only for their long survival but also for the risk of delayed recurrencies, a system for organized aftercare system is necessary. This system is based on regular clinical examinations, evaluation of tumour markers, ultrasonography, positive tumor scintigraphy. In medullary cancers, iCT is the most useful tumor marker, accompanied in some cases by CEA measurements and possibly by other markers. For differentiated (follicular and/or papillary) cancers the most useful tumor marker is plasma thyroglobulin level. Methods, used in the follow up of differentiated cancer are listed in table 1, those in medullary cancer in table 2. In spite of a very similar scope of these methods, there are some important differencies - patients treated for follicular/papillary cancers should be examined by repeated whole-body scans following withdrawal of thyroid suppression by relatively high radioiodine amounts. Such an examination must be performed on the in-patient basis in our country, especially as it may be followed by immediate therapeutic radioiodine administration. Similar examination in MCT patients is, however, performed on the outpatient basis.

All thyroid cancers in our group number about 2700 (table 3), out of them about 1500 are in the active evidence and need some form of aftercare.

Table 1: Thyroid cancer - aftercare diagnostic measures

clinical evaluation
AJT
plasma TG levels
plasma TSH levels
plasma autoantibodies
sonography
Tl-201 scans
I-131 scans
CT

Table 2: Thyroid cancer - aftercare MCT

clinical evaluation
iCT level
iCT after stimulation
CEA level
sonography
Tl-201
Tc-99m a-DMSA
CT

Table 3: Thyroid cancer - aftercare

2700	all patients
1500	pt. in active evidence
200	new cases yearly
150	treated with radioiodine

We have at our disposal 29 beds with maximum 600 admissions per year - we need in new patients to administer 120 radioiodine ablative doses and in 100 of them we must confirm absent uptake. In about 20, we administer further radioiodine therapy to tumorous tissue. That leaves about 300-350 admissions in the aftercare system, about 100 for a known disease, and 200-250 in regular check up.

Most of aftercare is performed in outpatients, admissions are limited to whole-body radioiodine scans (table 4).

We know that most thyroid cancer recurrencies are encoutered in the first five years after initial treatment (total thyroidectomy, thyroid radioiodine ablation, and confirmation of absent radioiodine uptake). We originally planned to stop the aftercare 20 years following initial treatment, but we found in this interval some unexpected recurrencies. Now, we are prepared to follow up our patients without limitation, with difference in intensitiy after the 5-year duration of remission.

Table 4: Thyroid cancer - aftercare

29	beds, maximum 600 admissions per y.
600	admissions
120	for radioiodine ablation
100	for confirmation of absent uptake
20	for I-131 therapy to tumorous tissue
300-350	aftercare admissions
100	for known disease
200-250	in regular check up

The aftercare system in differentiated cancers is more detailed and patients are divided according to the stage of the disease at the diagnosis.

Most simple is the follow up in patients with minimal thyroid cancers, where the risk of recurrence is near zero. No repeated surgery and no radioiodine therapy are indicated and clinical evaluation yearly for the first 5 years is necessary, in the late phase even once in 2-3 years. No further tests are indicated.

In patients T_2 N_0 M_0 the risk of recurrence is real while low. These patients are subjected to total thyroidectomy and thyroid ablation, sometimes called preventive thyroid ablation. Plasma TG levels form the basic method of the aftercare, followed in 5 years by I-131 scan with a neck sonography. In the late intervals, studies are made yearly and radioiodine is administred at the 10 years interval (table 5).

Table 5: Thyroid cancer - aftercare T_2 N_0 M_0

Test	before 5 years	after 5 years
clinical	6 M	1 Y
TG	6 M	1 Y
TSH	1 Y	2 Y
sono	5 Y	-
Tl-201	-	-
I-131	5 Y	10 Y
CT	-	-

In patients with T_{0-2} N_1 M_0 syndrome the risk of local (namely nodal) recurrencies is much higher while not necessarily followed by shortened survival (when proper treatment is administred). These patients need clinical and TG evaluation in shorter intervals (3 months). We know, however, that thyroglobulin evaluation miss many patients with nodal metastases. Therefore, sonographic evaluation of the neck is indicated, at least once yearly. Radioiodine evaluation may show the presence of metastases silent both by TG and sonography (Fexa et al. 1990), and is indicated at 3-years. Surveillance may be less tight after the first 5 years (table 6).

The group of locally advanced tumor (T_{3-4} N_{0-1} M_0 deserve an even closer follow up namely by sonography. I-131 scans are usually repeated yearly for the first 5 years. In this group, Tl-201 scans may be useful for detection of local recurrence without radioiodine uptake (table 7).

Table 6: Thyroid cancer - aftercare T_{0-2} N_1 M_0

Tests	before 5 Y	after 5 Y
clinical	3 M	6 M
TG	6 M	1 Y
TSH	6 M	1 Y
sono	12 M	2-3 Y
Tl-201	-	-
I-131	3 Y	5 Y
CT	-	-

Table 7: Thyroid cancer - aftercare T_{3-4} N_{0-1} M_0

Tests	before 5 Y	after 5 Y
clinical	3 M	6 M
TG	6 M	1 Y
TSH	6 M	1 Y
sono	6 M	1 Y
Tl-201	2-3 Y	-
I-131	1 Y	3 Y
CT	1 Y	-

In patients with distant metastatic T_{0-4} N_{0-1} M_1 is the clinical and TG examination the most useful and I-131 scans should be performed in 6-month intervals followed by treatment whenever possible. Sonography is much less useful and need not be indicated. In patients with longer survival, the intervals for I-131 wholebody scans are longer, but TG levels are needed at least twice a year (table 8)

Table 8: Thyroid Cancer - aftercare T_{0-4} N_{0-1} M_+

Tests	before 5 Y	after 5 Y
clinical	3 M	6 M
TG	3 M	6 M
TSH	6 M	1 Y
sono	-	-
Tl-201	-	-
I-131	6 M	1-2 Y
CT	-	-

Positive finding in this follow up system is indication for further treatment - radioiodine, repeated surgery, external irradiation or even chemotherapy.

In patients with medullary cancers, our therapeutic interventions are less specific and grading might be less important. Therefore, we divided our patient according to the iCT levels following the primary treatment. Patients with low iCT levels need further iCT evaluation twice a year, and once in one to 2 years stimulation test with pentagastrin and calcium is performed. Sonography is less important and no information is gained from positive scintigraphy (as discussed in more detail by Neradilová et al., Vlček et al. and Holub et al.). On the other hand, the search for the source of iCT in patients with high levels is necessary (sonography, Tl-201 and

Tc-99m DMSA scans) but in many patients it failed to localize the source of iCT even by repeated examinations.

Reference

Fexa, J., J. Němec et al.: Neoplasma **37** (1990), 461.

Discussion

Reiners: Why don't you do sonography in your patients, especially with medullary carcinoma in each time?
Němec: Sonographic capacities are limited, they should be performed in shorter intervals but it is dependent on limited capacity of sonographists who are experienced. Informations recieved from usual sonographs (department of radiology) are less informations.
Deckart: If it is possible one should perform the ultrasound control once a year in these patients to see if there are nodules. But do you think, that we could take the whole body uptake measurement and control with I-123 too?
Němec: I-123 diagnosis in the aftercare system is possible, but not advantageous. Normally many patients need immediate treatment following diagnosis.
Reiners: A disadvantage of I-123 is, that one can not perform the important late scans because of the short half life.

Medullary carcinoma of the thyroid - own experience

M. Neradilová, J. Némec, P. Vlček, V. Holub, J. Bednář,
M. Soutorová
Institute of Endocrinology and Dept. Nucl. Med.
Faculty Hospital Praha 5-Motol, CSFR

Until the end of 1990, 2821 patients with various types of thyroid malignancies were seen in our department. MCT therefore accounted for 180 of all thyroid carcinomas (6.4 %). Of course, when we consider the fact that till 1979 in the group of 1018 persons MCT accounted 35 patients only (the correct diagnosis was made retrospectively) and family screening was iniciated after 1980, the percentage of MCT in the period of 1979 - 1990 is substantially higher (8 %) and in some last years increases over 10 % (table 1).

One hundred thirty-three patients had sporadic variety of the disease (73.9 %), forty-seven familial form MCT (26.1 %). The females were more frequently affected than males in all subgroups.

In the subgroup of 110 surviving patients of both variants the ratio M:F is 1:2.23. In sporadic variety the disproportion is more relevant (M:F = 1:2.57), in familial one (with autosomal dominant trait) is the M:F ratio lower (1:1.69). In the subgroup of 70 dead patients, on the contrary, M:F ratio in the sporadic variety was 1:1.42 and in the familial one 1:2 (in all the dead persons M:F = 1:1.5).

The mean age at diagnosis in the subgroup of 70 dead patients was in all patients 53.2 y for men (13-86), 59.3 y for women (33-84), in familial variety for men 31.2 y (13-48), for women 51.9 (36-73) with the highest incidence in the sixth decade for sporadic and the third decade for familial /1/ (table 2).

In surviving persons, the mean age at diagnosis was in all patients 42.5 y (range 9-75). In 21 individuals diagnosed through regular screening program of affected families, the mean age was 27.5 y (8-51).

Table 1: Number and percentage of all MCT in the group of all thyroid malignancies

year	all thyroid tumors	MCT n	MCT %
to 1978	1018	35	3.4
1979	110	6	5.5
1980	123	5	4.1
1981	142	7	5.0
1982	160	10	6.2
1983	158	13	8.2
1984	149	12	8.0
1985	164	19	11.6
1986	177	19	10.7
1987	167	10	6.0
1988	133	12	9.0
1989	170	11	6.5
1990	150	17	11.3
		+ 4 lost of our control	
total	2821	180	6.4
1979-1990	1803	145	8.5

In familial variety (47 patients) the most frequent form in our country is non-MEN MCT (33 persons), while MEN type 2 is

Table 2: The group of all 180 MCT patients (by the end of 1990)

	patients (n)	type of MCT sporadic n	(%)	familial n	(%)	MCT n	(%)
male (62)	surviving	21	(15.8)	13	(27.7)	34	(18.9)
	dead	24	(18.0)	4	(8.5)	28	(15.6)
female (118)	surviving	54	(40.6)	22	(46.8)	76	(42.2)
	dead	34	(25.6)	8	(17.0)	42	(23.3)
all		133	(100)	47	(100)	180	(100)
M:F ratio							
survival		1:2.57		1:1.69		1:2.23	
dead		1:1.42		1:2.00		1:1.5	
all		1:1.95		1:1.76		1:1.90	

relatively rare (table 3). All affected individuals in MEN 2 had MCT or C-cells hyperplasia. The extrathyroidal location was known in 8 cases before MCT was diagnosed. It is necessary to note that in all our MEN 2a with pheochromocytoma, the adrenal tumor was the first manifestation of disease in the first member of certain affected family. Usually, patients came to our clinic after adrenalectomy. It is probable that the number of MEN type 2 will increase in our material in future. The relatively small number to this time is, perhaps, the result of insufficiently thorough screening of pheochromocytoma in our condition. Although the sporadic variety appears to be more common, clinical studies of the pedigrees of presumed sporadic patients have revealed large number of familial form. A variable expression of genetic information is very important in the epidemiology of MCT. For this reason it is necessary to examine family members of all new diagnosed patients /2/.

Table 3: Familial variety of MCT - number of various types

variant MCT \ sex		Number of patients				
		male	female	total n	total %	ratio M:F
MEN	2a	3	5	8	(17)	1 : 1.66
	2b	5	1	6	(12.8)	1 : 0.20
non-MEN MCT		9	24	33	(70.2)	1 : 2.66
all patients		17	30	47	(100)	1 : 1.76

Most of our 70 dead patients came late to treatment, often with large tumour burdens, cervical lymphadenopathy, respiratory pressure symptoms or diarrhoea (table 4). The extent of surgery varied markedly dependent on the stage of the disease and on the availability of pre- and intraoperative diagnosis and on the erudition of surgeon teams. In some persons the tumour was incurable in the time of initial surgery. After a very detailed analysis of anamneses of all dead persons we can show that there was surprisingly long period to diagnoses (on the average 10.5 years for males and 12.7 years for females). The survival from the beginning on the treatment until the death was 5.5 years in men and 8.1 years in women - on the average - in both cases with very large scatter (table 5). Nevertheless, in the majority of patients, MCT represents an indolent course compatible with prolonged survival. The disease appears to be less aggressive in certain lines without any explanation at the present time.

It is not theme of this report to assess in detail the prognostic factors of MCT. In a good agreement with all authorities we confirm that the most important factors influencing the prognosis are the stage of disease, the sex and the age

Table 4: Distribution of various stages of MCT in 70 dead patients according to international TNM classification at the time of diagnosis

	T		N			M	
	T_1-T_2	T_3-T_4	N_0	N_{1a}	N_{1b}	M_0	M_1
number of patients	11	59	16	17	17	46	24
%	15.7	84.3	22.9	24.3	52.9	65.7	34.3

Table 5: The period of origin of the first disease feature and from the beginning of the treatment until death

MCT	n	to beginning of		until death	
		years		years	
		mean (n)	from to	mean (n)	from to
male	28	10.5 (19)	2 - 16	5.5 (24)	1 - 32
female	42	12.7 (30)	1 - 49	8.1 (38)	1 - 27

Comment: Patients with occult MCT tumors found at autopsy and those died during surgery for pheochromocytoma are not uncluded

of the patients. Our clinical material show markedly higher morbidity with contemporary better prognosis in women. The high incidence of MCT in females - incomparable higher than in data of other authors - is, perhaps, connected with high incidence of thyropathies in Czechoslovak area with endemic goiter.

A half of the group of surviving patients are after adequate surgery (total bilateral thyroidectomy) at this time in good condition and have permanently low serum calcitonin levels after stimulation tests (after simultaneously calcium and pentagastrin administration in our modification). For a quarter of surviving persons who had appropriately adequate initial surgical treatment, no clinical features of the disease were demonstrable. However persistently elevated calcitonin levels were observed (table 6). This situation persists in some individuals for 6-10 years. In general, it is accepted that not only the presence but also the actual levels of basal and stimulated calcitonin values are important for prognosis. Some authors suggest that the levels following stimulation had a direct relationship to the prognosis /3,4/.
We emphasize in some cases the discordance between low calcitonin levels and large tumor mass. Some patients with low calcitonin levels might have a poor prognosis - anaplastization of tumour cells /5/. On the contrary, those with hypercalcitoninemia with a little tumor remnant, but well differentiated C-cells, have a favourable prognosis. Nevertheless, hypercalcitoninemia is the indisputable manifestation of persistent tumor or metastatic lesion and so we have to search these patients for the source of hormone secretion /6/.
We control repeatedly in short intervals (3-6 months) biochemical findings with noninvasive localizing modalities, above all high-resolution ultrasonography (Dr. Vlček), Tc-99m-DMSA scintigraphy and scanning with Tl-201 (Dr. Holub), even with computerized tomography. The discovery of malignant tissue signify, of course, the further surgical intervention. The aggressive surgical philosophy is in all cases recommanded, because neither radiation nor chemotherapy provide effective curative therapy.

The early diagnosis and treatment of MCT patients - familial form above all - is the single most important factor in assuring long-term disease-free survival. This fact emphasizes the importance of family screening for all persons at risk. We hope that in near future, reliable genetic marker will be available.

Table 6: Number of surviving patients according to iCT levels and type of MCT

Type MCT / iCT	Surviving patients					
	sporadic		familial		total	
	n	(%)	n	(%)	n	(%)
low	35	(46.7)	22	(63)	57	(52)
mild or intermittent increase	20	(26.7)	6	(17)	26	(23.5)
continuously	20	(26.7)	7	(20)	27	(24.5)
all patients	75		35		110	(100)

References

1. Saad, M.F. et al.: Medicine **63** (1984), 319. - 2. Ponder, B.A.J. et al.: Ann. D'Endocrinologie **49** (1988), 4. - 3. Wells, S.A.Jr. et al.: Ann. Surg. **188** (1978), 377. - 4. Brunt, L.M. et al.: Surg. Clin. N. Amer. **67** (1987), 263. - 5. Trump, D.L. et al.: New Engl. J. Med. **301** (1979), 253.

Discussion

Dralle: What was the incidence of Cushing syndrome in all patients? And is there a difference between sporadic and familial?

Němec: As far as I know it was the only one case with Cushing syndrome and is was a sporadic patient.

Neradilová: There were in all cases three patients with sporadic MTC in a terminally stage of the disease. All died in the end.

Prevalence of medullary thyroid cancer in the endemic goiter area

Z. Szybiński, E. Mazurek
Department of Endocrinology Nicolaus Copernicus
Medical School in Kraków, Poland

Medullary thyroid Cancer (MTC) accounts for 3-10 % of all thyroid malignancies /3/. However, information about its incidence in general population and about iodine deficiency as a risk factor of MTC is still scanty. The aim of this study is to answer the question of iodine deficiency modifies MTC in terms of its type and frequency.

Method

The Department of Endocrinology of Medical School in Kraków has developed the thyroid cancer register since 1976 in two welldefined iodine deficient areas. These are Nowy Sącz district - the carpathian endemic goiter area, mainly rural with about 600 000 inhibitants and Kraków district having 1.2 million people being mainly urban population in the subcarpathian highly industrialised area. Both districts are iodine deficient areas with extremely low level of iodines 0-1 /ug/l in portable water, low excretion of iodines in urine and high prevalence of goiter /6/.

The register of thyroid cancer has been developed basing on two independent sources: National Cancer Register carried out by the Division of the Institute of Oncology in Kraków, and registers of all histologic laboratories working in Kraków town and providing its services to Nowy Sącz district. All notifications arriving at the main register of the Department, were coded and collected in the computer. The following data were registered for each cancer case: identification of patients, place of residence, date of birth, date of diagnosis, date of surgery, date of death, clinical diagnosis, histological type of the cancer.

The incidence rate was calculated on the population basis by sex and 10^5 people yearly. Classification of the thyroid cancer was as close as possible to the International Classification of Diseases accepted by the WHO classification /4/. Calcitonine in the follow up studies was determined by means of RIA method.

Results and discussion

During a follow up of 14 years from 1976 to 1989 we collected 384 cases of thyroid malignancies including 251 in Kraków and 133 in Nowy Sącz. Diagnostic effectiveness measured as the percentage of cancer with microscopic verification has remained constant in the Kraków's region i.e. over 80 %, whereas it increased in Nowy Sącz from 58 % in the time from 1976 to 1980 to 64 % in the period 1980-1989. Effectiveness of the register measured as the percentage of death certificate accounted for less than 10 % - in both areas was over 90 % (table 1).

A mean incidence rate of the thyroid cancer in the period from 1976 to 1989 in both areas shows figure 1. In the Kraków district the incidence rate is 1.53 (SD = 0.49), in the Nowy Sącz district 1.67 (SD = 0.42); in females 2.3 and 2.33, respectively - in comparison with the mean incidence rate of the thyroid cancer in Poland it is over 50 %. It supports our hypothesis that iodine deficiency and endemic goiter are the main risk factors of the thyroid cancer in the carpathian endemic goiter area. A similar male female ratio in patients with thyroid cancer was observed by other authors /1,2,5/.

Histopathologic diagnoses are presented in table 2. The most interesting feature is lack of MTC in the carpathian endemic goiter area in Nowy Sącz. All the 5 cases of MTC were registered in the Kraków district. Both areas are similar in terms of iodine deficiency, prevalence of goiter and mean incidence rate of the thyroid cancer. The only difference is

Table 1: Prevalence of thyroid cancer in Kraków and Nowy Sącz districts from 1976 to 1989

	1976-1989				1976-1980				1981-1989			
	N	M	F	M/F	N	M	F	M/F	N	M	F	M/F
Total number cases registered	384	90	294	0.31	136	37	99	0.38	258	53	205	0.26
Number of thyroid cancers verified in pathological examination	281 73.2 %	65	211	0.31	100 73.5 %	26	74	0.35	193 74.8 %	35	158	0.22

evaluated. A similar uneven distribution of thyroid cancers including MTC among endemic and out of endemic areas was observed by other authors /1,5/. Table 3 presents characteristics of the patients with MTC. All the patients were not related to one another, were inhibitants of the Kraków town and presented male female ratio 1:4 - rather different from other authors' data. It is interesting that high malignancy with metastatic diseases was observed in three patients over 45 years old. In the follow up study we selected a patient after two operations of the thyroid gland with a still elevated level of calcitonine and then suspected for metastasis of MTC. This patient is actually hospitalized to find out a metastatic area.

The present data lead to a conclusion that deficiency of iodine and endemic goiter are not the risk factors for sporadic MTC. Etiologic factors of this type of MTC are still not clear however an industrial pollution as a risk factor may be taken into consideration. This hypothesis should be verified in further studies.

Conclusions

1. In rural carpathian endemic goitre area during 14 years observation no case of Medullary Thyroid Cancer (MTC) was registered.
2. In industrial iodine deficiency area in the same time of observation 5 cases of MTC were registered. In the patients with MTC M/F sex ratio was 1:4 and incident rates 0.012 and 0.05 respectively.
3. Uneven distribution of MTC among rural and industrial iodine deficiency areas raises the question about etiologic risk factors of sporadic Medullary Thyroid Carcinoma.

Mean incidence rate of the registered thyroid cancer in Krakòw and Nowy Sącz districts in the years 1976 - 1989 by sex.

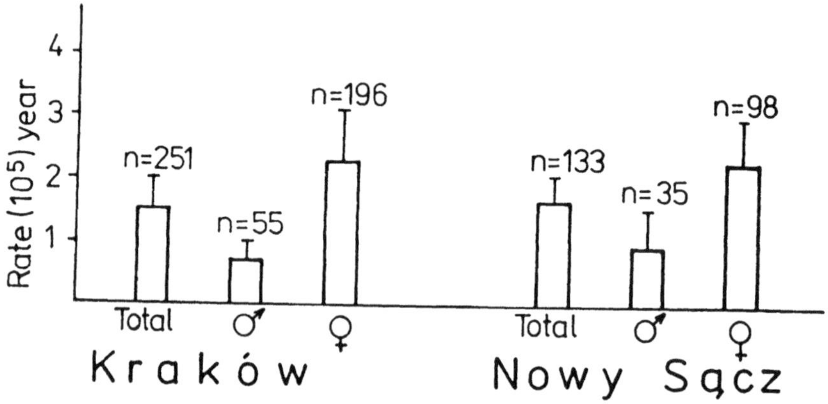

Figure 1

industrialization in the Kraków region which is characterized by an increased emission of CO_2 and SO_2 and metals like lead, chromium, cadmium and zinc deposition. Prevalence of others types of the thyroid cancer is typical for the endemic goiter areas. A percentage of the follicular cancer is higher than a papillary one in both regions and anaplastic cancer in males is much more frequent in Nowy Sącz. We did not notice during 14 years of observation a significant tendency to an increase in the incidence of the MTC and other types of the thyroid cancer, however more exact trend analyses in the groups of age and sex are actually being

Table 2: Histopathological examination of thyroid cancer in Kraków and Nowy Sącz districts from 1976 to 1989

Histopathological diagnosis	N	%	Kraków M	%	F	%	N	%	Nowy Sącz M	%	F	%
Follicular carcinoma	67	33.0	10	23.8	57	35.4	27	33.7	7	30.4	20	35
Papillary carcinoma	56	27.6	10	23.8	46	28.6	18	22.5	2	8.7	16	28
Anaplastic carcinoma	26	12.8	6	14.3	20	12.4	18	22.5	7	30.4	11	19.5
Medullar carcinoma	5	2.5	1	2.4	4	2.5	-		-		-	
Others	49	24.1	15	35.7	34	21.1	17	21.0	7	30.4	10	7.5
Total	203	100	42	100	161	100	80	100	23	100	57	100

Table 3: Patients with Medullary Carcinoma in Kraków district in the years 1976-1989

Patients	Sex	Age at diagnose	Age at surgery	Age at chemo-therapy	Age at death	Metastatic disease	Calcitonin pg/ml	Incidence rate (10^5) yr
S.M.	M	25	25	-	-	-	-	0.012
N.A.	F	28	28	-	-	-	-)	
M.M.	F	89	-	-	89	+	-)	0.05
S.N.	F	56	-	56	56	+	-)	
S.F.	F	48	48 52	-	-	+	1828.0)	

References

1. Belfioro, A., G. La Rosa, G. Padova, L. Sava, O. Ippolito, R. Vigueri: Cancer **60** (1987), 3096. - 2. Hakulinen, T.,A.A. Andersen, B. Malker, E. Pukkalo, G. Schon, H. Talinius: Acta Pathologica Microb. et Immunol. Scand. Suppl. **288** (1986), 94. - 3. Hazard, J.B., W.A. Hawk, G. Cvile: J. Clin. Endocrin. **19** (1959), 152. - 4. Hedinger, C.H.R., L. Sobin: Histological Typing of Thyroid Tumors. In: Roto-Sadag, SA, ed. International Histological Classification of Tumors, vol. 11 Geneva: World Health Organization, 1974, p. 17. -
5. Saxen, E: Acta Chir. Scand. Suppl. **156** (1959). -
6. Szybiński, Z., D. Korzeniowska, A. Przybyszowski, J. Przybylowski, M. Skalski, F. Golkowski, H. Stanuch, Z. Wiśniowski: Endokrynol. Pol. 1991 (in press).

Discussion

Deckart: Who has collected all these patients, have they been centralized in one hospital verified by a pathohistologist in the one center?
Szybinski: The main register is in the department of endocrinology in Krakow. They have their own computer and a subunit collecting all the data. There are fore collaborating laboratories in Krakow town. And in Krakow is a subunit: of the Institute of Oncology as an other source of data.
Deckart: But it is moustly a problem of pathologists, we know this from our own experience. We received specimens from pathologists in different towns and ten years ago pathologists had difficulties to define these as medullary carcinomas.
Szybinski: All our pathologists are in university, so the level of the judgement is rather the same. But I agree, still we have only 70 % of effectiveness of our register.

Family screening in Medullary Thyroid Carcinoma (MTC)

P. Groth, Ursula Zarmstorf, Irmtraud Stoll, R. Reincke
Nuklearmedizinische Abteilung der Radiologischen Klinik
der Universität Rostock, Germany

According to literature, MTC follows a hereditary predisposition in 20 to 26 p.c. of cases, often associated with tumors of further internal glands (MEA Typ 2).
The risk of developing MTC in young relatives of such patients is as high as 50 p.c. and dies out after the 60th year of life /1/. Every new case of MTC can be a familiar form. Thence the need for family screening.

We examined 45 bloodrelatives of 14 MTC patients, all of them were subjected to a Calcitonin test (CT). Calcitonin levels were estimated before and after stimulation with Calcium. Blood samples were initially examined using a kit from Mallinkrodt and later on by Medgenix in the Department of Nuclear Medicine of the "Städtisches Klinikum Berlin-Buch". If the results were abnormal, a scintigraphic examination of the head, neck, thorax and abdomen was done following the application of 150 to 350 MBq of alkaline TC-DMSA. Those who were screened included parents, 17 brothers and sisters, 15 children and 11 2nd grade relatives (table 1). The average age of MTC patients and their brothers and sisters was similar. Clinical signs were found more often in brothers and sisters as well as in children than in the other groups. The CT was abnormal in 18 cases, mostly in brothers and sisters and in 2nd grade relatives.

In the cases of unequivocal results, repeated CT was done after an average period of 5 months, thus a total of 76 such tests were carried out.
A distinct increase in calcitonin levels was evident in most patients on comparison of values of the first and repeated estimations (figure 1). Because of the short interval a sensibilization of hormone delivery should be more likely rather

Table 1: Clinical findings and calcitonin levels in 45 bloodrelatives

Relatives	N	Age (years)	Clinical findings	Calcitonin normal	Calcitonin abnormal
parents	2	65.5 (65-66)	2	1	1
brothers/ sisters	17	48.8 (34-58)	11	8	9
children	15	30.3 (6-51)	9	13	2
other	11	11.8 (6-37)	1	5	6

other: grandchildren, nieces and nephews

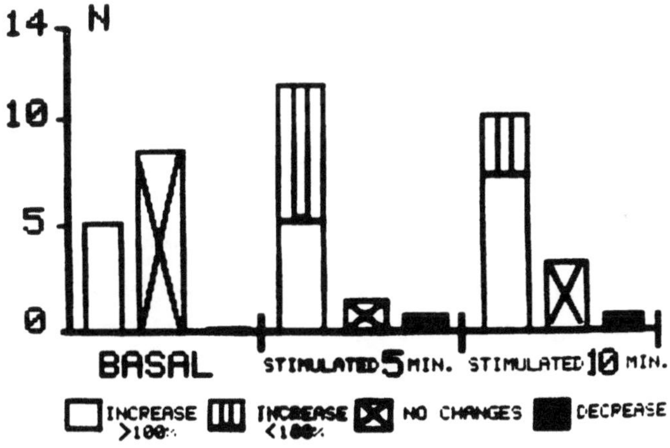

Figure 1

Comparison of calcitonin values at first and repeated calcitonin testing

than an acutal increase in tumor size.
In 97 p.c. of cases, the highest calcitonin levels were attained in 5 minutes after stimulation so that bloodwithdrawels after this period were not required.

In brothers and sisters, clinical findings and results of calcitonin evaluation were often in accordance (table 2). Those with abnormal calcitonin values were subjected to DMSA scintigraphy. Abnormal scintigrams were evident only in one half of the 18 examinations using alkaline Tc-DMSA.
Probands with clearly raised basal calcitonin levels always had an abnormal DMSA scintigram.

Table 2: Clinical findings and calcitonin values in brothers and sisters

Clinical findings	N	Calcitonin normal	abnormal
yes	11	4	7
no	6	4	2

Two families stood out during our screening. The most striking findings relating to one of these families will be presented. MTC (T_3 N_1 M_0) was diagnosed in a female patient 5 years ago, at age 21 years (figure 2). Her parents, brothers and sisters, as well as nieces and nephews subsequently underwent an estimation of calcitonin.
Whereas the fathers calcitonin values lay within the normal range, those of the mother, 2 sisters and one brother were clearly abnormal. The mothers and brothers CEA values were found to be abnormal too (table 3).
DMSA concentrated diffusely in the mothers thyroid, markedly so in the left lobe, where a defect was demonstrable on Tc-scintigraphy. She was found to be suffering from MTC on surgery.

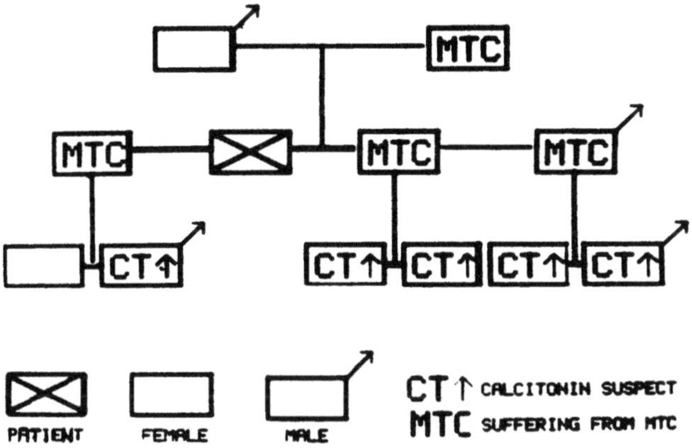

Figure 2
MTC in one family

Table 3: Calcitonin levels in 1st grade relatives relating to one family

Member of family	Ca^{++} (mg)	basal	Calcitonin (ng/l) stim.5 min	stim.10 min	CEA (/ug/l)
father	160	3	14	10	--
mother	160	1800	>2000	>2000	41
sister	150	204	>2000	>2000	--
sister	146	>2000	>2000	>2000	4
brother	180	>2000	>2000	>2000	105

Although DMSA scintigraphy of the neck was normal in the case of the 2 sisters, higher concentration of DMSA were detected in the liver. We found lesions in the thyroid on Tc-scintigraphy. Both were found to have MTC, once in the stage T_{2b}. Significantly high DMSA concentrations were detected in 2 regions of the brothers thyroid, which were obvious as defects on scintigraphy with Tc. He was also found to be suffering from MTC (T_{3b}) (figure 3).

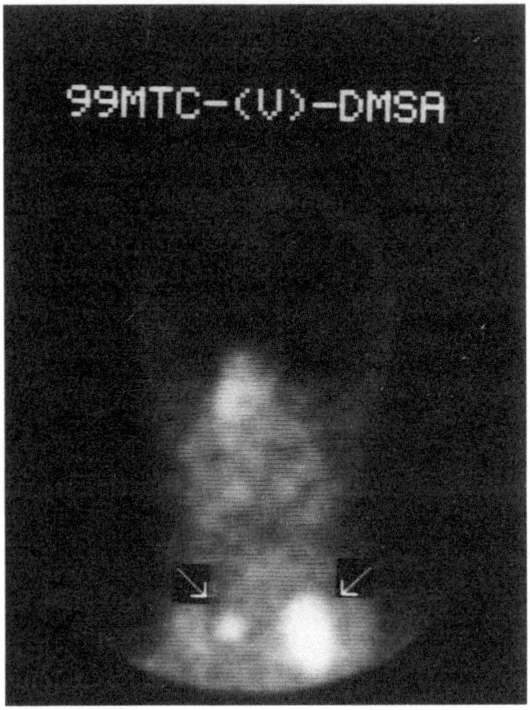

Figure 3

Positive DMSA scintigraphy in cold lesions of thyroid by Tc-scintigraphy and MTC

5 of 6 nieces and nephews had abnormal calcitonin levels. DMSA scintigram, however, showed no evidence of possible pathological changes.

Our results support the necessity of family screening in MTC. The exclusion of genetic affection by gene mapping could confine the number of bloodrelatives, which we have to screen by calcitonin. The others we would save from life-long insecurity and worry.

Reference

Ponder, B.A.J.: J. of the Royal Society of Medicine **77** (1984), 585.

Results of therapy in patients with medullary carcinoma of thyroid gland

(Poster)

D. Gottschild, Gabriele Zinner, Carmen Luck, N.M. Granzow
Nuklearmedizinische Abteilung der Klinik für Radiologie, Friedrich-Schiller-Universität Jena, Germany

Medullary carcinoma of thyroid gland is a very rare tumor. In Jena we treated from 1958 to 1985 367 patients with carcinoma of thyroid gland (table 1). 31 of them (9 %) had a medullary carcinoma. Age and sex of all patients and of patients with medullary carcinoma are shown in figure 1 a and 1 b. We found nearly the same distribution in age groups and a prevailing of female sex. In 2 patients (mother and daughter) the medullary carcinoma was part of an syndrome of Multiple Endocrine Neoplasia. In more than 50 % of the patients we found metastatic formations in regional lymphatic nodules and in distant organs (see table 2) at the time of diagnosis.

The treatment included operation, external radiation therapy, therapy with radioiodine, and application of thyroid hormones. The following combinations were used:

Operation and external radiation therapy	in 17 patients
Operation and therapy with radioiodine	in 2 patients
Operation, external radiation therapy, and radioiodine therapy	in 10 patients
External radiation therapy	in 1 patient
No therapy	in 1 patient

For all patients we prescribed thyroid hormones to suppress the secretion of TSH.

The radioiodine therapy was applied in 8 patients to eleminate functioning thyroid tissue and in 4 patients with a minimal accumulation in metastatic formations.

Table 1: Frequency of medullary carcinoma in relation to other histological types

Type of histology	patients	%
folliculary carcinoma	101	30
papillary carcinoma	98	29
differentiated carcinoma without classification	43	13
anaplastical carcinoma	48	14
medullary carcinoma	**31**	**9**
oncocytoma	10	3
sarcoma	7	2
carcinomasarcoma	1	0.3
metastatic eosinophile adenoma	2	0.6

Table 2: Frequency and localization of metastatic formations in patients with medullary carcinoma

Lymphatic nodules of neck	6 patients	19 %
distant localizations:	13 patients	42 %
lung	7 patients	
bone	6 patients	
liver	3 patients	
other localizations	2 patients	

The long-time follow up shows the following results: From all 31 patients with medullary carcinoma of thyroid gland were living 5 years after the beginning of therapy 16 (52 %). From 13 patients with distant metastatic formations were living 4 (31 %), and from 18 patients without distant metastatic formations were living 12 (66.7 %).

In evaluation of our experiences we recommand the following therapeutic regime:

1. Operation with removing of the primary tumor and subtile examination of the lymphatic nodules
2. External radiation therapy
3. Long-term follow up with control of thyroid hormones, TSH, calcitonin, and administration of thyroid hormones.

The place of ultrasonography in the evaluation of medullary thyroid cancer

P. Vlček, M. Neradilová, J. Němec, J. Bednář, Z. Novák
Institute of Endocrinology and Dept. Nucl. Med.
Faculty Hospital Prague-Motol, CSFR

Medullary thyroid cancer arises from parafollicular C cells of the thyroid and produces a variety of biologically active compounds. One of them is calcitonin, which is used as a biochemical marker for presence of disease.
Observation after surgery with determination levels of plasma calcitonin and ultrasound examination play important role in diagnosis of this disease.

Materials and methods

In our department were examined 49 patients with medullary thyroid carcinoma with high-frequency ultrasound. Neck and liver were imagined during 15 months (January 90 - March 91). The age of the 49 patients (20 men and 29 women) ranged from 17 to 78 years (mean 37.3 years). All patients had undergone previous thyroidectomy. The interval between surgery and ultrasonography ranged from 6 months to 8 years. In all patients plasma immunoreactive calcitonin levels were measured basally and after pentagastrin and calcium stimulation.

Sonography of the neck and the liver were performed using diagnostic apparatus Hewlett Packard and Ultramark IV, Medata, equipped with ATL system. Sectorial probes with changeable frequencies were used, for neck evaluation with crystals with frequency 7.5 MHz and for liver examination with frequency 3 MHz. Very short focusation range 10-40 mm in 7.5 MHz frequency allowed the differentiation of superficially located structures also.
Plasma calcitonin levels was measured with sets Diagnostic System Laboratories, Texas, USA. The upper level in this system is a 1000 ng/l. Normal levels are lower than 130 ng/l.

Table 1: Sonographic findings and levels of plasma calcitonin in 49 patients with medullary thyroid carcinoma

Sonographic findings	No. of patients	levels of plasma low	high
Negative findings after TTE	22	15	7
Remainder of thyroid	12	10	2
Lymph nodes	6	1*	5
Lymph nodes and remainder of thyroid	3	-	3
Calcified tissue in thyroid bed	3	-	3
Hepatic metastases	3	-	3

*Inflammatory node

Results

The table shows, that in 22 patients from 49 observed were not found thyroid tissue, lymph nodes or distant metastases in liver. In 15 cases the plasma calcitonin levels were low testifying this the eradication of tumor. In 7 cases, however, the ultrasound findings were negative and levels of calcitonin were enhanced. 3 patients had MEN IIb syndrome and 1 patient was classified as non-MEN syndrome.

In 12 patients remainders of thyroid were found. These patients had not undergone total thyroidectomy. Enhanced levels of calcitonin were detected in 2 cases.

In 6 patients enlarged lymph nodes were seen, in 5 cases the levels of calcitonin were high. The size of cervical lymph nodes detected by ultrasound ranged from 5 to 22 mm. In 3 cases in these nodes calcifications were found. In 1 case hypoechogenic node 14 x 6 mm was evaluated as an inflammatory one, as the level of calcitonin was very low.

In 3 patients both lymph nodes and remainders of thyroid were found. The size of the lymph nodes were about 8-28 mm, remainders of thyroid about 10-25 mm. Calcifications were seen only in 1 patient. The levels of calcitonin were over 1000 ng/l in all cases.

In 3 patients calcified tissue in thyroid bed was seen, in all were extremely high plasma calcitonin levels. These findings we evaluated as primary tumor.

In 3 patients (6 %) were detected hepatic metastases. Lymph nodes in 2 of theses cases were also present. 1 patient with MEN IIb syndrome had undergone total thyroidectomy with negative ultrasound of the neck, but we found hepatic metastases with calcifications. In all cases the levels of calcitonin were over 1000 ng/l.

Discussion

The treatment of choice for medullary thyroid cancer is a total bilateral thyroidectomy and modified neck dissection. Surgery may be incomplete in some patients if the diagnosis is not known at the time of surgery. In these patients enhanced levels of calcitonin may be explained by sonographic detection of remaining thyroid tumors tissue. Sonographic findings of high echogenic foci often associated with acustic shadows were found in our patients with mass in thyroid bed and with lymph nodes. These calcifications within thyroid tissue are nonspecific. In our group, however, enhanced levels of calcitonin were found in all patients with calcifications. Patients who underwent total thyroidectomy for medullary cancer and have elevated plasma calcitonin levels present clinical problem. The persistent hypercalcitonemia indicates residual secretion in extrathyroidal localization or distant metastases. We saw with ultrasound distant metastases of the liver in 3 cases (6 %). The levels of calcitonin were always over 1000 ng/l. In our study we had 5 patients with MEN II syndrome - only in 1 patient calcitonin level was low.

We have patients where palpable, sonographic and scintigraphic findings are negative and calcitonin levels remain high. These patients need to be carefully followed up.

Sonography is a modern noninvasive method in the evaluation of findings of the neck and liver, where palpation is especially difficult in the presence of postoperative scaring or after radiation therapy. Ultrasound with measurement of the plasma immunoreactive calcitonin levels rank among basic diagnostic methods in this disease.

References

1. Gorman B. et al.: Radiology **162** (1987), 147. 2. VanBeers et al.: Am. J. og Radiology **11** (1990), 107. - 3. Růžek et al.: Prakt. lék. (Praha) **67** (1987), 835. - 4. Telander, R.L. et al.: Arch. Surg. **124** (1989), 841.

Medullary thyroid carcinoma - results of some diagnostic procedures used at our institute

D. Bergant, M. Auersperg, M. Us-Krasovec, F. Pompe, J. Petric, T. Movrin, Z. Zemva*, N. Bešič
The Institute of Oncology, Ljubljana, Yugoslavia/Slovenia
*University Clinic of Nuclear Medicine, the University Clinic Center, Ljubljana, Yugoslavia/Slovenia

Diagnostic procedures used in 42 patients with medullary thyroid carcinoma (MTC) diagnosed and/or treated at the Institute of Oncology in Ljubljana between 1978-1989 are reviewed. The value of routine procedures such as tumor marker assay (calcitonin (TC), CEA), fine needle biopsy (FNAB) and radionuclide tracers imaging (Tc-99m(V) DMSA, I-131-MIBG, In-111-anti CEA) was assessed.
The accuracy of the diagnostic methods was: TC assay 97.3 % (36/37 pts), FNAB 89.7 % (35/39 pts), Tc-99m(V) DMSA scintiscan 83.3 % (15/18 pts), CEA assay 82.1 % (23/28 pts), I-131-MIBG 27.2 % (3/11 pts) and In-111-anti CEA scintiscan (2/3 pts).

Medullary thyroid carcinoma (MTC) originates from calcitonin (TC) producing parafollicular cells (C-cells) /35/.
Relatively few cases of MTC, great clinical /26,27,30/ and histological variability /15,28/32/ genetic aspects of MTC /21,24/ diagnostic and therapeutic problems with advanced MTC call for multivarious diagnostic workup for recognition of the disease and its extent /1,8,13/ prior to any treatment planning /3,22,26,27,36/.
This report is intended to present the results of some diagnostic procedures for MTC used at our Institute, such as: tumor marker assays (TC and CEA), fine needle aspiration biopsy (FNAB), radionucleid tracers imaging (Tc-99m(V)-DMSA (DMSA), I-131-MIBG (MIBG), In-111-anti-CEA (anti-CEA) and screening programme.

Material

During 1978-1989, 478 patients (pts) with thyroid carcinoma were diagnosed and/or treated at the Institute of Oncology, Ljubljana. Medullary thyroid carcinoma was diagnosed in 42 patients (8.7 %), 20 males and 22 females, mean age 40.0 years, range 16-78. Out of 42 pts thirty-six had the sporadic variety of MTC. MEN IIa was observed in 3/42 pts (23.33 and 34 years); MEN IIb in 1/42 pts (17 years), non-familial MEN IIb in 1/42 pts (16 years) and non-MEN familial form of MCT in 1/42 pts (37 years). Three families (5 patients) with hereditary form of MTC were diagnosed.
All of our 42 pts with MTC had a palpable neck tumor. Distant metastases were present in 11/42 pts on the first admission. Ten/42 pts were referred to this Institute from other hospitals. Eight of them were misdiagnosed and treated already. MTC was diagnosed on revision of the histologic tissue specimens.

Methods

The clinical records of 42 pts with MTC who attended our Institute during the referral period were studied. FNAB was performed by conventional technique. Cytologic smears were routinely stained by Giemsa, and Papanicolaou methods. Grimellius method was used for the determination of neurosecretory granules whereas and immunoreactive TC and CEA cells were determined by the ABC method and antibodies produced by DAKO-Denmark.
Serum TC was measured by radioimmunoassay for human TC. A commercial kit RIA-mat calcitonin I produced by BYK-Sangec Diagnostica, FRG was used.
Serum CEA was determined by enzyme immunoassay method using a CEA-EIA-Duomab 60 "Roche" kit. The DMS compound and I-131-MIBG were produced by the Boris Kidric Institute, Vinca, Yugoslavia. Afterwards DMS was labelled in our laboratory with Tc-99m(V) at pH 8.0.

Anti-CEA antibodies and In-111 were provided by Internatio-nal-CIS, France.
Only standard scintigraphy was performed.

Results

1. FNAB
   FNAB (blind or US controlled) was performed in 39/42 patients with the following results (table).

   Table

FNAB diagnosis	number of patients
MTC or suspected MTC	35/39
Anaplastic thyroid carcinoma	2/39
Poorly differentiated follicular carcinoma	2/39

   Four cases were not recognized as MTCs before treatment; there were no clinical features of MTC present, the FNAB results were misleading and tumor markers (TC, CEA) were not determined, so that MTC was diagnosed by histology.

2. Tumor marker assays
   Tumor marker assays were introduced in the diagnostic workup as late as in 1978, and were limited to the determination of TC and CEA owing to laboratory conditions.
   On admission, TC was determined in 37/42 patients and was pathological in all but one.
   In our series CEA was analysed less regularly (33/42). Pathological levels were obtained in 28/33 patients, borderline levels in 4/33 and normal levels in 1/33 patients. In the latter case TC was significantly elevated.

3. Radionuclide tracers

Tc-99m(V)-DMSA (DMSA), I-131-MIBG (MIBG) scintiscan have been used from 1986 on and In-111-anti-CEA (anti-CEA) since 1989, as an additional diagnostic methods for imaging primary, residual, recurrent or metastatic MTC.

On admission, DMSA scintiscan was performed in 18/42 patients. Specific uptake by MTC was demonstrated in 15/18 pts (thyroid tumor 11/15, several tumor sites 4/15). In 2/18 cases the results were false negative and in one case false positive. In latter case DMSA specific cumulation was demonstrated in the thyroid MTC and liver metastases, whereas false positive cumulation was demonstrated in a brain haemangioma later found on autopsy.

MIBG was used in 11/42 cases. Specific imaging of MTC was found in 3/11. False negative results were obtained in 8/11 cases; there were no false positive results.

Immunoscintigraphy with anti-CEA was performed by conventional scintigraphy in 3 cases. MTC was imaged twice.
All but one site, where DMSA, MIBG, and anti-CEA specific uptake was demonstrated, were confirmed to be MTC by FNAB or histology.

4. Screening

Screening used at our Institute since 1969 was initially limited to physical examination of the registered family members who were informed about MTC and screening. Tumor marker (TC, CEA) determination was not available at that time. These methods were added to our screening programme later. Since the beginning of 1990 our screening programme comprised:

- register of affected families
- consulting of family members about MTC and the benefit of screening

- physical examination
- basal TC and CEA assay
- provocative tests with pentagastrin and determination of TC serum levels after it.
- follow up

Altogether three families with familial form of MTC were found.

Discussion

Although MTC represents only 2-12 % of thyroid cancers, it should always be considered in the thyroid pathology /8,26, 27,36/. In our series the incidence was 8.7 %.

The fact that 8/10 cases referred to our Institute from elsewhere were initially misdiagnosed, probably owing to the clinical and the histological variability of the tumor, limited experience of the diagnostician and cramped laboratory conditions does indicate that MCT is still a diagnostic problem /29/.
TC /8,9,11,15/ and FNAB /8,16,18,26/ enable a reliable preoperative diagnosis of MTC. The results of these diagnostic procedures were equally reliable in our series as reported /12,15,16,19,25/.

The value of CEA assay for diagnosis and follow up in patients with MTC is great, though CEA is a less specific and less sensitive tumor marker for MTC then /5,20,26,36/.
CEA is not useful in familial screening because it is not elevated in C-cell hyperplasia /4,5,20,29/.

Favourable results were obtained using DMSA for MTC imaging. They were possibly influenced by relatively great number of patients with advanced MTC, though similar result were observed for residual, recurrent and disseminated disease too. These findings correspond well to the reported ones /14,17, 23,31/.

Using MIBG for MTC visualisation we did not achieve as good results as those obtained with DMSA /6,17/. Nevertheless, MIBG whole body scintigraphy should be performed on admission. Possible coexisting pheochromocytoma can be demonstrated and, when a specific uptake by MTC is found, additional therapy with MIBG is possible /2,17/.

Anti-CEA scintigraphy poses some immunological problems, the main being specificity and sensitivity of the method, sensibilisation and consequential allergic reactions /10/.
Our experience with this method is very limited (3 cases) and no conclusions can be drawn.
According to literature, the incidence of the familial form of MTC is 20-30 % /22,24,26,36/. Only in 5/42 (11.9 %) of our cases familial MTC was observed, possibly owing to incomplete familiar screening, also due to poor family members compliance.

In general, the prognosis in patients with MTC depends above all on early diagnosis and an adequate therapy. Prior to any treatment planning, a multidisciplinary diagnostic workup is needed to identify MTC and possible coexisting MEN (especially pheochromocytoma).
Family screening is mandatory for early MTC detection /7,11, 24,33/. When subclinical MTC or even C-cell hyperplasia is diagnosed and is treated correctly, the best chances for cure are achieved /24,25,30/.

References

1. Baulieu, J.L., D. Guilloteau, F. Bauilieu, J.C. Besnard, L. Pourcelot: Bull Cancer **71** (1984), 182. - 2. Baulieu, J.L., D. Guilloteau, M.J. Delisle et al.: Cancer **60** (1987), 2189. - 3. Ben Mrad M.D., P. Gardet, A. Roche et al.: Cancer **63** (1989), 133. - 4. Busnardo, B., M.E. Girelli, N. Simioni, D. Nacamulli, E. Busetto: Cancer **53** (1984), 278. -

5. Calmettes, C., M.S. Moukhtar, G. Milhaud: Cancer Immunol. Immunother. **4** (1978), 251. - 6. Clarke, S.E., C.R. Lazarus, P. Wraight, C. Sampson, M.N. Maisey: J. Nucl. Med. **29** (1988), 33. - 7. Deckart, H., E. Deckart, Ch. Koloc et al.: Radiobiol. Radiother. **28** (1987), 714. - 8. Delisle, M.J.: Ann. Endocrinol. **49** (1988), 51. - 9. Duh, Q.Y., J.J. Sancho, F.S. Greenspan et al.: Arch. Surg. **124** (1989), 1206. - 10. Edington, H.D., C.G. Watson, G. Levine et al.: Surgery **104** (1988), 1004. - 11. Emmertsen, K., H.E. Nielsen, L. Mosekilde, H. Hvid Hansen: Acta Radiol. Oncol. **19** (1980), 85. - 12. Garcia, A., F. Martin, C.F. Garcia, F.J. Cavanzo: Surg. Pathol. **3** (1990), 19. - 13. Gorman, B., J.w. Charboneau, E.M. James et al.: Radiology **162** (1987), 147. - 14. Guerra, U., C. Pizzocaro, A. Terzi, R. Giubbini, M. Bestagno: J. Nucl. Med. Allied Sci. **32** (1988), 242. - 15. Guliana, J.M., E. Modigliani: Ann. Endocrinol. **49** (1988), 34. - 16. Hawkins, D. Bellido, C. Bernal et al.: Cancer **59** (1987), 1206. - 17. Hoefnagel, C.A., C.C. Delprat, D. Zanin, J.B. van der Schoot: Clin. Nucl. Med. **13** (1988), 159. - 18. Kopald, K.H., L.J. Layfield, R. Mohrmann, L.J. Foshag, A.E. Giuliano: Arch. Surg. **124** (1989), 1201. - 19. Lowhagen, T., J.S. Williems, G. Lundell, R. Sundblad, P.O. Granberg: World J. Surg. **5** (1981), 61. - 20. Mendelsohn, G., S.A. Wells, S.B. Baylin: Cancer **54** (1984), 657. - 21. Nelkin, B.D., A.C. de Bustros, M. Marby, S.B. Baylin: JAMA **261** (1989), 3130. - 22. Neradilová, M. J. Němec, V. Nahodil: Radiobiol. Radiother. **28** (1987), 722. - 23. Patel, M.C., R.B. Patel, P. Ramanathan, N. Ramamoorthy: Eur. J. Nucl. Med. **13** (1988), 507. - 24. Ponder, B.A., N. Finer, R. Coffey et al.: Int. J. Radiat. Oncol. Biol. Phys. **9** (1983), 161. - 26. Saad, M.F., N.G. Ordonez, R.K. Rashid et al.: Medicine **63** 81984), 319. - 27. Sizemore, G.W.: Semin. Oncol. **14** (1987), 306. - 28. Sobol, R.E., V. Memoli, L.J. Deftos: Engl. J. Med. **320** (1989), 444. - 29. Takami, H., T. Bessho, T. Kameya et al.: World, J. Surg. **12** (1988), 572. - 30. Telander, R.L., D. Zimmerman, J.A. van

Heerden, G.W. Sizemore: J. Pediat. Surg. **21** (1986), 1190. - 31. Udellsman, R., O.A. Mojiminiyi, N.D.W. Soper, I.D. Buley, B.J. Shepstone, N.E. Dudley: brit. J. Surg. **76** (1989), 1278. - 32. Uribe, M., C.M. Fenoglio-Preiser, M. Grimes, C. Feind: Am. J. Surg. Pathol. **9** (1985), 577. - 33. Wells, S.A., S.B. Baylin, W.M. Linehan, R.E. Farrell, E.B. Cox, C.W. Cooper: Ann. Surg. **188** (1978), 139. - 34. Wheeler, M.H.: Surgery **104** (1988), 1477. - 35. Williams, E.D.: J. Clin. Pathol. **19** (1966), 114. - 36. Williams, E.D.: In: Polak, J., S.R. Bloom eds. Endocrine Tumor: the pathobiology of regulatory peptide-producing tumors. Edinburgh: Churchill Livingstone (1985), 229.

FREE PAPERS

Tumor markers in thyroid diseases

J. Bednář, J. Němec, M. Neradilová, M. Soutorová
Institute of Endocrinology, Prague and Department of Nuclear Medicine, Faculty Hospital, Prague-Motol, Czechoslovakia

In the last ten years' period two in vitro diagnostic parameters have been commonly considered as tumor markers: serum thyroglobulin (TG) concentration in the diagnosis of differentiated thyroid cancer, and serum immunoreactive calcitonin (iCT) concentration in the diagnosis of medullary thyroid carcinoma.

Serum thyroglobulin determination has been performed in our laboratory since 1981 /1/. Up to the end of the last year (1990) we have made nearly 22 000 determinations in blood serum of patients investigated in our institute. In the last years, at about 3000 determinations have been made yearly on the average.

Since the time we have begun to use our own new specific antiserum against TG (the working dilution 1:90000 i.e. the final dilution 1:270000 is used), the resulting TG values decreased to a certain degree. Nowadays, the TG concentration of 60 /ug/l is regarded as the upper limit of "normal" values in healthy persons with an eufunctional thyroid gland.

The distribution of results of the thyroglobulin determination in patients with differentiated thyroid carcinoma after total thyroid ablation (by surgical and radioiodine treatment) without proved residual tumors or metastatic lesions, and in patients with differentiated thyroid carcinoma with an active tumor or metastatic lesions and/or where the suspicion of them could not be excluded, is given on figure 1a and 1b. In addition to the basic division at 100 /ug/l intervals, another division is used depicting in detail the distribution between 0 and 100 /ug/l. In the subgroup with metastases (figure 1b) nearly half of patients (47.4 %) had lymph node metastases proved or suspected. Only a quarter of patients (24.6 %) had highly elevated concentration of thyroglobulin (over 100 /ug/l). Patients with lymph node metastases (suspected or confirmed, isolated or in combination with a rest of tumor, some of which accumulated I-131) had the TG concentration below the limit 60 /ug/l or above it.

The optimal result of treatment is the decrease of TG concentrations to the values close to zero. This limit differs according to the laboratory method. Now, we regard the value 20 /ug/l as a limit between normal and enhanced TG concentration in our patients under thyroid suppressive treatment and 35-40 /ug/l in patients after the withdrawal of this treatment in hypothyroidism with negative result of whole body scintigraphy. Fully athyroid patients have usually considerably lower values.

In patient with distant metastases of differentiated thyroid cancer, more than 95 % have increased or high TG values. Also in our group of patients with distant metastases and with negligible uptake of radioiodine who have been treated by radioiodine without dose measurement, more than 85 % had an increased TG concentration. In comparison with that, only 15 % of patients with local dissemination on the neck in metastatic nodules and/or with the recurrence of primary tumor, and with suppressed uptake, had enhanced TG concentration. In spite of the fact that this group of patients is not wholy typical, because it includes also patients with dedifferentiation of the original tumor, these circumstances represent a strong warning against the overestimation of low thyroglobulin values. In cases, where the concentration of TG lies in the limits of athyroidism, the whole body scintigraphy should be made each 5-7 years (see the scheme of monitoring of differentiated thyroid carcinoma on this symposium).

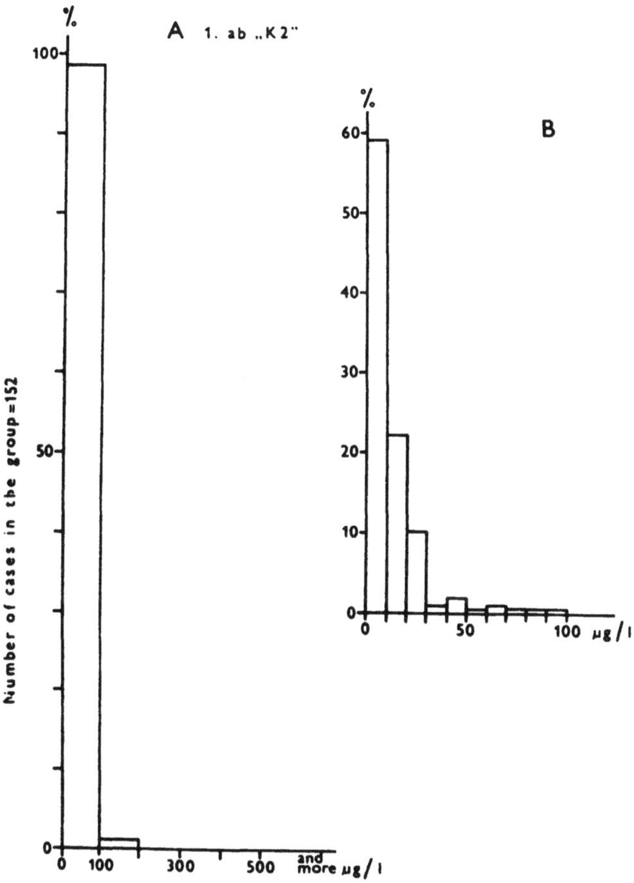

Figure 1a

Thyroglobulin concentration in patients with differentiated thyroid carcinoma after total thyroid ablation without tumor or metastases

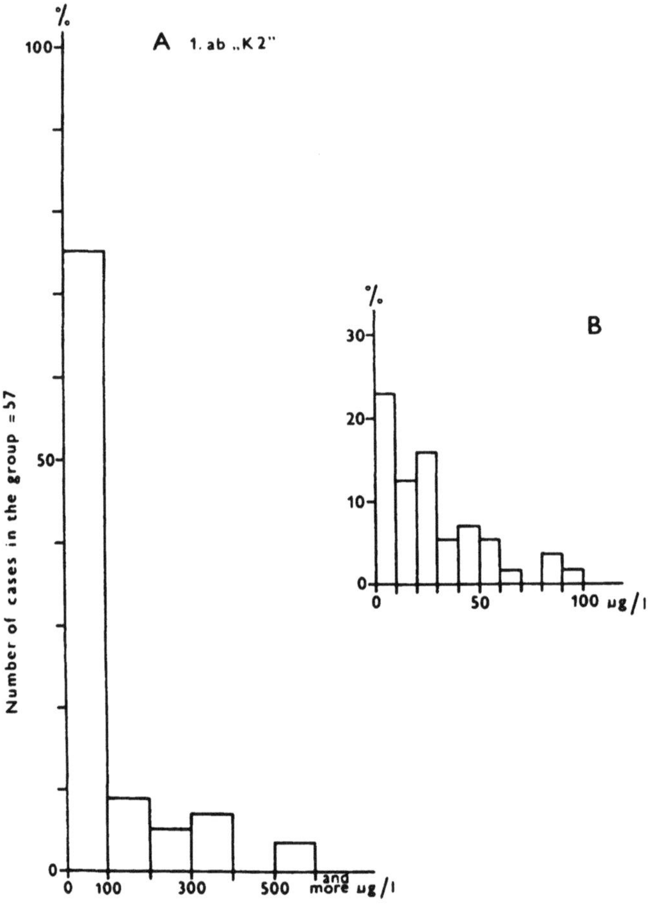

Figure 1b

Thyroglobulin concentration in patients with differentiated thyroid carcinoma with metastases or tumor

The termination of thyroglobulin has only negligible value for screening of thyroid carcinoma because in every case of goiter regardless of its function the TG concentration can be enhanced, often very considerably. By retaining the thyroid in situ the TG concentration cannot be used reliably to the follow up of patients. Only in cases, where we look for the primary source of distant metastases high TG value can serve to an objective diagnosis. This may be effective especially where the gland is not enlarged as proved by palpation.

Medullary thyroid carcinoma always produces enormous quantities of calcitonin. Up to 30 % of cases with MCT are the so-called familiar variant characterized by an autosomal dominant type of heredity. In subclinical period calcitonin secretion in endangered individuals can be enhanced on the basis of hyperplasia of C-cells. Enhanced calcitonin secretion in persons from those families appears as an indicator of the illnes or a menace of it. It is sufficient to the estimation of diagnosis and enables to indicate surgery even in the subclinical stage which influences very positively the prognosis of disease (importance of the familiar screening). In addition, the control of the dynamics of iCT secretion during the treatment and in the follow up of patients can serve for testing the effect of treatment and indicates also possible recurrence of the disease (i.e. recurrence of the primary tumor or the presence of distant metastases).

On figure 2 the results of serum iCT determination in four subgroups from our group of 410 patients investigated, are demonstrated (RIA-mat Calcitonin II test kit). According to the manufacturer, the upper limit of "normal" iCT concentrations is 130 pg/ml. A normal (Gaussian) distribution cannot be generally proved, therefore the value of median has been calculated. The upper limit of normal values has been 100 pg/ml.

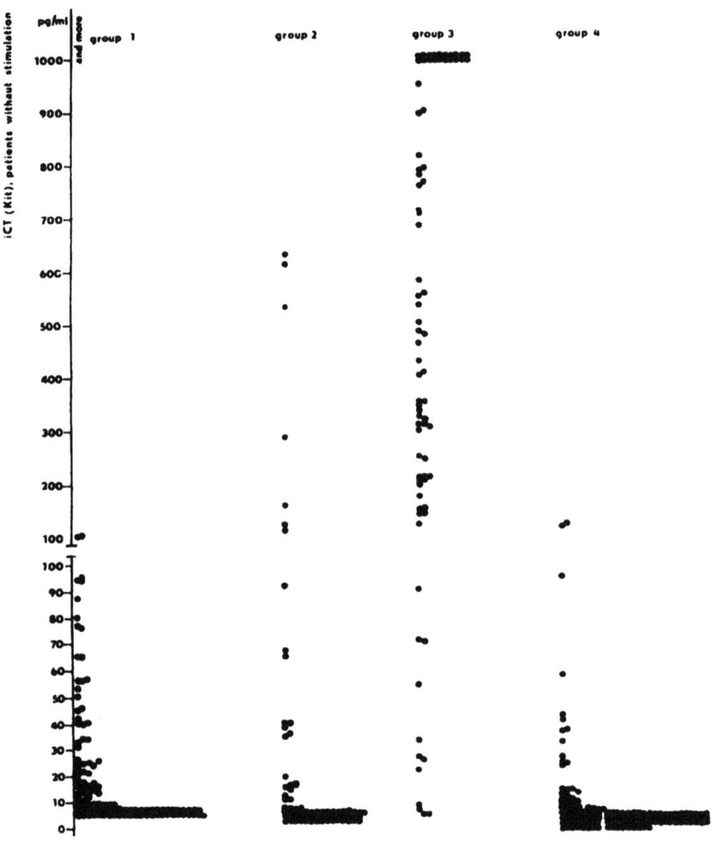

Figure 2
Results of serum iCT determination

The individual subgroups involve: 1. Patients examined for the suspicion of MCT, where the disease has not been clinically or in other ways proved and/or individuals examined for another thyroid disease (with exception of MCT) or for a non-thyroidal disease. 2. Patients with MCT after thyroidectomy and/or external irradiation, and on hormonal substitution without any clinical suspicion of the presence of an active tumor or metastases. 3. Patients with MCT as in previous group, but suspected of metastatic lesions and/or with metastases clinically proved (lymph nodes, liver, lung, bones). 4. Patients after complete ablation of the thyroid (i.e. after TTE and radioiodine treatment) for differentiated thyroid carcinoma. A survey of the most important results of serum iCT determination before and 5 min after i.v. application of calcium (3-4 mg/kg) and pentagastrin (Peptavlon, ICI, 5-7 /ug/kg of body weight) is presented on table 1. The differences between the concentration of iCT before and after stimulation were diverse. The difference of their means between the subgroup with and without metastases was statistically significant.

A similar picture has been obtained from parallel iCT determination in the same group of patients by means of a proprietary method using our own specific antiserum against iCT and labelled iCT (I-125) which has been prepared in our laboratory /2,3/. With this method, the concentrations of iCT were generally higher, and therefore the limit of "normal" values has been raised up to 300 pg/ml. Our own specific antiserum against iCT shows probably cross-reactions with circulating related peptides, whose spectrum is owing to the process of calcitonin biosynthesis very large and whose source may not be only in the thyroid.

Mutual overlapping of iCT concentration values before stimulation of calcitonin secretion in patients with and without metastases of MCT has been mild (about 10 % in the test-kit

Tab.1. Serum calcitonin (iCT) determination in healthy subjects and in patients with medullary and/or differentiated thyroid cancer

Subgroup of patients investigated	Serum iCT concentration (pg/ml) before stimulation of calcitonin secretion (basal values)					Serum iCT concentration 5 min after calcium and Peptavlon injection			
	No. of analyses	iCT median	% of values in the subgroup			No. of patients	% of values after stimulation		
			iCT < 7.8	iCT > 100.0	iCT > 1000.0		> basal value (positive result)	equal or < basal value (negative result)	> 1000.0 pg/ml
1. Healthy persons (familiar screening)	109	9.0	45.9	2.7	0.0	57	71.9	28.1	0.0
2. Patients with MCT partially thyroidectomized without tumour or metastases	78	7.8	55.1	9.0	0.0	73	45.2	54.8	1.4
3. Patients with MCT after total thyroid ablation, with metastases	79	493.6	2.5	84.8	29.1	41	97.5	2.5	36.6
4. Patients with differentiated thyroid cancer after total thyroid ablation	144	7.8	75.7	1.4	0.0	-	-	-	-

and 11-13 % in the proprietary method). It has been confirmed that iCT determination is very helpful tool for the differential diagnosis of MCT in the follow-up of patients with MCT.

References

1. Bednář, J., D. Pichová, J. Němec, S. Rohling, V. Stankov, J. Holušová: Českoslov. Farm. **30** (1981), 294. - 2. Bílek, R., M. Soutorová, J. Bednář, M. Pechová, M. Neradilová, J. Němec, J. Havelka: Českoslov. Farm., in press. - 3. Bednář, J., M. Neradilová, M. Soutorová, R. Bílek, J. Němec, M. Pechová, J. Havelka: Czechoslovak Medicine, in press.

Effects of Propranolol enantiomers in hyperthyroidism

(Poster)

B. Obermayer-Pietsch, C. Stiegler, H. Warnkroß, G. Obermayer, S. Sager*, W. Lindner*, G. Leb
Department of Internal Medicine, University of Graz,
*Institute of Pharmaceutical Chemistry, University of Graz, Austria

Racemic propranolol is known to inhibit the conversion of thyroxine (T_4) to triiodothyronine (T_3) with a simultaneous increase of reverse-triiodothyronine (rT_3). The levorotatory (S-) enantiomer has 179 times more beta-blocking activity than R-propanolol.

22 hyperthyroid patients with recent onset of disease and nine euthyroid healthy controls received 40 mg R-prop. t. i.d. for 5 days; 10 patients and the euthyroids also s-prop. after a placebo-pause. We recorded cardiac parameters, peripheral thyroid parameters and serum-levels of the prop. enantiomers using HPLC.

There was a wide range of individual propranolol values; S-prop. levels were about 40 % higher than R-prop. levels.

T_3 and fT_3 decreased significantly (p 0.01) in both groups, rT_3 increased markedly (p 0.01; 50 %); the T_3/T_4-ratio decreased in both groups during R-prop. indicating lower conversion from T_4 to T_3.

Since beta-blocking effects of R-prop. are negliable at the dosage used, we assume a stereospecific inhibition of 5'-deiodeinase in the conversion-step from T_4 to T_3 and the accumulation of rT_3. We conclude that a benefit for hyperthyroid patients especially for those with contraindications for beta-blockers (congestive heart failure, obstructive airway disease etc.) is evident.

Thyroglobulin pattern in hyperthyroidism factitia (Case report)

Eva Deckart
Klinikum Berlin-Buch, Clinic for Nuclear Medicine and Endocrinology

A female patient, 22 years of age, was transferred to our outpatient department with suspicion on hyperthyroidism. Her complaints: headache, nervousity, tachycardia (115/min). The clinical examination: no goiter, no vascular murmur, but hyperthyroid impression. No pertechnetate uptake of the thyroid gland (figure 1a) normal echopattern in thyroid sonography (figure 2). In vitro parameter: high TT_3- and TT_4-serum level, no thyroid antibodies detectable, extreme low thyroglobulin concentration, normal TBG serum level despite estrogen pill intake (table 1).
The patient was asked to take thyrostatic drug (Methimazole), but no treatment effect was seen during the following three months. The strong intervention on her bad compliance led her to consult a physician in Vienna, who confirmed the diagnosis of hyperthyroidism.

The appelation to her common sense to stop the dangerous intake of high doses of thyroid hormone (as technician employed in a thyroid hormone tablets producing company she could get these tablets without recipe) and the surveillance during a stay on our ward finally normalized the situation: After withdrawal of tablets the thyroid hormone serum level began to normalize since December 1990 (table 1).
The eumetabolic state can be observed by the increase of body weight (24 kg within 2 months), the change of sinus-tachycardia with a heart frequence of 115/min to normal frequence of 69/min and by normalization of bone metabolism (alkaline phosphatase was increased to 8.1/uMol/ml (normal range 1.4 - 2.8) during thyroid hormone abusus), and normal pertechnetate uptake in thyroid gland (figure 1b).

Table 1: Thyroid hormone and immunparameter in the course of disease

Date	TT_3 nmol/l	TT_4 nmol/l	TSH mU/l	MAK	TAK mg/l	TRAK U/l	Tg /ug/l
18.09.90	5.3	196	< 0.1	1:< 100	< 0.1	> 5	11
26.10.90	18	246	< 0.1				6
13.11.90	> 20	421					7
04.12.90	11	112	< 0.1				
		ward					
18.12.90	5.3	107	< 0.1				> 500
20.12.90	2.4	152					
27.12.90	1.2	60					
02.01.91	1.1	44	< 0.1				
31.01.91	1.8	104	0.5				14 49

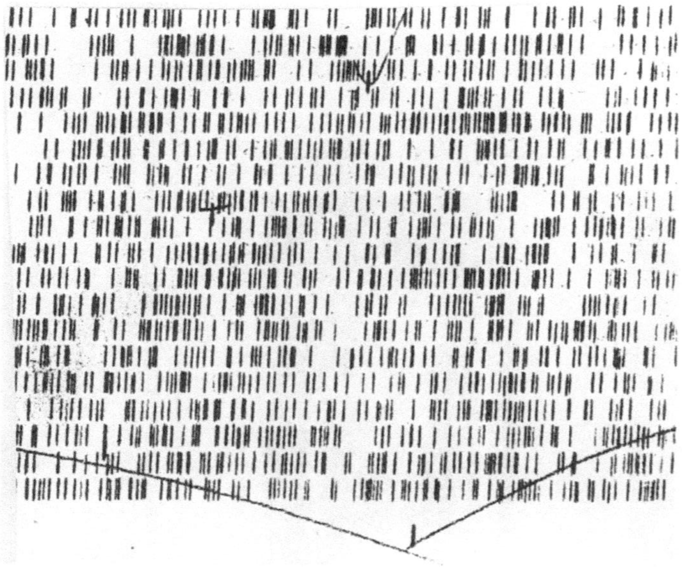

Figure 1a

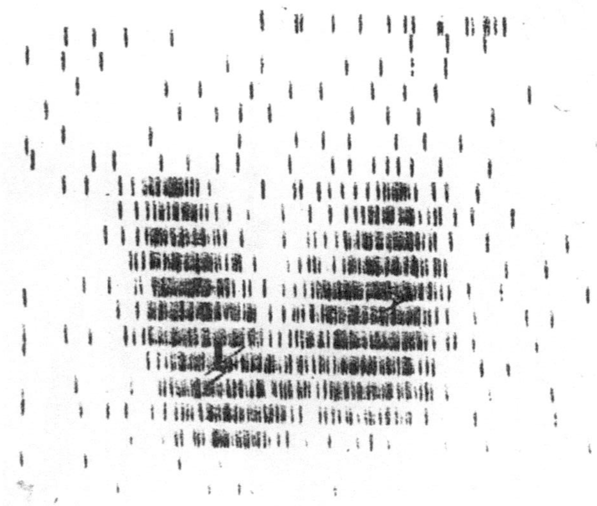

Figure 1b

Figure 1

Thyroid scan with Tc-99m-pertechnetate

1a: Suppression of pertechnetate-uptake, low basal TSH and low thyroglobuline serum level caused by high thyroid hormone intake, September, 10, 1990

1b: Normal Tc-99m-pertechnetate-uptake after withdrawal of thyroid hormone drug. Activation of thyroid cell function represented by high thyroglobulin-level (table 1), December, 18, 1990

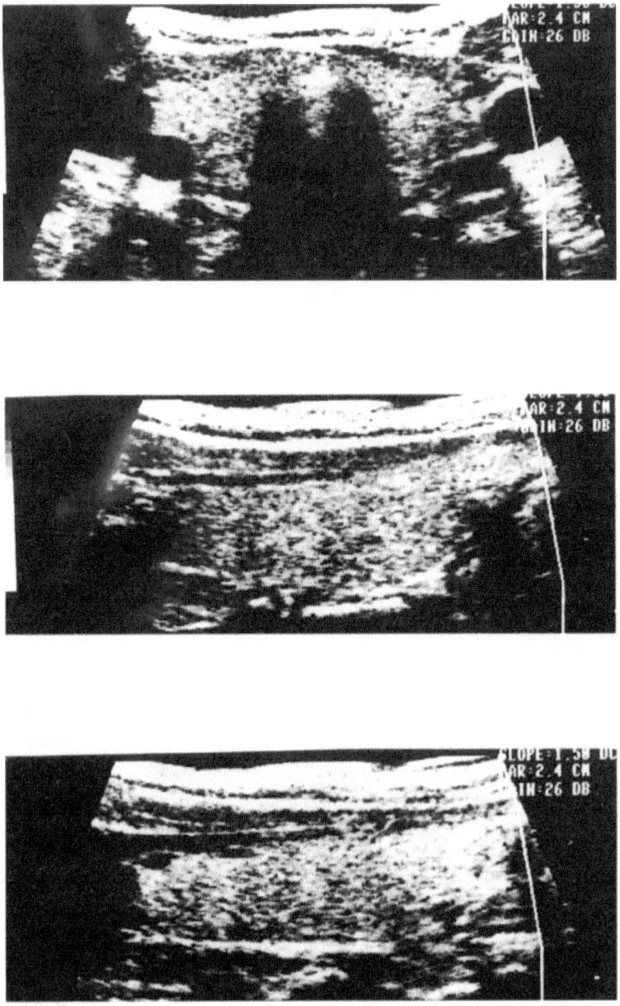

Figure 2

Thyroid ultrasound, transverse section (above), longitudinal section of left and right lobe (middle, lower fig). Normal echo pattern. Normal thyroid size

Thyroid function was suppressed by high doses of thyroid hormone (TSH 0.1 mU/l, thyroglobuline 6/ug/l).
The high serum level of thyroglobuline (above 500/ug/l) after drug release indicated the reactivation of thyroid cell function followed by a normalization within six weeks.

Conclusion

Report on a psychopathic female patient who induced herself hyperthyroidism by thyroid hormone consumption in high doses keeping secret to the physician she consulted.
Thyroglobulin- and TSH-serum level reflected the suppression of pituitary-thyroid axis. Thyroglobulin was the first parameter showing reagibility of thyroid cell system after withdrawal of thyroid hormone drugs.

References

1. Alzawa, T., M. Ishihara, Y. Koizumi, K. Hashizume et al.: Amer. J. Med. **89** (1990), 175. - 2. Deckart, H., A. Blottner, W. Lobers, E. Deckart, W. Rüchel: Thyroglobulin - a diagnostic parameter in Hyperthyroidism and in its follow-up. Radioaktive Isotope in Klinik und Forschung, Vol. 19 (Hrsg. H. Höfer, H. Bergmann, H. Sinzinger), Schattauerm Stuttgart, New York 1991, p. 514, Radiol. diagn. **26** (1985), 119.

Parameters of bone-metabolism in patients with hyperthyrosis
(Poster)

P. Dietel, H.J. Heberling, D. Lohmann
City Hospital Leipzig, Germany

The occurrence of hypercalcemia in a thyrotoxic patient may present an interesting problem.
A moderate elevated serum calcium level may be noted during the course of hyperthyroidism in about 2.2 %.
Excess of thyroid hormones is thought to produce hypercalcemia and hypercalcuria by activating osteoclastic bone resorption. Furthermore, thyroid hormone has been shown to increase the responsiveness of bone to administrated PTH, but whether endogenous PTH plays a role in the exaggerated osteoclastic activity of hyperthyroidism remains controversial, since PTH values have been reported to be elevated, diminished or normal. Primary hyperparathyroidism has also been reported in several hyperthyroid patients, but probably accounts for hypercalcemia in no more than 1 % of thyrotoxic patients. In such cases however it could be desirable to detect the parathyroid lesion before definitive therapy of hyperthyroidism is chosen.

Parathyroid hormone levels, electrolytes, phosphatases and thyroid function were monitored during therapy with antithyroid medication in a group of patients with different forms of hyperthyroidism (n = 36).

In average there was no significant change in serum calcium and AP after normalization of thyroid function, but a small significant increase of PTH-levels. However, in patients with elevated serum calcium levels at presentation, a significant decrease of serum calcium was found. That's why it may be, that the primary effect of thyrotoxicosis is the stimulation of osteoclastic bone resorption and that the resulting small increase in serum calcium tends to suppress PTH secretion.
In contrast to reports in the literature we had no diagnostic

problems in the one patient with confirmed pHPT. He revealed clearly elevated calcium- and PTH-values even in the phase of active hyperthyroidism.

PARATHYROID

Clinical experience in parathyroid carcinoma

G. Knappe, Helga Gerl, M. Ventz
Clinic of Internal Medicine, Humboldt-University,
Charité Berlin, Germany

Primary hyperparathyroidism due to parathyroid carcinoma is a rare disease. According to McCance et al. (1987) about 120 cases have been reported in the literature during nearly 40 years since 1948. 2 to 5 % of all cases of primary hyperparathyroidism are estimated to be malignant, although the incidence found by various authors differed from 0.2 to 5.3 % (Gottswinder et al., 1984; Rapado et al., 1988). The most common presenting signs and symptoms are hypercalcemia, bone disease, renal stones and a palpable neck mass. Local recurrence or metastatic spread are to be expected in 30 % in each case, and less than half of the patients die within 5 years (Schantz and Castleman, 1973). The following report is a retrospective evaluation of five cases we observed since 1973.

Case reports

Case 1
This young man suffered from multiple bone fractures beginning at the age of 18. 6 years later he presented a palpable mass on the right side of the neck which corresponded to local uptake of selen-methionin in the scintiscan. The total serum calcium was excessively elevated up to 4.8 mmol/l. The patient presented with typical clinical signs of primary hyperparathyroidism which was later proved by successful removal of a parathyroid adenoma and subsequent hypocalcemia. Two years later hypercalcemia recurred and the reoperation three tumors, one of which was a histologically proved carcinoma with invasion of thyroid gland tissue. Although three adenomas and one carcinoma had been removed serum calcium remained elevated. A new surgical exploration revealed

inoperable conditions with tumor invasion of the entire ventral neck region. The clinical course was characterized by severe disease deterioration of osteopathy and loss of nearly all teeth due to the development of a large epulis-like tumor in the right maxillar region. X-ray irradiation of the neck region did not delay the fatal course. It is not known if only hypercalcemia and renal failure but also distant metastases contributed to the death in the following year. Unfortunately, autopsy was not carried out.

Case 2

The second patient, a man of 20 years of age, presented with excessively high serum calcium (4.8 mmol/l) and elevated parathyroid hormone (880 μmol/l). A firm palpable nodule from the left neck region was extirpated, and after diagnosing malignancy by frozen section examination the operation was completed with total thyroidectomy. Additionally, a hyperplastic parathyroid gland was found in the lower pole of the right thyroid lobe. The final tumor diagnosis was anaplastic parathyroid. After transient hypocalcemia the patient was feeling well. He was treated for postoperative hypothyroidism, but a correction of serum calcium was not further needed. 20 months later calcium and parathyroid hormone were found to be in the normal range. Five years after surgery the patient was free of complaints and in good health. Unfortunately, follow up examinations of serum calcium, parathyroid hormone and neck ultrasound were not carried out. This patient was the only case of carcinoma in a series of 55 patients with primary hyperparathyroidism published by Wendt and Geipel (1989).

Case 3

A similar good outcome was observed in a 37 years old woman presenting with typical primary hyperparathyroidism and a palpable firm nodule, nearly 4 cm in diameter, at the level of the left upper thyroid pole. Sonography showed a solid nodule with irregular echo structure. The serum calcium ranged between 3.25 and 3.75 mmol/l, and PTH was elevated to 580 pg/ml (C-terminal assay). After removal of the tumor and histologic diagnosis of a partly trabecular parathyroid carcinoma with multiple and in part atypical mitoses a second operation with total thyroidectomy was carried out. Four years later the patient was seen in good health and without any evidence of recurrence. Calcium and parathyroid hormone were found normal, and only thyroid hormone replacement was needed. 10 years after surgery the patient was free of complaints and normocalcemic.

Case 4

A 51 years old woman suffered from nephrocalcinosis and severe cystic osteopathy with bone fractures. The serum PTH was elevated to 836 pmol/l (midregional assay), and serum calcium ranged from 3.45 to 3.59 mmol/l. A nodular goitre was palpable and solid nodules were found on both sides on sonography. The Tc-99m-scintiscan showed the maximal uptake in the right nodule whereas a cold nodule was found in the left lobe. A fine needle biopsy of the cold nodule revealed oncocyte-like cells. After surgery this nodule was judged to be a parathyroid adenoma. Additionally in the right thyroid lobe a follicular thyroid carcinoma was diagnosed. After subsequent thyroidectomy no malignancy was found in the removed tissue.
Because of thyroid carcinoma the treatment was completed with radioiodine irradiation. Nevertheless, the disease advanced, X-ray examinations revealed multiple osteolytic lesions and very small pulmonary nodules, and hypercalcemia persisted with values exceeding 3 mmol/l. An oral treatment with WR-2721, an organic thiophosphate compound, normalized the serum calcium as well as the elevated magnesium levels and ameliorated the clinical condition. A clear-cut decrease of parathyroid hormone could not be observed.

No recurrent goitre or lymph nodes were palpable. An attempt of tumor localization with thallium scintiscan was negative in the neck and chest. Some thallium uptake in the left metatarsal bones remained obscure. Finally, a long term treatment with WR-2721 was carried out for several months which again lowered serum calcium but without normalization.

The patient returned to her family and died in her regional hospital. At autopsy scattered clusters of parathyroid cacinoma were found in the paratracheal scar tissue showing fibrous bands, mitotic figures and capsular and blood vessel invasion. No thyroid tissue could be detected. No systemic metastases were found in the lungs and bones, but brown giant cell tumors and other signs of hyperparathyroidal osteopathy were present in the skeleton.

Case 5

This female patient, now 63 years of age, seemed to be cured from primary hyperparathyroidism by removal of a chief cell adenoma. During a ten year follow up calcium and parathyroid hormone remained normal but after that hypercalcemia up to 3.0 mmol/l reappeared. A nodule of 12 mm in diameter was found on sonography and computed tomography. At first the patient was treated with WR-2721 which normalized the serum calcium. Later the tumor and right thyroid lobe were removed. The histologic investigation revealed in part normal parathyroid tissue as well as tumor tissue with invasion of surrounding structures and blood vessels. The patient is now in good health but after transient normocalcemia the serum calcium increased again possibly indicating persisting carcinoma.

Discussion

It is well known from literature that the clinical picture in patients with hormone secreting parathyroid carcinomas does not differ substantially from the findings in benign primary hyperparathyroidism. There are the same biochemical findings, and the excess of parathyroid hormone causes the same organ manifestations in kidneys and bones. Nevertheless, some special aspects which agree with other reports are remarkable in our cases (table 1). Corresponding to other reports (Cohn et al., 1985; Wahl et al., 1988) three of our patients were younger than 40 years of age whereas primary hyperparathyroidism due to adenoma occurs predominantly in older people. Several authors (McCance et al., 1987; Gotteswinter et al., 1984) refer to relatively high serum calcium in malignancy which was proved true in three of our patients with calcium levels exceeding 4 mmol/l. The experience with parathyroid hormone levels and with tumor markers seems too limited up to now to permit conclusions although some authors noticed striking high PTH values (McCance et al., 1987; Shapiro et al., 1989; Rapado et al., 1988; Wahl et al., 1988). The carcinomas have been found palpable in four of our patients which confirms the general experience of a high frequency of palpable tumors (McCance et al., 1987; Pollack et al., 1961; Schantz and Castleman, 1973).

Recurrent hyperparathyroidism has been described in both genetic and sporadic forms but predominantly adenomas are involved in this situation. Two of our patients seemed at first cured but 2 to 10 years later relapsed with a malignant tumor. According to Mazzuoli et al. (1987) recurrent hyperparathyroidism is a very rare event and in their case reports only one of three patients had carcinoma. On the other hand, hyperparathyroidism associated with differentiated thyroid carcinoma is found more frequently though generally the coindidental parathyroid tumors are benign. Niederle et al. (1982) reviewed 151 cases which were 2.9 % in a series of more than 5000 cases of primary hyperparathyroidism.
The prognosis of parathyroid carcinoma is relatively good though only the initial operation represents the only chance of cure and chemotherapy and radiotherapy failed to improve

survival (Cohn et al., 1985). Weather WR-2721 contributes to a more favourable course cannot be concluded from our two cases. Results of long-term treatment with WR-2721 have not been reported up to now whereas short time studies with intravenous application led to significant decrease of serum calcium (Glover et al., 1985; Morita et al., 1985).

Table 1: Remarkable findings in parathyroid carcinoma

Patient	1	2	3	4	5
age < 40	+	+	+	-	-
Ca > 4 mmol/l	+	+	+	-	-
osteopathy	+	+	+	+	+
tumor palpable	+	+	+	+	-
multiple tumors	+	-	-	+	+
first histology	ad	ca	ca	ad	ad
remission with first treatment	+	+	+	-	+
remission of hyperparathyroidism in years	2	5	10	0	10

Acknowledgement

The parathyroid operations (case 1,3-5) were performed in the Clinic of Surgery, Humboldt-University/Charité (Director: Prof. Dr. Dr. h.c. H. Wolff); case 2 was operated on in the I. Clinic of Surgery, Klinikum Buch, Berlin (Director: Prof. Dr. F. Wendt). The autopsy of case 4 was carried out in the Institute of Pathology, Bezirkskrankenhaus Halle/Saale (Head: Dr. sc. med. Knolle).

References

1. Cohn, K., M. Silverman, J. Corrado, C. Sedgewick: Surgery **98** (1985), 1095. - 2. Glover, D.J., L. Shaw, J.H. Glick, E. Slatopolsky, C. Weiler, m. Attie, S. Goldfarb: Ann. Intern. Med. **103** (1985), 55. - 3. Gottswinter, J.M., R. Ziegler, H.J. Weise, K. Baczako, B. Heymer, Ch. Herfarth: Klin. Wochenschr. **62** (1984), 613. - 4. Mazzuoli, G., S. Minisola, A. Scarda, A. De Matteis, S. Tabolli, F. Bigi, C. Valtorta, E. D'Erasmo: Postgrad. Med. J. **63** (1987), 201. - 5. McCance, D.R., B.D. Kenny, J.M. Sloan, C.F.J. Russel, D.R. Hadden: J. Roy. Soc. Med. **80** (1987), 505. - 6. Morita, M., K. Higashi, J. Tajiri, T. Sato: Ann. Intern. Med. **103** (1985), 961. - 7. Niederle, B., R. Roka, K. Klaushofer, J. Kowarik: In: A. Fritsch und G. Geyer (Hrsg.): Hyperparathyreoidismus, Urban & Schwarzenberg, Wien-München-Baltimore, 1982, 76. - 8. Pollack, S., R.R. Goldin, M. Cohen: Arch. Intern. Med. **108** (1961), 583. - 9. Rapado, A., G. Renedo, J.M. San Román, H. Oliva, J.M. Castrillo, V. Soné, M. Velo, F. Rurrión: Rev. Clin. Esp. **182** (1988), 407. - 10. Schantz, A., B. Castleman: Cancer **31** (1973), 600. - 11. Shapiro, D.M., W. Recant, M. Hemmati, T. Mazzone, R.H. Evans: Surgery **106** (1989), 929. - 12. Wahl, R.A., M. König, H. Schmidt-Gayk, H.D. Röher: Wien. med. Wochenschr. **138** (1988), 461. - 13. Wendt, F., D. Geipel: Exp. Clin. Endocrinol. **94** (1989), 163.

Discussion

Gembicki: My congratulation for so excellent presentation - may I ask you for some comments on two following subjects:

1. I am sure you performed bone scintigraphy in majority of your cases. Does this method, which usually is demonstrating bone changes much earlier then X-ray method, help you in evaluation of cases pathology as well as to monitor the progress of the treatment?
2. You mentioned that you treated one patient with radioactive iodine - may I ask you what was the reason of such a

treatment?

Knappe: Bone scintigraphy was not made in all patients, and only in the one who had first presented an adenoma and long term remission for ten years there was some evaluation of osteopathy. But now we look for before severe disease and I can not give an answer.

To your second question - it was the treatment of the coincidence of follicular thyroid carcinoma. This patient two carcinomas - one thyroid carcinoma and parathyroid carcinoma.

Peschel: Remarks to the difficulties in establishing the definitive diagnosis if you find solid trabecular patterns with mitosis but no vascular invasion as it has been demonstrated in case number three.

Knappe: In all cases we have this extensively discussed with our pathologists and regularily they made the diagnosis of carcinoma when capsular and blood vessel invasion is found. In the problematic case (No. 3) they have only found clusters of irregular mitosis but no blood vessel invasion.

Rink: Did you observe some ECG changes in this patients with hypercalcemia?

Knappe: I don't remember exactly, but some ECG changes are related to hypercalcemia, may be.

Unusual course of primary hyperparathyroidism

R. Hehrmann
Medizinische Klinik, Abteilung I,
Diakonissenkrankenhaus Stuttgart, Germany

As an introduction into the subject of primary hyperparathyroidism (I.HPT) an unusual case is being reported, showing, that even today I. HPT can be mistaken for metastatic cancer.

A 69 year old women came into our hospital by chance, when she visited her husband, who was treated as an inpatient because of a transitory ischemic attack in November 1990. She suffered severe pain in her back, her pelvis and her right leg, and she could only walk using two crutches.
An X-ray of her pelvis and vertebral column was made showing a spontaneous fracture of the right pelvis and all signs of low bone mineral content.

The patient became now hospitalized and the retrospective case history revealed the following:
Hypertension and hyperlipidaemia were known since 1985 and peripheral arterial vessel disease was treated by catheter dilatation of the right superficial femoral artery.
In 1988 cerebral ischemia with left hemiplegia was treated in another hospital with complete neurological recovery.
Since January 1990 she suffered from increasing back pain and inconsistant pain in both legs. Multiple X-rays over the year and a bone scan in September 1990 led to the diagnosis of multiple osteolytic bone lesions. An extensive search for a primary tumor was without success.
In September 1990 a bone biopsy was performed on one of the osteolytic lesions at the dorsal processus of the 7th cervical vertebra, but a definite histological diagnosis could not be made, however bone metastases could not be verified.

In October 1990 palliative radiation of the osteolytic lesions of the spine and the right calcaneous was performed.

There was only little relief of pain, the use of analgetics remained high.

After the visit of her husband in our hospital the patient was also hospitalized and the relevant laboratory parameters showed the following results:
Calcium was repeatedly normal with 4.8 mVal/l, PO4 was slightly decreased to 1.8 mg/dl. Kidney function was normal as well as total protein, albumin and electrophoreses. Urinary calcium excretion was normal.
Alkaline phosphatase was extremely elevated to 1075-1300 U/l.
Parathyroid hormone (PTH) was clearly elevated:
- PTH C-terminal was 322 pMol/l (normal 10-55)
- PTH intact was 22 pMol/l (normal 1-6).

Bone density was as low as 48 % of young normals (DPA of left femoral neck).
Ultrasonography of the neck revealed a small bilateral nodular goitre (right lobe 24 ml, left lobe 15 ml) and a small echo-poor nodule in right inferior position measuring 11 x 11 x 13 mm.
The diagnosis of primary hyperparathyroidism seemed to be sufficiently safe.
On December 7th, 1990 parathyroidectomy was carried out. In right inferior position a parathyroid adenoma of 0.6 g was removed as well as one normal parathyroid in right upper position. A third, normal parathyroid was identified in left upper position, a fourth gland could not be found.
In addition nearly total thyroidectomy of the right lobe was performed.

Postoperatively calcium fell to 3.7 mVal/l without symptoms of tetany. Oral calcium substitution was initiated, the patient discharged from the hospital 1 week after operation.
4 weeks later she reported dramatic improvement of symptoms, back and joint pain had almost vanished, she could walk without support.

Calcium was now normal (4.4 mVal/l) as well as phosphate (2.8 mg/dl) but surprisingly, alkaline phosphatase was still markedly elevated (636 U/l). C-terminal PTH (105 pMol/l) and intact PTH (8.5 pMol/l) were clearly lower than preoperatively, but were not normalized. Oral calcium substitution was discontinued.
3 months after operation the patient felt very well, was practically without complaints.
Calcium had further increased to 4.8 mVal/l, PO4 was low (1.9 mg/dl), alkaline phosphatase was unchanged (641 U/l). PTH remained moderately elevated (PTH C-terminal 104 pMol/l, intact PTH 14 pMol/l).

Despite dramatic clinical improvement after removal of a parathyroid adenoma the diagnosis of

residual hyperparathyroidism due to
"multiple gland disease"

must be suspected.
Computertomography and magnetic resonance tomography could not clearly demonstrate the site of a further parathyroid adenoma, ultrasound shows a small echopoor area parattracheally and dorsal to the residual left thyroid lobe. A second operation os planned.

References

1. Hehrmann, R.:Plasma-Parathormon, Methodik, Pathophysiologie und Klinik. Urban & Schwarzenberg (1980). -
2. Freyschmidt, J., R. Hehrmann: Röntgen-Bl. **31** (1978), 495.-
3. Hehrmann, R., E. Keck: Dt. Ärztebl. **79/28** (1982), 42.

Long-term results of operated hyperparathyroidism

U. Krause*, Ch. Jeziorowski*, Th. Olbricht**
Abteilung für Allgemeine Chirurgie* und Abteilung für Klinische Endokrinologie** der Medizinischen Klinik der Medizinischen Einrichtungen der Universität, Gesamthochschule, Essen, Germany

The natural history, diagnosis, treatment modalities and early post operative results of primary hyperparathyroidism (pHPT) are well described in the literature /1-4,6/. Also, the indication for surgical treatment as well as the operative procedure are generally accepted /1,7/. On the other hand, reports about long-term results after successful surgical treatment are rare. Rates of true recurrences are reported to be about 1 % /5/.

From July 1990 till March 1991 we performed a retrospective study of all patients who were operated on for primary hyperparathyroidism at our institution from 1979 through 1989. There were 225 patients with the diagnosis of pHPT. The majority has been operated between 1985 and 1989. Mean age at time of operation was 60.4 years (range 21 to 85). Most of the patients were between 51 and 70 years old (135 or 60 %) (see figure 1). The sex ratio was 3:1 in favour of the females.
Thirty patients had no symptoms of their disease (13.3 %), whereas the rest of 195 patients were symptomatic. Of these, 57 % had nephrolithiasis, 29 % had bone disease, 14 % had gastric or duodenal ulcer and 9 % had psychiatric disturbances. The total percentage is more than 100 because of multiple symptoms in about 1/3 of patients (table 1).

Operative results

1. Localization diagnostics
   As a standard method of localization we performed ultrasound in all cases. In 123 patients we obtained a positive

preoperative image of the suspected adenoma, resulting in a sensitivity rate of 55 %. In 102 patients (45 %) ultrasound was negative. In these cases correct negative results are included, however (approximately 10 %).
Computed tomography we did not use routinely. Most of the patients with CT-scans were referred to us after diagnosis elsewhere. Of 59 patients there were 36 with positive imaging (61 %). In 23 patients or 89 % CT-scan was negative.
We do not recommend any localization diagnostics before initial surgery for pHPT, except ultrasound. Like most other active groups in this field we perform the first operation regardless of the result of preoperative localization diagnostics.

2. Intraoperative findings
Enlarged glands could be detected in 214 patients (95 %). The localization was nearly equally distributed between the upper and lower position (43 versus 39 %). In 12 % of the patients adenomas were found in both positions, in only one patient a mediastinal adenoma was removed.
Regarding pathology, in 11 patients only normal tissue was removed corresponding to a failure rate of 5 %. In 183 patients (81 %) one adenoma was found. in 17 patients (7.6 %) two adenomas were removed, three in eleven patients or 5 % and four in 3 patients or 1.3 %. For the purpose of this study we did not distinguish hyperplasia and multiple adenomas. The majority of patients with more than one adenoma had multiglandular disease, whereas true double adenomas were rare.

3. Perioperative morbidity
Permanent recurrent nerve paralysis - the major complication of parathyroid surgery - occurred in 7 patients or 3.3 %. Five patients had unilateral lesions and two patients suffered from bilateral injury. One patient required

tracheostomy. This rate of recurrent nerve paralysis compares to other authors, who report recurrent nerve injuries in 0.5 to 10 % of cases /1/.

4. Immediate postoperative results (table 2)
The serum calcium levels were normalized at time of dismission from hospital in 134 patients (95.5 %). 78 patients were hypocalcemic, requiring oral substitution of calcium. These two groups of patients add to a total number of 212 patients who can be regarded as being successfully operated (94.5 %). Thirteen patients (5.5 %) remained hypercalcemic. In these number 4 patients with reoperation are included, as well as two patients who had malignant disease of parathyroids, which was recognized in further operations.

Table 1: Symptoms of 225 patients with pHPT

Symptoms	frequency	percent
without symptoms	30	13.3 %
with symptoms	195	86.7 %
- nephrolithiasis	129	57.3 %
- bone disease	65	28.9 %
- ulcer disease	30	13.3 %
- psychiatric disturbance	20	8.9 %

n = 225

Table 2: Immediate postoperative results of 225 operated patients: Serum-calcium levels

Serum calcium	frequency	percent	
normal	134	59.5 %)	=94.5 %
hypo	78	34.7 %)	
hyper*	13	5.8 %	
(*n = 4 reoperations)			

Results of follow up examination (table 3)

In 1990 till March 1991 we could examine 129 of 225 operated (57 %) in our policlinic. Of additional 50 patients we received information by a questionnaire sent to the patients and their doctors. Mean follow up time was 4.8 years (minimum was 1.1 and maximum was 11.1 years). The majority of patients (57 % had a follow up time of 3 to 6 years. Among the 179 evaluable patients there was no symptomatic recurrence of hyperparathyroidism, except four patients with persisting hypercalcemia who could not be cured after initial and follow up surgery (s. chapter III, 4.). Of 129 patients who were reexamined we have exact laboratory data (see table 3). Three patients with biochemical recurrence of hyperparathyroidism were detected during re-evaluation 83, 8, 10 years after initial surgery). True recurrence was defined as elevated calcium level as well as elevated parathormone after originally achieved normocalcemia lasting at least one year after surgery. All of the three patients had no symptoms. One of these we have operated on again in the meantime, and found a local recurrence. Fourteen patients or 10.8 % were normocalcemic, without symptoms, but had elevated pTH-levels. In our opinion, these patients have a considerable risk of developing a recurrence later on. These patients will be carefully observed in the future.

Table 3: Results of follow up examination (mean time 4.8 years): three patients developed recurrences

n = 129 examined)
n = 50 by questionnaire) 175 (cured after initial surgery)

	n =	%
recurrence (Ca↑, PTH↑)	3	2.3
normocalcemic, PTH↑	14	10.8
hypocalcemic	3	2.3
normal PTH, normal Ca	109	84.6
	129	100 %

n = 129

Three patients or 2.3 % were hypocalcemic, but without symptoms.

The rest of the patients, that means 109 (85 %) had normal PTH and normal calcium levels. However, fifteen of these or 11 % were substituted with oral calcium.

Among the 50 patients asked by questionnaire there was no symptomatic recurrence. The laboratory data referred to us did not reveal any more recurrence, these are incomplete, however.

Summarizing the results of follow up examination, we found 3 of 129 evaluable patients with recurrent hyperparathyroidism, that means 2.3 %. Regarding the total of 175 patients evaluable, the recurrence rate would be 1.7 %. If we assume, the same recurrence rate in the group of patients who are lost to follow up there might be one more patient with recurrent disease.

Most interesting is a group of normocalcemic patients with elevated PTH (14 or 10.8 % of evaluable patients). Theoretically, these patients have an increased risk to develop recurrent hyperparathyroidism later on.

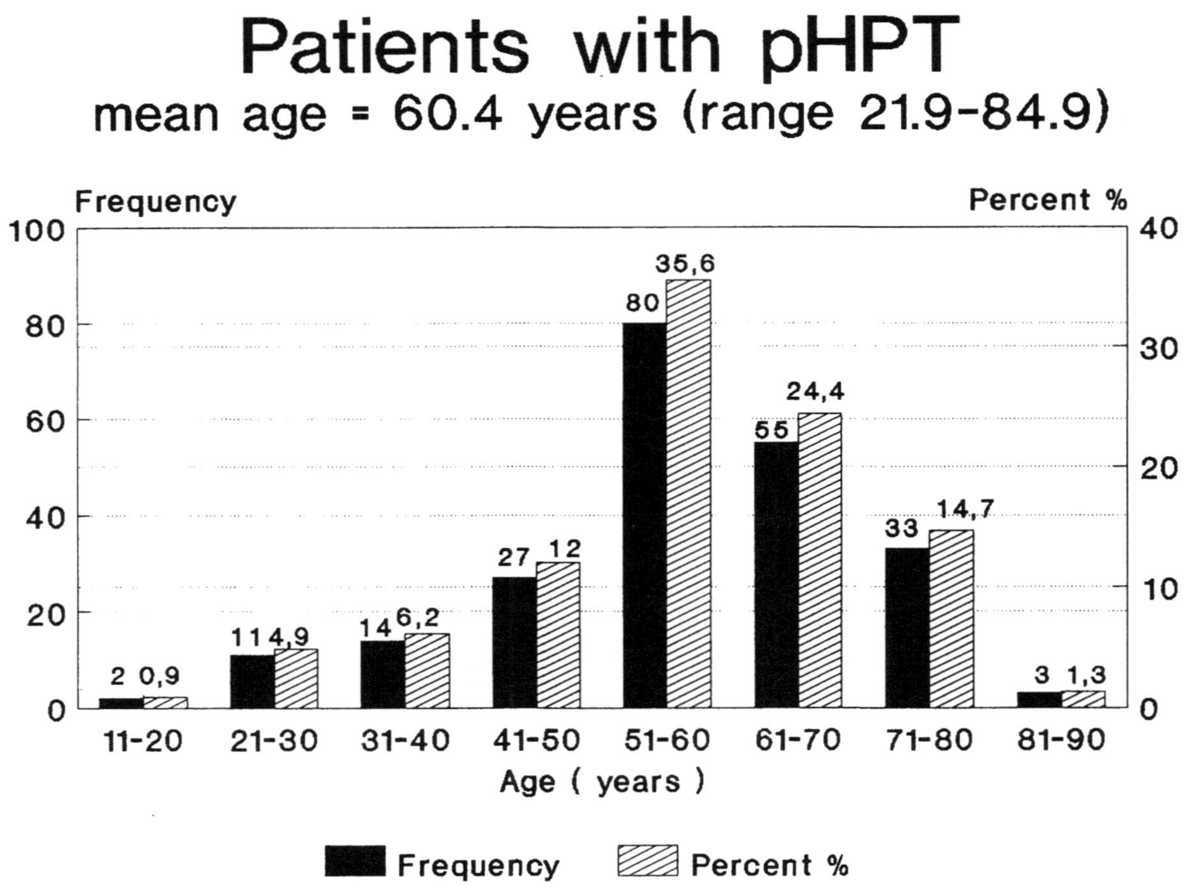

Figure 1: Age distribution of 225 patients, operated for pHPT, 1979-1989

Conclusion

Our data suggest a higher percentage of recurrent primary hyperparathyroidism than reported in the literature up to now /5/. The consequence should be to recommend regular follow up of operated patients with pHPT at least ten years after surgery and preferably life-long.

References

1. Aun, F., R.H. Egdahl:World. J. Surg. **1** (1977), 721. - 2. Dotzenrath, C., P.E. Goretzki, H.D. Röher: World. J. Surg. **14** (1990), 660. - 3. Grant, C.S., J.A. van Heerden, J.W. Charboneau, E.M. James, C.C. Reading: World. J. Surg. **10** (1986), 555. - 4. Harness, J.K., S.R. Ramsburg, R.H. Nishiyama, N.W. Thompson: Arch. Surg. **114** (1979), 468. - 5. Müller, H.: Brit. J. Surg. **62** (1975), 556. - 6. Niederle, B., R. Roka, G. Schernthaner: Dt. med. Wochenschr. **113** (1988), 163. - 7. Wagner, P.K.: Langenbecks Arch. Chir. Suppl. **II** (1990), 971.

Diagnostic problems of primary hyperparathyroidism (pHPT) - own experiences

H.J. Heberling, B. Bierwolf, P. Dietel, E. Kuhlmann, D. Lohmann
City Hospital Leipzig, Germany

Nowadays there is no doubt that after diabetes mellitus and hyperthyroidism, pHPT is at least the third frequent endocrine functional disorder. The prevalence is about 0.12-0.52 % /1-8/. From the clinical point of view there are two reasons to look for pHPT. On the one hand the clinical suspicion and on the other hand the increased calcium level found by chance. On the basis of our own experiences in this field we performed the diagnostic in the following manner.
In the first table it is shown the basic programme. It centres around the clinical aspects the repeated determination of serum- and urine-electrolytes. A typical constellation would be: hypercalcemia, hypercalciuria and hypophosphatemia. Up to date serum calcium estimation is the most valuable parameter in screening for primary hyperparathyroidism, but other causes must be excluded. The determination of urine calcium may be helpful, but hypercalciuria must not necessarily be present. The serum phosphate is only second ranking if compared with the calcium value.
The first figure demonstrates the serum calcium in dependence on the clinical predominant features. It is evident that patients with predominant renal features have not always clearly elevated serum calcium values in contrast to the other forms.
Only in 40 % of the patients we found decreased phosphate-values. There are no differences in the various mode of presentation (figure 2). Besides the electrolytes serum phosphatases should be determined. In bone implication the alkaline phosphatase is increased in contrast to the acid bone. However, the isoenzyme pattern of alcaline phosphatase must be considered.

Table 1: Diagnostic programme for patients of pHPT

Step I (Basic programme)	
<u>obligatory:</u>	serum calcium and phosphate
	urine calcium and phosphate
	serum protein
	serum creatine
	alcaline and acid phosphatases
	x-ray photograph of hand skull
	x-ray photograph of abdomen
<u>additional:</u>	bone biopsy
	x-ray photograph of kidneys, of skeleton system or gastrointestinal tract
	serum chloride
	acid-base status

Table 2: Diagnostic programme for patients suspicious of pHPT

Step II	
<u>obligatory:</u>	PTH in serum
<u>additional:</u>	(preoperative localization)
	sonography
	computed tomography
	scintigraphy
	phlebography with selective blood sampling for PTH

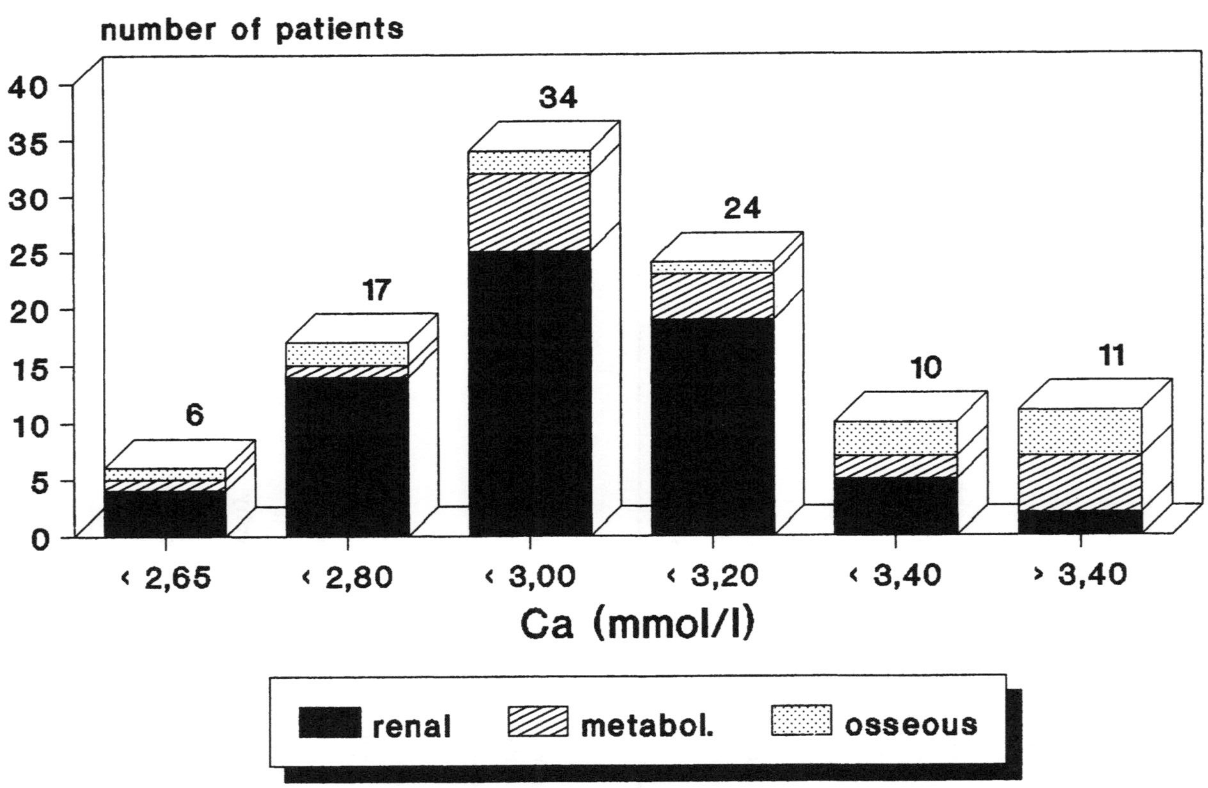

Figure 1
Serum calcium values in patients with pHPT (n = 102)

From the clinical point of view the examination of the bile-duct specific LAP or y-GT is sufficient for differentiation. We have found elevated levels of AP in patients with and without radiological evidence of bone disease, although the proportion of those with an distinct elevated level was greater, in patients with bone changes. For proof of minimal bone changes conventional radiological procedure is insufficient (figure 3).

Attention has been called to the x-ray films of the hand and skull. An x-ray film of abdomen is helpful to find out kidney stones, nephrocalcinosis or calcification of pancreas. The other investigations of the basic programme depend on the clinical findings. They are not always required directly for confirming the diagnosis. Table 2 is showing the second step of our diagnostic programme. The most reliable method is the determination of PTH. In most cases we have used the C-terminal or C-regional assay from Henning.
Both are suited for PTH measurement in peripheral blood. It is confirmed that the Kidneys takes part in the metabolism of PTH. In patients with renal insufficiency therefore PTH-levels are elevated. Now, the question arises, in which cases is the PTH estimation absolutely indicated from the clinical point of view and necessary for discrimination?

In the figure 4 you see the serum calcium in relation to the PTH levels in the own material. If the serum calcium values are clearly elevated (like or above 2.8) than we found certain elevated PTH levels. In this situation there will be no doubt in the diagnosis of pHPT. But the problem becomes interesting in the many calcium stone formers with marginal or borderline hypercalcemia. Considering the regulatory system two situations are distinguishable. On the one hand in cases of calcium levels in the upper marginal range and normal, that means suppressed PTH levels, primary hyperparathyroidism may be excluded. On the other hand in the case of marginal calcium and

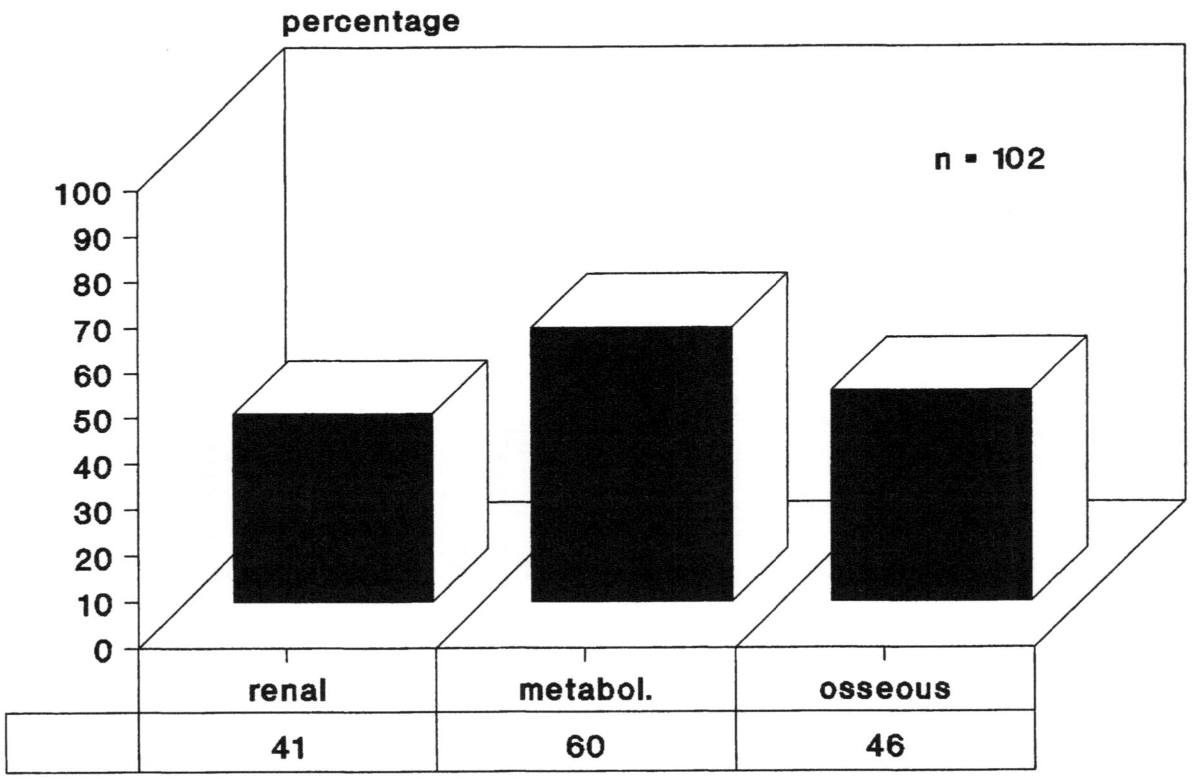

Figure 2: Decreased serum phosphate values (%) in patients with pHPT (n = 102)

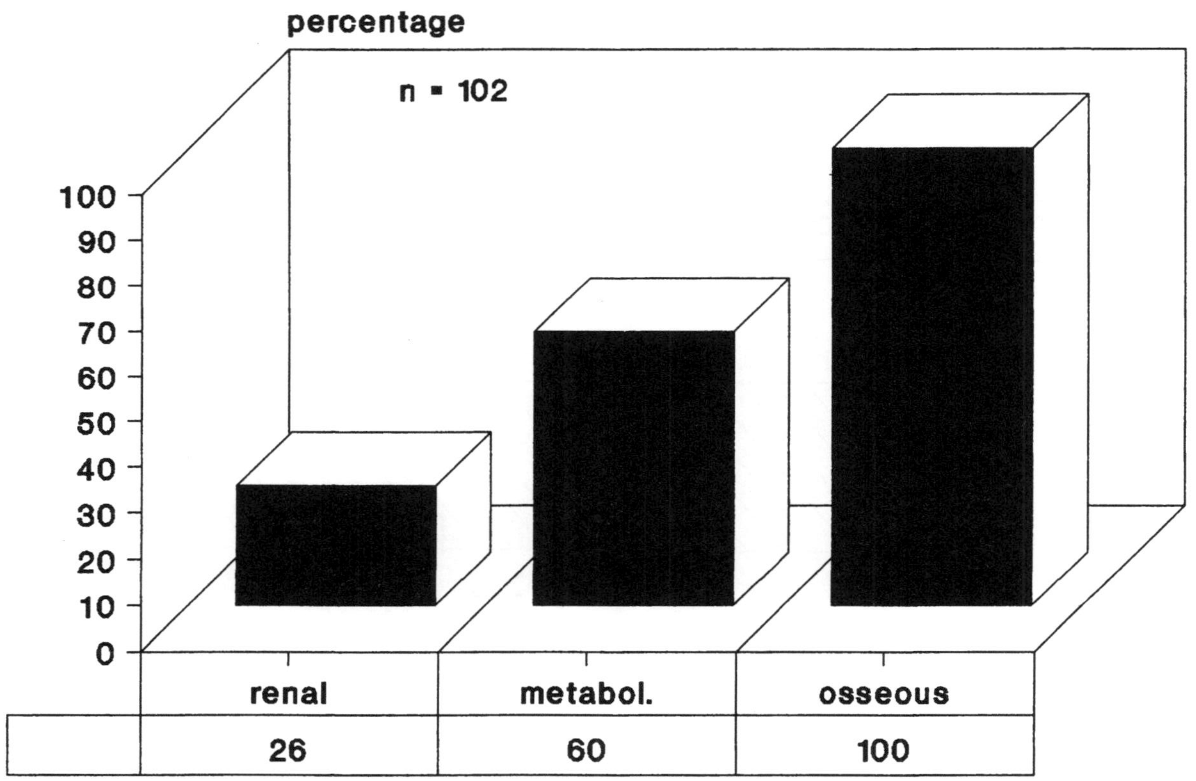

Figure 3: Increased alcaline phosphatase in patients with pHPT (n = 102)

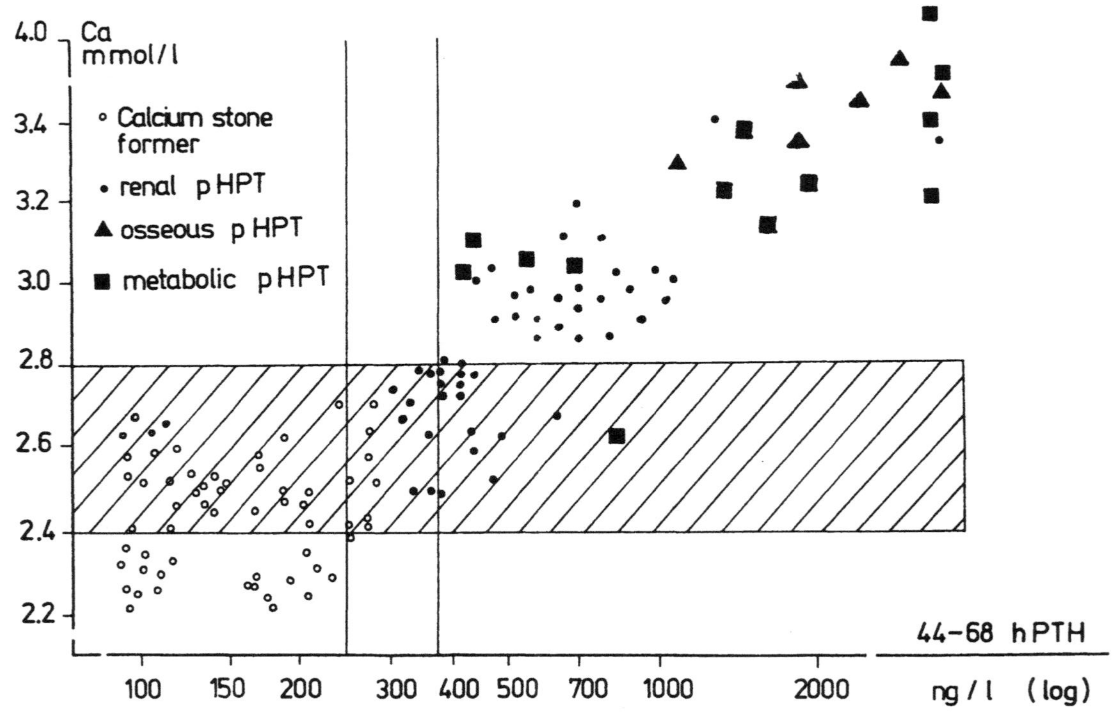

Figure 4: Relation between serum calcium and PTH in patients suspicious of pHPT

marginal or elevated PTH levels, suspicion of pHPT must be assumed, if renal function is normal.

Because of location anomalies of the parathyroid adenomas exactly preoperative localization would be desirable. Many techniques have been described (table 2).

It is generally agreed that these are not necessary before an initial parathyroid operation, which in experienced hands is successful in more than 94 % of cases. Only ultrasound should be performed preoperatively in all cases.

Summary

Primary hyperparathyroidism is one of the most common endocrine disorders in adults. The prevalence is about 0.12-0.52%. 2/3 of our patients had predominant renal signs. The repeated determination of serum calcium is the most suitable method for confirmation of pHPT. PTH measurement is not suitable for screening. In the rule the clue for diagnosis is the clinical suspicion, the persistent hypercalcemia with and without hypercalciuria, hypophosphatemia and the exclusion of other causes of hypercalcemia. Especially in patients with recurrent stone formation and borderline serum calcium values, PTH-estimation is useful for confirmation of the diagnosis primary hyperparathyroidism.

References

Boonstra, C.E., C.E. Jackson: Amer. J. clin. Pathol. **55** (1971), 523. - 2. Boyd, M.J.: Brit. med. J. **290** (1985), 378. - 3. Christiansson, T., K. Hellström, B. Wengle, A. Averyd, B. Wikland: Acta med. Scand. **200** (1976), 355. - 4. Heath, H., S.F. Hodgson, M.A. Kennedy: New Engl. J. Med. **302** (1980), 189. - 5. Jamieson, M.J.: Brit. med. J. **290** (1985), 378. - 6. Lafferty, F.W.: Arch. intern. Med. **141** (1981), 1761. - 7. Mundy, G.R., D.H. Cove, R. Fisken: Lancet I (1980),1317. - 8. Niederle, B., R. Roka, W. Woloszczuk, G. Schernthaner, E. Schubert, E. Borek, A. Kaiser, E. Hirsch, F. Seidl, E. Pesendorfer, Th. Matzinger, G. Lindtner, R. Kaiser: Dt. med. Wochenschr. **113** (1988), 163.

X-ray-morphologic and radiomorphometric results in patients with primary hyperparathyroidism

(Poster)

K . P. Schröder, P. Dietel, H.J. Heberling, D. Lohmann
City-Hospital Leipzig, Germany

The diagnosis of primary hyperparathyroidism (pHPT) can be established by typical clinical symptoms, characteristically changed labor parameters, bone histology, demonstration of parathyroid adenoma and X-ray findings.
Methods of radiomorphometry and microradioscopy will be presented. The combined cortical thickness (CCT) of the metacarpale II was measured radiomorphometrically on the basis of X-ray examinations of the hand skeleton; the subperiosteal resorption of the phalanges of the hand, pathognomic for a pHPT, were assessed with the microradioscopy (degree of striation 0-3 according to Meema and Schatz (1970).
66 patients were included in a period of 10 years. 39 female and 27 male patients (mean age 47.6) were classified into three types according to their main manifestation (renal, osseous and metabolic).

Results

54.5 % of the patients showed a pathologically enhanced degree of striation. Prior to that only in 15.1 % the radiological diagnosis of a pHPT was established.
21 out of 22 patients showed a significant improvement of the degree of striation in the follow up after successful parathyroid surgery.
Preoperativ we found in 65.1 % of the patients data of radiomorphometry under the norm value.

Conclusions

- The estimation of the degree of striation is a significant diagnostic advantage and it is useful for the follow up.

- Low radiomorphometric values are additional indications for a pHPT. The estimation of the CCT seems to be sufficient.
- Participation of the bones could be demonstrated in the main groups of manifestation of the disease.

A strategic scheme for the radiological diagnosis of a pHPT will be presented. It includes also X-ray examinations of other parts of the skeleton.

Reference

Meema, H.E., D.L. Schatz: Simple radiologic demonstration of cortical bone loss in thyrotoxicosis.

Authors' Index

Auersperg, M., 337
Bakó, Gy., 96
Baumann-Antczak, A., 1
Bednář, J., 309, 333, 345
Beňová, M., 265
Bergant, D., 337
Bešič, N., 337
Bierwolf, B., 380
Birke, Susanne, 280
Blažek, T., 265
Blottner, Annemarie, 23, 32, 184
Damm, J., 228
Deckart, Eva, 23, 32, 193, 210, 280, 355
Deckart, H.F., 23, 32, 184, 253, 280
Dietel, P., 360, 380, 389
Djakowa, Katharina, 253
Dralle, H., 228
Duntas, L., 89
Finková, M., 165
Fórisz, E., 8, 46, 96
Fülöp, T., 46
Gembicki, M., 18
Gerl, Helga, 362
Gerlach, Sabine, 23
Gottschild, D., 330
Granzow, N.M., 330
Groth, P., 324
Gryczyńska, M., 1
Haerting, J., 73
Heberling, H.J., 360, 380, 389
Hehrmann, R., 370
Hniková, O., 165
Hnilica, P., 145, 205
Holub, V., 265, 309
Jenei, Zs., 46
Jeziorowski, Ch., 31
Karányi, Zs., 177

Keck, F.S., 89, 101
Knappe, G., 161, 362
Koloc, Chr., 280
Kosowicz, J., 1
Krause, U., 373
Kuhlmann, E., 380
Łacka, K., 18
Ladurner, D., 272
Leb, G., 354
Leövey, A., 46, 96, 118, 177
Limanová, Z., 134
Lindner, W., 354
Lobers, W., 280
Lohmann, D., 360, 380, 389
Loos, U., 101
Luck, Carmen, 330
Marciniak, H., 253
Mazurek, E., 316
Meinhold, H., 54
Mende, T., 1
Mezösi, E., 8, 46, 96
Mühr, G., 32
Murin, J., 83
Movrin, T., 337
Němec, J., 142, 172, 265, 302, 309, 333, 345
Neradilová, M., 265, 302, 309, 333, 345
Nilius, R., 73
Novák, Z., 142, 333
Nyulassy, S. 145
Obermayer, G., 354
Obermayer-Pietsch, B., 354
Olbricht, Th., 373
Oravec, S. 111
Otto, L., 38
Panyige, A., 46
Pechář, J., 83
Peschel, H.G., 127, 241
Petric, J., 337
Pilz, R., 193, 280

Podoba, J., 145, 205
Pompe, F., 337
Raue, F., 216
Reincke, R., 324
Reiners, Chr., 291
Riccabona, G., 272
Rink, Chr., 73
Sarközi, S., 8
Schenk, Susanne, 38
Scheumann, G.F.W., 227
Schmid, K., 272
Schmidt, K.P., 193
Schneider, G., 38
Schröder, K.P., 389
Seres, I., 46
Siersleben, U., 73
Simova, Nina, 152
Sorger, Dietlind, 38
Soutorová, M., 309, 345
Srbecký, M., 205
Stiegler, C., 354
Stöger, A., 272
Stoll, Irmtraud, 324
Štrbák, V., 145
Strehlau, E., 32, 193, 253, 280
Szabó, J., 8, 46
Sztankay, A., 96
Sztojka, I., 177
Szücs, S., 8
Szybiński, Z., 316
Us-Krasovec, M., 337
Ventz, M., 161, 362
Veres, I., 83
Vlček, P., 142, 265, 309, 333
Wardius, Claudia, 280
Warnkroß, H., 354
Weiss, Marie-Luise, 184, 246, 253, 280
Wieberneit, J., 101

Wolf, Ch.-F., 89, 101
Wünsche, Angelika, 38
Zamrazil, V., 142, 172, 302
Zarmstorf, Ursula, 324
Zemva, Z., 337
Ziegelitz, D., 161
Zikmund, J., 170
Zinner, Gabriele, 330

Index

Addison's disease 1
amyloid 241, 247, 259
anemia, pernicious 1
APUD cell system 241 247
Askanazy cells 128
Autoantibodies 1
" - adrenal 2
" - microsomal 1, 8, 15, 20, 24, 32, 123, 174, 177, 184, 193, 210, 356,
- - pituitary 2
- - antithyroglobulin 1, 20, 24, 32, 123, 174, 177, 184
- - antiTSH-receptor 1, 32, 38, 124, 174, 193, 210, 356
- - TPO 1, 8

Basedow's disease, see Graves' disease
Boyden test 9, 19
calcitonin 217, 233, 251, 257, 261, 272, 289, 303, 324, 345, 352
antagonist 101, 225, 265, 324, 333, 351
C-cell hyperplasia 243, 251, 273, 278, 341
CEA 242, 247, 257, 261, 272, 289, 303, 337
chemotherapy (cytostatic drugs) 220, 288, 307, 315
cholera toxine 47
cholesterol 116
chromogranin 242, 248, 257
computed tomography (CT) 255, 261, 263, 291, 303, 365, 374, 380
contrast media 57
Cushing syndrome 315
cytostatic drug, see chemotherapy
deiodinase, deiodination 55, 68, 89, 108
diabetes 1
DIT (deiodothyronine) 56, 62, 65, 66

ETR 84

fasting 59
fibrous retroperitonitis, mediastinitis 171
fine needle aspiration biopsy (FNA) 177, 185, 197, 209
(MTC) 224, 246, 253, 337

FT_4 (FT_3) 66, 102
Ga-67-citrate 261
glucocorticosteroids 161, 174, 193
Graves' disease 1, 8, 23, 32, 38, 46, 96, 119, 172, 210
GTPase 46
Guajakol assay 8
Guanylnucleotides 46
Hashimoto's thyroiditis, see thyroiditis
Hashitoxicosis 126
hemagglutination test, see Boyden
HLA 23, 119, 145
Hürthle cells 128
hyperthyroidism, autoimmune 1, 23, 32, 38, 96, 157, 172, 174, 210, 354, 360
- iatrogenic (factitia) 122, 172, 355
- T_3- 23
hyperparathyroidism 282, 360, 362, 365, 370, 373, 380, 389
hypoparathyroidism, autoimmune 3, 21, 38, 96, 111, 175, 177, 193, 210
hypoparathyroidism 287, 375

iodine-supplementation 80
I-131-therapy 38, 172, 174, 220, 273, 303, 330

LDL 111
lipoprotein 116
liver cirrhosis 59, 73
lymphadenomectomy, see dissection
lymphocytes (B-, T-cells) 99, 129, 130, 184
lymphoma, malignant 128, 281
Non Hodgkin - (NHL) 139

Marine-Lenhart-syndrome 32
marfanoid habitus 283
MEA-, MEN syndrome 216, 242, 249, 265, 273, 277, 284, 311, 337
MIBG (I-123, I-131) 261, 266, 289, 294, 337
MIBG - I-131 treatment 288
MIT (monoiodotyrosine) 56
MRT 219
MTC, see thyroid cancer: medullary
MTC Study Group Registry 17

myocardial infarction 59, 83
myxedema 1
neck dissection 219, 228, 335
N. recurrens, lesion of 287
neuron specific enolase (NSE) 257
Nitrendipine 101
oncocytes, thyroid 128, 140, 186, 331
orbitopathy, endocrine 174
osteopathy 360, 362, 370, 373, 385
parathormone (PTH) 360, 364, 370, 377, 380
parathyroid 360, 362, 370, 377, 380
- carcinoma 362, 370
pentegastrin stimulation test 220, 225, 265, 289, 324, 333, 351
pertussis toxine 47
pheochromocytoma 219, 227, 282
propranolol 59, 354
radiation therapy (external) 220, 273, 288, 307, 314, 330
rheumatoid arthritis 1, 19
scintigraphy 250, 253, 261, 270, 280, 289, 357, 380
- I-131 272, 303, 337
- immune (anti-CEA) 261, 262, 277, 289, 294
- see also Ga-67, Tl-201, Tc-99m(V)DMSA, MIBG, somatostatin
Sipple's syndrome, see MEA, MEN
Somatostatin 243, 257, 261, 272
survival courves (MTC) 222, 229, 235, 286, 311
synovial fluid 18
struma ovarii 201
T_3, low T_3 syndrome 59, 79, 83
rT_3 (T_3 reverse) 55, 59, 66, 73, 89, 98, 102
TBG 102
Tc-99m(V)DMSA 261, 265, 270, 289, 291, 303, 314, 324, 337
Tetrac 56
thiamazole 38, 81, 91, 174, 210
thyroid ablation, total 347
thyroid C-cell 241, 243
thyroid carcinoma anaplastic 251, 281, 321, 331, 339
differentiated 177, 248, 256, 281, 302, 321, 331
medullary 216 - 344

thyroid medullary histopathology 241, 276, 277, 282, 315
- cytology 246
- metastases 216 - 345
- prevalence 316
thyroidectomy, subtotal 174, 287
total 219, 229, 260, 273, 287, 289, 304, 330, 335
thyroiditis 118, 127, 172, 177, 184, 193, 205
focal nonspecific 131, 136, 140
Hashimoto's 1, 18, 118, 122, 128, 134, 142, 152, 165
postpartum 120, 152, 175
silent, painless 119, 175, 177
subacute de Quervain 118, 127, 142, 145, 173, 177, 193
Riedel's 131, 161, 182
thyroid peroxidase (TPO) 1, 8
thyroid volume 207
thyroglobulin 242, 257, 272, 277, 302, 345, 355 (hyperthyroidism)
thyrotoxicosis, see hyperthyroidism
Tl-201- chloride 261, 262, 265, 291, 303, 314
TNM classification 229, 282, 305
TRAK assay 32, 38, 99, 174, 193, 210
trapping, Tc-99m-pertechnetate - 32
TRIAC 56
triglycerides 113

ultrasonography
- Graves' disease 210
- thyroiditis 23, 32, 38, 142, 169, 189, 193
- thyroid cancer 219, 250, 253, 258, 263, 277, 280, 289 303, 314, 333
- parathyroid 365, 380

Bei Fragen zur Produktsicherheit wenden Sie sich bitte an:
If you have any questions regarding product safety,
please contact:

Walter de Gruyter GmbH
Genthiner Straße 13
10785 Berlin
productsafety@degruyterbrill.com